NUTRITIONAL CARE
of the
OLDER ADULT

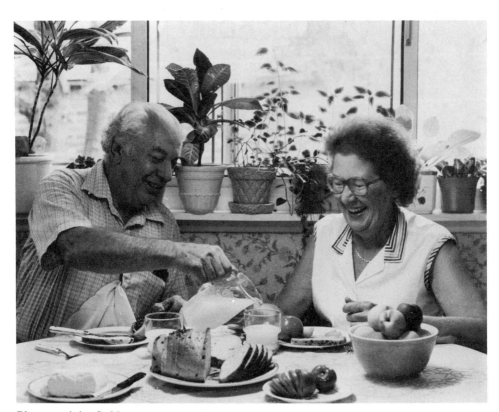

Photograph by S. Natow

NUTRITIONAL CARE
of the
OLDER ADULT

Annette B. Natow, Ph.D., R.D.
Professor
Coordinator of Nutrition Courses
School of Nursing
Adelphi University
Garden City, New York

Jo-Ann Heslin, M.A., R.D.
Nutritionist
Multidisciplinary Center on Aging
Adelphi University
Garden City, New York

With the assistance of
Allen J. Natow, M.D.
New York University Medical Center
New York, New York

Macmillan Publishing Company
NEW YORK

Collier Macmillan Canada, Inc.
TORONTO

Collier Macmillan Publishers
LONDON

Macmillan Publishing Company
866 Third Avenue, New York, New York 10022

Collier Macmillan Canada, Inc.

Collier Macmillan Publishers • London

Library of Congress Cataloging-in-Publication Data

Natow, Annette B.
    Nutritional care of the older adult.

    Includes bibliographies and index.
        1. Aged—Diseases—Nutritional aspects.   2. Aged—
Diseases—Diet therapy.   3. Age factors in disease.
4. Nutrition disorders—Age factors.   I. Heslin, Jo-Ann.
II. Natow, Allen.   III. Title.   [DNLM: 1. Nutrition—in
middle age.   2. Nutrition—in old age.   3. Preventive
Medicine.   QU 145 N2795n]
RC952.5.N38   1986   613.2'0880564   85-24112
ISBN 0-02-386200-9

Printing: 1 2 3 4 5 6 7 8   Year: 6 7 8 9 0 1 2 3 4

Preface

Old age is a positive period in life if accompanied by the continued respect of younger people and a minimum of physical decline and loss of status. The founding fathers of this country recognized and respected the wisdom that comes with age by stipulating in the Constitution that a president must be at least 35 years of age. In practice, most presidents have been in their fifties and sixties when they served. Ronald Reagan served as president when well into his seventies.

We view life as a continuum, with no single factor, event, or combination of these clearly separating the older adult from others. Thus, we have chosen to refer to persons over age 40 as older adults, admitting from the outset that this group is extremely heterogeneous, and that this demarcation is artificial.

As preventive medicine continues to assume a greater role in the life-style of Americans, there is increasing awareness of the value of nutritional intervention in disease. Virtually all disease processes affecting the older adult have nutritional implications—in the prevention of disease, treatment of disease, relating to medication, or relating to specific disabilities caused by disease. Thus, all health care workers need to be well versed in the nutritional implications of disease and need to be able to put this knowledge into practice.

In reading this book, it will become obvious that we stress *moderation* and *individualization*. We are enthusiastic about the role of nutrition in disease prevention and treatment, but are skeptical of claims that are poorly substantiated. Except for a few special situations, we do *not* advocate strict diets. Nutrition is an ongoing pleasurable part of life, but is only one of several factors important in disease, though a major one. Also, we feel that every patient must be treated as an individual, *not* as a "case."

v

Very few older adults have simple single medical problems, and although written information is useful to help patients to remember instructions, printed sheets can never substitute for careful and ongoing evaluation and re-inforcement of treatment plans by a concerned *person*.

Eating is a central part of life, and now, nutrition is beginning to assume the importance it deserves in the treatment and prevention of disease. We hope that this book will make it possible for health care professionals to address the nutritional needs of their adult patients and thereby offer the highest quality of care.

ANNETTE B. NATOW
JO-ANN HESLIN
ALLEN J. NATOW

Acknowledgments

Chapter 18, Psychosocial Factors and Societal Systems that Affect Nutritional Care, was contributed by:

Elaine B. Jacks, M.S., R.N.
Director
Multidisciplinary Center on Aging
Adelphi University
Garden City, New York.

We would also like to acknowledge the help of Dr. Martin Lefkowitz, University of Pennsylvania Hospital, Dr. Irene Rosenberg, New York Hospital-Cornell Medical Center, Elizabeth Linnehan, R.D., Professor, Department of Nursing, Molloy College, Laura Lefkowitz for typing the manuscript and, as always, our families for their support and encouragement.

A.B.N.
J.H.
A.J.N.

"Good feeding is one of the greatest factors in maintaining health but . . .
. . . there is no magic diet for any disease."

Mary Swartz Rose
FEEDING THE FAMILY
The Macmillan Company
1916

Contents

Preface   v

Acknowledgments   vii

Part I: FUNDAMENTALS OF GERIATRIC NUTRITION   1

Chapter 1   Aging and Body Systems   3
Factors influencing longevity   6
The aging body   7
Changes in body systems with age   8

Chapter 2   Nutritional Assessment   19
Anthropometric measurements   19
Laboratory measurements   27
Clinical examination   28
Diet assessment   28

Chapter 3   Nutrient Needs as People Age   43
Energy   43
Energy nutrients   44
Fiber   47
Water   49
Vitamins and minerals   50
Use of nutrient supplementation   51

Part II: NUTRITIONAL INTERVENTION IN DISEASE   63

Chapter 4   Counseling and Compliance   65
            Counseling techniques to improve compliance   66
            Aging factors that affect compliance   68
            Physical limitations that affect compliance   70

Chapter 5   Alcohol   77
            Effects of alcohol   78
            Alcohol and drugs   83
            Alcohol in pharmaceutical products   83
            Alcohol in long-term care   84
            Alcohol use in therapeutic diets   85

Chapter 6   Digestive Disorders   89
            Conditions of the gastrointestinal tract   90
            Liver disease   102

Chapter 7   Renal Disease   105
            Aging and the kidney   105
            Chronic renal disease   106
            Kidney stones   111

Chapter 8   Diabetes Mellitus   115
            Complications   116
            Management   117
            Diabetic diet in long-term care facilities   121
            Diabetic foods   122
            Alcohol   124
            Drugs that affect diabetes management   124

Chapter 9   Cancer   129
            Diet and cancer risk   130
            Aging and cancer risk   130
            Nutritional support   132
            Nutritional assessment in cancer care   137
            Feeding the cancer patient   141
            Nutrition misinterpretation   149

Chapter 10 Cardiovascular Disease   157
            Hyperlipidemia   159
            Hypertension   170
            Nutritional management of myocardial infarction   177

Chapter 11 Osteoporosis, Gout, and Arthritis   183
            Osteoporosis   183
            Gout   190
            Arthritis   191

Chapter 12   Neurologic Disease   197
              Dementia   198
              Stroke   200
              Parkinson's disease   201
              Feeding the person with a movement disorder   203

Chapter 13   Nutritional Anemias   209
              Microcytic anemia   210
              Macrocytic anemia   212

Chapter 14   Infectious Disease   217
              Nutritional deficiency   219
              Nutritional requirements in infectious disease   220
              Feeding considerations in infectious disease   222

Chapter 15   Skin   229
              Aging skin   229
              Decubitus ulcers   232

Chapter 16   Respiratory Disease   243
              Ventilator-dependent patients   244
              COPD (Chronic obstructive pulmonary disease)   248

Chapter 17   Nutritional Considerations with Drug Use   251
              The impact of drugs on nutritional status   252
              The effects of nutrients on drug activity   255
              Over-the-counter medication   259
              Compliance with medication   263

              **Part III: PSYCHOSOCIAL FACTORS THAT
                            AFFECT NUTRITIONAL INTAKE**   **265**

Chapter 18   Psychosocial Factors and Societal Systems that
              Affect Nutritional Care   267
                    by *Elaine B. Jacks, M.S., R.N.*

              Economic status   268
              Educational status   268
              Male vs. female accommodation to aging   270
              Social isolation   271
              Disordered behaviors   273
              Food as a positive social factor   274
              Cultural, religious, and regional food practices   277

Appendix A.   Progressive Hospital Diet   283
Appendix B.   Diabetic Exchange Lists for Meal Planning   287
Appendix C.   Interpreting Nutritional Research   293

Index   297

Part I

FUNDAMENTALS OF GERIATRIC NUTRITION

Chapter 1

AGING AND BODY SYSTEMS

In many traditional cultures, age has long been admired, and the elderly have been honored and respected for their wisdom and achievements. The same cannot be said of the United States and most other highly industrialized countries, in which older citizens have been shunted out of society's mainstream. However, in recent years, because of their increasing numbers, education, and sophistication, mature adults have become a significant political and economic force in this country. Each day, more than 5000 Americans reach age 65, and more than 3500 over age 65 die(1). Thus, those over 65 constitute the most rapidly changing segment of the U.S. population, with an annual increase of over a half million. By 1990, the baby boom population, post-World War II babies, will be 40 or older, further swelling the ranks of the mature adult population. In 1970, 40% of those over 65 had completed high school; by 1978, 85% had done so (2).

The proportion of older adults in this country is steadily increasing. The elderly of today have more purchasing power and are more comfortable with activism than their counterparts of a decade ago. In the future, the elderly will attract an increasing amount of attention from manufacturers, merchants, and politicians (see Tables 1-1 and 1-2). However, in spite of their presently increasing numbers and influence, older people in the United States still live in a society that puts a premium on a youthful appearance and attitude. Aging adults often have an increased need for health care, both preventive and interventional. Ideally, this care will be provided by practitioners who appreciate the biological and social changes experienced by older adults, and which affect the type of care they need.

Table 1–1   Population 1981 (40 years and older) thousands

Age	Total	Male	Female
40–44	12,043	5896	6147
45–49	10,985	5342	5643
50–54	11,545	5546	5999
55–59	11,600	5474	6126
60–64	10,335	4782	5553
65–74	15,893	6892	9000
75 and over	10,361	3668	6693

Source: U.S. Bureau of Census, Census of Population: 1970, vol. 1, and Current Population Reports series P-25, No. 917.

At all ages there should be the expectation of continued life. Mortality statistics support this expectation (see Table 1–3). Recently, a new terminology has been proposed that attempts to remove the stigma of growing old and to more clearly define the stages of aging (3). It is based on the theoretical life-span of 115 years for humans.

Aged: persons 86 years old and older
Elderly: persons 77 through 85 years
Aging: persons 69 to 76 years
Mature adults: persons 68 years and younger

Table 1–2   Projections of the United States Population (in the Thousands): 1985 to 2025

Age (yr)	Date			
	1985	1990	2000	2025
All ages	238,648	249,731	267,990	301,022
40–44	14,107	17,841	21,982	19,612
45–49	11,642	13,973	19,753	17,539
50–54	10,819	11,418	17,341	17,241
55–59	11,261	10,451	13,285	18,046
60–64	10,946	19,639	10,494	19,508
65–69	9,227	10,006	9,110	18,314
70–74	7,635	8,048	8,583	14,774
75–79	5,534	6,224	7,242	11,103
80–84	3,482	4,060	4,965	6,767
85 +	2,794	3,461	5,136	7,678
62 +	35,136	38,151	41,086	70,429

Adapted from Current Population Reports, Populations Estimates, and Projections Series P-25, No. 922 Issued October 1982. U.S. Dept. of Commerce Bureau of the Census.

Table 1-3 Life Expectancy

Female		Male	
Age (yr)	Expected years of life remaining	Age (yr)	Expected years of life remaining
50	30.5	50	24.6
60	22.1	60	17.1
65	18.4	65	14.0
70	14.7	70	11.1
75	11.5	75	8.7
80	8.9	80	6.9
85	6.9	85	5.5

Vital Statistics of the United States 1978 Volume II—Mortality Part A, U.S. Dept. of Health and Human Services Public Health Service, National Center for Health Statistics.

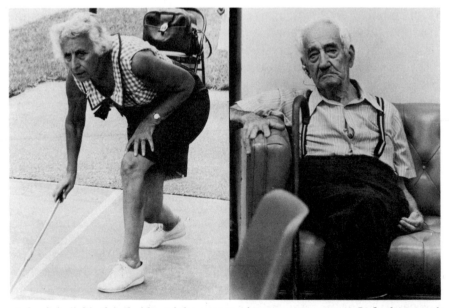

Aging is individual and older adults are not a homogeneous group. Left photograph by L. Miller; right photograph by R. Rudman.

This helps to give a longitudinal focus to the stages of older adult life and may help prevent health care personnel from lumping all older adults into one category. The Census Bureau has also recognized the need to categorize the aged in a longitudinal way (4).

FACTORS INFLUENCING LONGEVITY

Although our present understanding of aging offers little more than a hint at the extreme complexity of the process, it is widely agreed that the length of life is determined by an interplay of genetic and environmental factors. It is now accepted that humans have a finite life-span of approximately 115 years, with various factors such as the presence or absence of specific disease states, dietary habits, personality type, intelligence, and gender each having an influence. However, if all the killer diseases of later life were eliminated, it is estimated that no more than 10 years would be added to an average individual's life expectancy.

Inheritance of specific disease states may reduce life expectancy. Inheritance of hypercholesterolemia frequently shortens one's life-span. Noninherited diseases such as organic brain syndrome may be predictive of a shortened life-span as well (5).

A sedentary life-style increases the risk of early death, while regular exercise appears to have a protective effect. It also appears useful to regulate body weight. Being overweight by 20% or more increases the risk of sudden death. Moreover, it has been suggested that occasional prolonged fasting will increase longevity (6). Moderate use of alcohol, 1–2 ounces daily, may be associated with prolonged life. However, excessive drinking may lead to inadequate nutritional intake, liver damage, violence, or even suicide (see Chapter 5).

Four of the major threats to longevity of the older adult are obesity, diabetes, cancer, and heart disease, which together account for 69.3% of deaths. All these disease processes may be modified by diet (7). Thus, in a medically advanced country like the United States, where infant mortality is relatively low, nutrition plays a major role in determining longevity.

High intelligence is associated with a longer life-span. Among college graduates, honor students have a higher life expectancy than other graduates. Also, people listed in *Who's Who* have a lower mortality rate than others in the population. Studies of personality type show that those people more affected by time pressure are more vulnerable to myocardial infarction and are more likely to have other serious disease.

Women generally live longer than men. This may be purely a biological phenomenon resulting from the "protective" effect of female hormones (or lack of male hormones) or may be of psychosocial origin. Women may be more concerned with weight control and smoke fewer cigarettes than men. Recent changes in the roles and behavior women are assuming may be shown in the future to adversely affect their life-span.

Though the interplay of the various factors is very complicated and not well understood, one general trend repeatedly emerges from study of the factors influencing longevity: the single most effective predictor of one's life-span is the life-span of one's biological parents.

THE AGING BODY

With aging defined as a change in the activity of living systems due to the passage of time, different organs and tissues age at various rates. A man of 40 may, for the first time in his life, need glasses to read the newspaper, while his lung function may be virtually unchanged from what it was 20 years before. On the other hand, the man's wife of 40 may still have perfect vision though her lung capacity may be only 90% of what it was when she was 20. Not only does aging affect different organ systems in different ways, but aging of specific organs also proceeds at different rates in different people.

Generally, with advancing age, there is an increased tendency of cells that normally divide to stop doing so, and there is a deterioration of specialized nondividing cells, such as nerve and muscle cells, leading to their death. Some physiological parameters such as blood volume and red cell count are unchanged with increasing age. However, the connective tissue proteins, such as collagen, which comprise more than 40% of the body's protein, become more rigid, causing blood vessels to be more resistant to flow. Therefore, blood pressure and tissue nourishment will change.

The organ systems of young adults are able to meet greater demands than are ordinarily placed on them. This *reserve capacity* of most systems gradually decreases with aging. Thus, the elderly are less able than younger persons to maintain a stable internal body environment when subjected to stress. For example, after a glucose load, the return of the blood sugar level to normal will take substantially longer in the elderly than it will in a 20-year-old (8).

Advanced age is associated with nonuniform changes in the various body tissues (see Table 1–4). Generally, all these changes result in a loss of cells and lower energy levels of the remaining cells. This is associated with a diminished reserve capacity of most organs, as discussed above, slowed reaction times, and an increased rigidity of connective tissues.

Table 1–4 Physiological Changes in Aging

---

1. Cardiovascular system—Decreased force of contraction
   Decreased stroke volume
   Declining cardiac output
   Reduced elasticity of blood vessels
2. Respiratory system—Loss of elasticity
   Decreased maximum breathing capacity
3. Renal system—Decreased blood flow
   Reduced glomerular filtration
   Decreased tubular excretion
   Reduced number of nephrons
4. Neuromuscular system—Decreased responses of receptor organs
   Decline in physical strength
   Decline in motor function
   Decline in muscle mass
5. Nervous system—Decline in reaction time
   Decreased speed of nerve impulses
   Decreased responses of receptor organs
6. Endocrine system—Reduced blood levels of some hormones
   Increased sensitivity in some tissues
   Declining glucose tolerance
7. Gastrointestinal system—Loss of teeth
   Decreased taste sensation
   Decreased saliva secretion
   Reduced hydrochloric acid in stomach
   Decreased secretion of digestive enzymes and mucus
   Loss of muscle tone in stomach
   Decreased peristalsis
   Formation of intestinal diverticula
8. Skin—Reduced subcutaneous fat
   Atrophy of sweat glands and hair follicles
   Skin discolored, thin, dry, wrinkled, and fragile
   Increased number of skin cancers

CHANGES IN BODY SYSTEMS WITH AGE

Cardiovascular Systems

After age 19, there is a decrease in the heart's force on contraction and stroke volume amounting to 1% per year. By age 65, cardiac output may decline by 40% (9). The body's circulation redistributes to compensate for the decreased cardiac output so that the blood supply to the heart and brain is decreased less than the blood supply to the kidney and liver. Decreased blood supply does not necessarily result in reduced function since the heart, kidney, and liver all have large reserve capacities.

The function of the heart valves may be impaired because of fibrosis and calcification, causing them to become more rigid (10). The collagen molecules in the heart wall and peripheral vessels become increasingly cross-linked so that all tissues containing collagen become rigid. The rigid blood vessels impede blood flow, with arterial resistance increasing about 1% per year after maturity. This leads to increased blood pressure, possibly to enlargement of the heart and a tendency toward congestive heart failure. Calcium is deposited in the wall of arteries as part of the process of atherosclerosis (11). Numerous dietary factors—amount and type of fat, amount of carbohydrate, and alcohol use—have been shown to influence the development of atherosclerosis.

Systolic blood pressure generally increases from age 20 to age 70 or 80, though there is not uniform agreement on this fact. Diastolic blood pressure increases gradually over the same time period, though again a variety of different time courses have been reported. Normal blood pressure at age 25 is about 120/75, whereas a level of approximately 160/90 is expected after age 65 (12). Those with blood pressure levels over these figures at these ages are considered to be hypertensive (13). However, it is difficult to define hypertension in mature adults. Its diagnosis should really be based on adverse effects to the eye, kidney, heart, and brain and not simply on elevated blood pressure measurements.

High blood pressure and congestive heart failure call for a reduction of sodium in the diet and possibly weight loss. There is not as much certainty about the value of other dietary modifications such as increasing potassium, calcium, and magnesium intake and manipulating the type and amount of fat eaten.

Reduced cardiac output limits the capacity for physical work, and it hinders the body's ability to adjust to physical stress. Exercise of the same intensity and duration raises the heart rate and blood pressure more in old age than in youth.

Respiratory System

Lung tissue has abundant collagen and elastin fibers. The changes in these fibers that lead to increased rigidity of blood vessels also occur in the lung and lead to progressive loss of elasticity of lung tissue with advancing age (14). In addition, similar tissue changes cause impaired oxygen delivery to the blood (15). The older person expends more energy breathing and is more susceptible to aspiration and other respiratory problems. Obesity may aggravate all of these; therefore, a reduce calorie intake may be warranted.

Renal System

All functions of the kidney gradually decline with age. The blood flow to the kidneys is reduced by an average of 55% between the ages of 35 and 80. The decrease averages about 0.6% per year in adults. The ability to form concentrated urine is reduced, as is the ability to excrete a salt load. This means that fluid intake must be carefully considered (16). Dehydration can result in confusion, and both dehydration and fluid retention can cause electrolyte imbalance.

Decreased renal function permits medication to remain present and active in the body of the older individual for longer periods, increasing the possibility of drug toxicity. In addition, reduced renal function may contribute to elevated blood pressure.

Neuromuscular System

Motor function declines with age, as does physical strength (17). For instance, a decrease in handgrip strength is detectable as early as age 30. Muscle size is reduced, and there may be degenerative changes in the joints, leading to pain, weakness, and stiffness. The older person has a reduced capacity for muscular work and requires a longer time to warm up to full working capacity. By age 75 the overall excitability of muscles decreases and the speed of nerve conduction is reduced by 10%. These neuromuscular changes often may reduce the older adult's ability to buy, prepare, and even eat sufficient nutrients to meet needs.

Nervous System

With age, there is a general slowing of responses to environmental stimuli. The functioning of sense organs becomes impaired, affecting taste, pain, touch, heat, cold, and point-position perceptions. The number of olfactory receptors markedly declines, causing a reduced sensitivity to odors. The elderly are found to require a threshold concentration at least 11 times as great as that of young persons to perceive a wide variety of odors.

This loss of taste and smell affects appetite as it diminishes the pleasure of eating. There is a reduction in visual and auditory acuity as well; this too adversely affects food intake.

The decreased conduction velocity of neurons associated with old age results in slowed voluntary movements, slowed reflex and reaction time, and increased time necessary for decision making. Also high blood pressure, a common problem in the elderly, is associated with a decline in memory and intellectual function. However, the reduced blood flow to the brain characteristic of advanced age does not tend to have any adverse effects if the individual is in good health. Thus, the absence of pathological conditions, long-term memory and reasoning ability may be only minimally affected. A high level of intellectual activity is often possible because of adaptive mechanisms that compensate for age-related changes in the nervous system.

Endocrine System

With aging, the amount of connective tissue in the endocrine glands increases, replacing secretory cells. Therefore, blood levels of many hormones decrease. Blood concentrations of testosterone in men and estrogen in women decrease with age. Blood levels of triiodothyronine are also decreased, and the functional activity of the thyroid gland diminishes. However, body tissues adapt to the lower hormone levels, and the body's metabolic homeostasis is preserved (18). Parathyroid hormone also shows a fall in blood concentration with a concomitant increase in tissue sensitivity.

There is a gradual and continuous decline of glucose tolerance with age (19). It has been theorized that mature adults may have an increased amount of insulin antagonists in the blood and thus a lower effective blood insulin level. Although the incidence of diabetes in the aged population may be overestimated because of a failure to appreciate the natural age-related changes in glucose tolerance, minimal dietary changes such as reducing the use of simple sugars and increasing the intake of foods that have less effect on blood sugar levels would be beneficial.

Gastrointestinal System

Not all studies on taste and smell sensitivity in the elderly are in agreement. Different measurement methods have led to different results (20). Sex differences, diseases, and the effect of smoking further complicate attempts at generalization. The reduced taste and smell perception that are reported to occur with advanced age may affect the appetite and desire for food. The loss of taste buds is believed to begin in middle age and primarily affects those buds that detect sweet or salty taste. Those that detect bitter or sour usually remain unaffected. This may explain why some older adults complain that all foods taste bitter or sour. Dentures that cover the palate further reduce taste sensation.

Deficiencies of niacin, vitamin A, and zinc may cause decreased taste acuity. Deficiencies of copper and nickel are also related to changes in ability to taste. Disease states such as cancer and treatment such as radiation, major surgery, and drugs also alter taste acuity (21). Improved oral hygiene in the elderly can improve taste perception, particularly for sweet and salty taste (22).

Diet is greatly affected by the loss of teeth and by ill-fitting dentures (23). Fifty percent of all Americans have lost all their teeth by age 65 (24). A study of 100 70-year-olds showed that 28 men and 38 women had lost all their teeth, and, of those, 80% either did not replace them or replaced them with dentures that did not fit properly (25). Even well-fitting dentures can cause problems, and dentures that fit well at one time may become loose owing to atrophy of the gingiva. We have all seen people who have few or no teeth at all "gum" foods and appear to handle even hard foods, such as nuts by mashing them with their gums. Despite these few, the loss of teeth leads to impaired chewing ability, often limits the choice of foods and even may decrease the desire to eat (26). Moreover, it has been shown that inadequate chewing of at least some food can result in malabsorption of certain nutrients (27). Thus, if one is edentulous, it is important to obtain and maintain well-functioning dentures.

With aging, there is a diminution in the secretory activity of the various sections of the gastrointestinal tract. Decreased salivary secretion may interfere with eating by causing difficulty in swallowing, which may already be impaired by slowed reflex muscular activity. Salivary secretion is reduced by the intake of tranquilizers and other drugs.

With aging, the parietal cells of the stomach lose their ability to secrete hydrochloric acid. The incidence of achlorhydria (the absence of hydrochloric acid in the stomach) increases after the age of 60. Hydrochloric acid has several functions: it provides the proper acidity for protein digestion; it converts the inactive form of the gastric protease pepsinogen to pepsin; it increases the solubility of iron and calcium; and it acts as a bactericidal agent. The reduction of hydrochloric acid in the stomach thus may interfere with protein digestion and mineral absorption as well as contribute to proliferation of bacteria that can cause digestive upsets. The incidence of pernicious anemia is associated with reduced hydrochloric acid secretion, but the reason for this association has not been clarified.

In the elderly, there is also a reduced secretion of mucus and of digestive enzymes, which thus impairs the digestion and absorption of foods. Salivary amylase, pancratic amylase, and lipase, as well as trypsin and pepsin secretion, are all decreased. For some enzymes, the reduction begins in one's teens. The decreased production of lactase with age is very prevalent in certain groups of people. The problem of lactose intolerance will be discussed in Chapter 6.

In spite of these gastrointestinal changes, there does not seem to be a marked decrease in the ability of the aged to digest most foods. However, there is some evidence that protein digestion is less efficient.

Loss of muscle tone in the stomach results in reduced gastric motility, which, in turn, causes delayed emptying of the stomach. Along with reduced gastric motility, there is a reduction of hunger contractions. In fact, there is a reduction in the motility of the entire gastrointestinal tract as well as a reduced blood supply to it and a lessened response to neural control.

Aging affects the integrity of the gastrointestinal tract. Medications such as steroids, aspirin, and reserpine, passing through a weakly motile tract, may predispose the elderly to ulcer formation. The prevalence of intestinal diverticula also is age-related and may result in bouts of diverticulitis. It has been theorized that increasing the amount of fiber eaten will reduce the tendency to form diverticula and reduce the incidence of inflammation in existing diverticula.

The type and numbers of intestinal microflora change with age, and more putrefactive and fever-producing bacteria are found in the intestine of older than younger people. This may cause flatulence and a greater susceptibility to food-borne illness.

D-Xylose, a carbohydrate, is used to study the intestinal absorption of food. No change in the absorption of xylose is found until after age 80 (28). However, there have been reports of impaired absorption of thiamin, folic acid, and fats in the aged. Poor absorption of fat is often linked to malabsorption of calcium because unabsorbed fat may form insoluble complexes with the calcium present in the gastrointestinal tract.

The loss of muscle tone and resultant reduction in peristalsis contributes to constipation. A study focusing on digestive disorders in older people found the most frequent complaint to be constipation in each of two age groups: those aged 45 to 64 and those over 65 (29). However, the prevalence of the complaint was three times as great in those aged 65 and over than in the younger group—hence, the common use of laxatives among the elderly.

Skin

Like most other organs in the body, the skin undergoes a gradual decrease in both size and function with age, becoming thinner and less elastic. There is a decrease in the number of functioning sweat glands and a slowed turnover of cells. This may be an important factor in the decreased ability of aged skin to heal well after injury. Furthermore, the skin becomes more permeable, making it less able to retain water and repel environmental substances.

The blood vessels of the skin become less able to dilate and constrict, making the aged less able to adapt to extremes of temperature. This is why older people are more susceptible to heat stroke and hypothermia than younger persons (30).

Immune System

The immune system, which acts to protect the body from foreign substances, infections, transplanted organs, and cancer, changes with age. Its function declines progressively after adolescence. It has been suggested that calorie restriction in adults may help prevent this decline in immune function and may also be protective against autoimmune phenomena (31).

On the other hand, in people suffering from protein malnutrition, certain functions of the immune system are markedly depressed, and they return to essentially normal after an adequate diet is reinstituted (32).

Body Composition

During the adult years there is a progressive decrease in lean body mass and an increase in body fat (see Figure 1–1). Studies have shown an average lean body mass of 59 kg at age 25, which decreases to 47 kg by age 65 to 70. During this same time, the average amount of body fat increases from 14 to 26 kg. This indicates a decrease of 12 kg lean body mass and an increase in body fat of 12 kg. This increased amount of fat is probably due not to an increased rate of fat deposition but rather to a reduced capacity of the body to mobilize fat. However, the biochemical basis of this is unknown. With age there is a decrease in the amount of body water along with a reduced oxygen consumption.

Bone loss also occurs later in life. Maximum bone density is found in women around age 40 and in men around age 50. Thus, men and women begin losing bone matter after these ages. Women lose far more bone than men do—about 8% per decade as opposed to 3% per decade for men. In addition, women do not have a leveling off of this rate as do older men. This bone loss can cause serious clinical problems in the elderly, and it does not seem to be easily corrected by nutritional means. Increasing the intake of calcium to 1.5 g/day does not seem to entirely

	Age 25 Percent	Age 70 Percent
Fat	20	36
Cell mass	47	36
Bone mineral	6	4
Other	27	24

Figure 1–1.   Body composition and age of men.

Source: Adapted from Gregerman and Bierman, *Textbook of Endocrinology*, 1974.

prevent it (33). On the other hand, evidence suggests that getting 1 hour of endurance exercise four times a week is sufficient to arrest bone loss in the elderly. Such exercise may also act to lower the proportion of body fat in the elderly to that which is characteristic of middle-aged individuals (34).

Body changes in aging have often been determined from cross-sectional, not longitudinal, studies. Therefore, estimates of change in body composition such as decreased lean tissue may be an artifact of the type of study and not really be representative of the situation in all older adults. Recent data from longitudinal studies suggest that the lean body mass may be unchanged as a person ages, but that persons with less body tissue tend to live longer (25).

REFERENCES

1. The National Council on the Aging, Inc., February, 1978. *Fact Book on Aging,* 1828 L. Street, N.W. Washington D.C. 20036.
2. *Newsday*, Monday, Nov. 10, 1980, Part II, p. 2.

3. Watkin, D.M., The physiology of aging, *Am. J. Clin. Nutr.* 36(4) (suppl.): 750, 1982.

4. Elderly choose retirement community living, *The New York Times*, April 5, 1984, p. C1.

5. Eisdorfer, C., *Some Variables Relating to Longevity in Humans. Epidemiology of Aging*, U.S. Dep't. Health Education and Welfare, DHEW Pub. No. (NIH) 77–711, 1972.

6. Pitot, H.C., Carcinogenesis and aging—two related phenomena. *Am. J. Pathol.* 87:444, 1977.

7. *Vital Statistics of the United States*, Annual, U.S. National Center for Health Statistics.

8. Insulin resistance and aging, *J. Clin. Invest.* 71:1523, 1581, 1983.

9. Shock, N.W., 1977 Biological theories of aging, in: *Handbook of the Psychology of Aging*, eds. J.E. Birren, K.W. Schaie. New York: Van Nostrand Reinhold Co., p. 103.

10. Sell, S., Scully, R.C., Aging changes in the aortic and mitral valves, *Am. J. Pathol.* 46:345, 1965.

11. Koch-Weser, J., Correlation of pathophysiology and pharmacology in primary hypertension, *Am. J. Cardiol.* 32:499, 1973.

12. Harris, R., Cardiovascular diseases in the elderly, *Med. Clin. North Am.* 67:379, 1983.

13. Franklin, S.S., Geriatric hypertension, *Med. Clin. North Am.* 67:395, 1983.

14. Boucek, R.J., Noble, N.L., Marks, A., Age and fibrous proteins of the human lungs, *Gerontologia* 5:150, 1961.

15. Candler, L., Mayer, J.H., *Aging of the Lung*. New York: Guine and Stratton. 1964.

16. Bowles, L.T., Portnoy, V., Kenny R., Wear and tear: Common biologic changes of aging, *Geriatrics* 36:77, 1981.

17. McQuillen, M.P., Neuromuscular fatigue in middle life, what it means and how to treat it, *Geriatrics* 34:67, 1979.

18. Davis, P.J., Aging and endocrine function, *Clin. Endocrine Metals* 8:603, 1979.

19. Andreas, R., Tobin, J.D., Endocrine systems, in: Finch, C.E., Hayflick, L., eds., *Handbook of Biology of Aging*. New York: Van Nostrand Reinhold Co., 1977, p. 357.

20. Krehl, W.A., The influence of nutritional environment on aging, *Geriatrics* 29:65, 1974.

21. Handvon, K.T., (letter) Taste, the unnecessary sense? *N. Engl. J. Med.* 308:529, 1983.

22. Engen, T., Taste and smell, in: *Handbook of the Psychology of Aging*, eds. J.E. Birren and K.W. Schaie. New York: Van Nostrand and Reinhold Co., 1977, p. 554.

23. Neill, D.J., Phillips, H.I.E., The masticatory performance, dental state and dietary intake of a group of elderly army pensioners, *Br. Dent. J.* 128:581, 1980.

24. Busse, E.W., How mind, body and environment influence nutrition in the elderly, *Postgrad. Med.* 63(3):118, 1978.

25. Masoro, E., Physiologic change with aging, in: *Nutrition and Aging,* ed. M. Winick. New York: John Wiley & Sons, 1976, p. 61.

26. Ettinger, R.L., Diet, nutrition and the elderly edentulous patient, *Edinburgh Dent. Hosp. Gaz.* 12:24, 1972.

27. Levine, A.S., Silvie, S.E., Absorption of whole peanuts, peanut oil, and peanut butter, *N. Engl. J. Med.* 303:917, 1980.

28. Masoro, E., Other physiologic changes with age, in: *Epidemiology of Aging*, eds. A.M. Ostfeld, and D.C. Gibson, DHEW Publication No. (NIH) 77-711, 1972.

29. Shank, R.E., Nutritional characteristics of the elderly—An overview, in: *Nutrition, Longevity and Aging*, eds. M. Rockstein and M.L. Sussman. New York: Academic Press, 1976.

30. Gilchrest, B.A., Aging of the skin, in: N.A. Soter and H.P. Baden, *Pathophysiology of Dermatologic Diseases.* New York: McGraw-Hill, 1984.

31. *Special Report on Aging 1980,* U.S. Dept. of Health and Human Services; NIH Publication No. 80-2135, Aug. 1980.

32. Watson, R.R., Nutrition, disease resistance and age, in *Food Nutr. News* 51(1): Oct.-Nov. 1979.

33. Thompson, D.L., Frame, B., Involutional osteopenia: Current concepts, *Ann. Intern. Med.* 85:789, 1976.

34. Sidney, K.H., Shephard, R.J., Harrison, J.E., Endurance training and body composition of the elderly, *Am. J. Clin. Nutr.* 30:326, 1977.

Chapter 2

NUTRITIONAL ASSESSMENT

The nutritional status of older adults reflects much more than their current food intake. Lifelong food habits must be considered, as well as all factors affecting those habits, such as pain medications used, allergies (real or imagined), medical illnesses, surgical procedures, and physical disabilities that interfere with obtaining, preparing, and eating food. One elderly woman developed malnutrition as a result of limited mobility, because of overgrown toenails that she could not cut. This surely is an extreme case but can serve to remind health care personnel to ask questions to uncover problems that might be otherwise overlooked. Nutritional status can be evaluated in a variety of ways. Usual methods include anthropometric measurements, laboratory measurements, clinical examination, and diet assessment.

ANTHROPOMETRIC MEASUREMENTS

Weight

Weight is considered the single most useful measurement of nutritional status and is the measurement most commonly recorded. It is best to weigh people after they have voided, and when they are wearing minimal clothing. There are several standards available for the assessment of weight.

Table 2–1 Metropolitan Life Insurance Company Height and Weight Tables 1983

Height		Men		
Feet	Inches	Small frame	Medium frame	Large frame
5	2	128–134	131–141	138–150
5	3	130–136	133–143	140–153
5	4	132–138	135–135	142–156
5	5	134–140	137–148	144–160
5	6	136–142	139–151	146–164
5	7	138–145	142–154	149–168
5	8	140–148	145–157	152–172
5	9	142–151	148–160	155–176
5	10	144–154	151–163	158–180
5	11	146–157	154–166	161–184
6	0	149–160	157–170	164–188
6	1	152–164	160–174	168–192
6	2	155–168	164–178	172–197
6	3	158–172	167–182	176–202
6	4	162–176	171–187	181–207

Weights at ages 25–59 based on lowest mortality. Weight in pounds according to frame (in indoor clothing weighing 5 lb, shoes with 1-in. heels).

Height		Women		
Feet	Inches	Small frame	Medium frame	Large frame
4	10	102–111	109–121	118–131
4	11	103–113	111–123	120–134
5	0	104–115	113–126	122–137
5	1	106–118	115–129	124–140
5	2	108–121	118–132	128–143
5	3	111–124	121–135	131–147
5	4	114–127	124–138	134–151
5	5	117–130	127–141	137–155
5	6	120–133	130–144	140–159
5	7	123–136	133–147	143–163
5	8	126–139	136–150	146–167
5	9	129–142	139–153	149–170
5	10	132–145	142–156	152–173
5	11	135–148	145–159	155–176
6	0	138–151	148–162	158–179

Weights at ages 25–59 based on lowest mortality. Weight in pounds according to frame (in indoor clothing weighing 3 lb, shoes with 1-in. heels).

Table 2–1   (Cont.)

How to Determine Your Body Frame by Elbow Breadth

To make a simple approximation of your frame size:

Extend your arm and bend the forearm upwards at a 90-degree angle. Keep the fingers straight and turn the inside of your wrist away from the body. Place the thumb and index finger of your other hand on the two prominent bones on *either side* of your elbow. Measure the space between your fingers against a ruler or a tape measure.* Compare the measurements on the following tables.

These tables list the elbow measurements for medium-framed men and women of various heights. Measurements lower than those listed indicate you have a small frame and higher measurements indicate a large frame.

Men

Height in 1-in. heels	Elbow breadth
5′2″–5′3″	2½″–2⅞″
5′4″–5′7″	2⅝″–2⅞″
5′8″–5′11″	2¾″–3″
6′0″–6′3″	2¾″–3⅛″
6′4″	2⅞″–3¼″

Women

Height in 1-in. heels	Elbow breadth
4′10″–4′11″	2¼″–2½″
5′0″–5′3″	2¼″–2½″
5′4″–5′7″	2⅜″–2⅝″
5′8″–5′11″	2⅜″–2⅝″
6′0″	2½″–2¾″

*For the most accurate measurement, have your physician measure your elbow breadth with a caliper.

The familiar Metropolitan Height-Weight Tables (1) (see Table 2–1), which were revised in 1983, may not be appropriate for use with older adults as they are based on weights of adults up to age 59. These tables represent weights associated with the lowest mortality for persons of various heights and body frames. A method for estimating frame size by measuring elbow breadth is suggested.

Another reference, published by the National Center for Health Statistics, includes weights for older adults up to the age of 74 (2) (see Table 2–2). For persons older than 74, an average height-weight table based on data from more than 5000 men and women is often used (3) (see Table 2–3).

Weight standards must be adjusted to compensate for loss of body parts owing to trauma or surgery. Table 2–4 gives the percentage of total

Table 2-2   Average Weights for U.S. Men and Women 1971–74[1]

Sex and height	Age group (yr)			
	35–44	45–54	55–64	65–74
Men	*Weight (lb)*			
62 inches	143	147	143	143
63 inches	148	152	147	147
64 inches	153	156	153	151
65 inches	158	160	158	156
66 inches	163	164	163	160
67 inches	169	169	168	164
68 inches	174	173	173	169
69 inches	179	177	178	173
70 inches	184	182	183	177
71 inches	190	187	189	182
72 inches	194	191	193	186
73 inches	200	196	197	190
74 inches	205	200	203	194
Women				
57 inches	125	129	132	130
58 inches	129	133	136	134
59 inches	133	136	140	137
60 inches	137	140	143	140
61 inches	141	143	147	144
62 inches	144	147	150	147
63 inches	148	150	153	151
64 inches	152	154	157	154
65 inches	156	158	160	158
66 inches	159	161	164	161
67 inches	163	165	167	165
68 inches	167	168	171	169

[1]Estimated values from regression equations of weight on height for specified age groups.

NOTE: Examined persons were measured without shoes: clothing weight ranged from 0.20 to 0.62 pound, which was not deducted from weights shown.

Adapted from Weight by Height and Age for Adults 18–74 years: United States, 1971–74, Office of Health Research, Statistics and Technology, National Center for Health Statistics, U.S. Dept. of Health, Education and Welfare.

body weight that should be subtracted from weight to compensate for the amputation.

Height

Obtaining accurate standing height measurement may be difficult because older persons may find it painful to "stand tall" or because of ar-

Table 2-3 Average Height-Weight Table for Persons 65 Years of Age and Over

Height (in.)	Men					
	Ages 65-69	Ages 70-74	Ages 75-79	Ages 80-84	Ages 85-89	Ages 90-94
61	128-156	125-153	123-151			
62	130-158	127-155	125-153	122-148		
63	131-161	129-157	127-155	122-150	120-146	
64	134-164	131-161	129-157	124-152	122-148	
65	136-166	134-164	130-160	127-155	125-153	117-143
66	139-169	137-167	133-163	130-158	128-156	120-146
67	140-172	140-170	136-166	132-162	130-160	122-150
68	143-175	142-174	139-169	135-165	133-163	126-154
69	147-179	146-178	142-174	139-169	137-167	130-158
70	150-184	148-182	146-178	143-175	140-172	134-164
71	155-189	152-186	149-183	148-180	144-176	139-169
72	159-195	156-190	154-188	153-187	148-182	
73	164-200	160-196	158-192			

Table 2-3 (Cont.) Average Height-Weight Table for Persons 65 Years of Age and Over

Height (in.)	Women					
	Ages 65–69	Ages 70–74	Ages 75–59	Ages 80–84	Ages 85–89	Ages 90–94
58	120–146	112–138	111–135			
59	121–147	114–140	112–136	100–122	99–121	
60	122–148	116–142	113–139	106–130	102–124	
61	123–151	118–144	115–144	109–133	104–128	
62	125–153	121–147	118–144	112–136	108–132	107–131
63	127–155	123–151	121–147	115–141	112–136	107–131
64	130–158	126–154	123–151	119–145	115–141	108–132
65	132–162	130–158	126–154	122–150	120–146	112–136
66	136–166	132–162	128–157	126–154	124–152	116–142
67	140–170	136–166	131–161	130–158	128–156	
68	143–175	140–170				
69	148–180	144–176				

Source: Arthur M. Master, et al., Tables of average heights and weights of Americans aged 65 to 84 years. *JAMA, 172:658, 1960.*

Table 2–4 Adjustment of Body Weight Standard for Amputation

Type of amputation	Percentages of total body wt.
Foot	1.8%
Below knee	6.0%
Above knee	15.0%
Entire lower extremity	18.5%
Hand	1.0%
Below elbow	3.0%
Entire upper extremity	6.5%

In order to use this information, you must know the patient's approximate height before the amputation. Use this height to calculate the desirable body weight for the normal adult. Then adjust the figures according to the type of amputation performed.

Example: To determine the desirable body weight for a 5'10" man with a below-the-knee amputation:

1. Calculate desirable body weight for a 5'10" man   166 lb
2. Subtract weight of amputated limb (6.0%)
   $166 \times .06 = 9.86$ (approx. 10 lb)   − 10 lb
3. Desirable weight of a 5'10" man with a below-the-knee amputation   156 lb

Source: Brunnstrom, S., *Clinical Kinesiology*. Philadelphia: F.A. Davis Co., 1972.

thritis, spinal curvature, or large fat deposits on the back, preventing body contact with the wall. Recumbent length has been suggested as a more accurate means of height measurement (4).

When standing measurement is impossible, as when a person is wheelchair bound, knee height (distance from bottom of heel to top of knee when knee is bent at 90 degrees) measured with the person in a recumbent position can be used to estimate height. This measurement correlates well with stature and changes little with increasing age. Values for midarm circumference and skinfold thickness are also similar for standing and recumbent positions (5).

Other Measurements

Arm circumference measurement, taken on the nondominant side if possible, is a good indication of muscle mass and a measure of available fat and protein stores (6) (see Table 2–5). Measurement of skinfold thickness by calipers may provide more information about available fat stores than weight and height alone because one-half of all body fat is found right under the skin. The triceps measurement is often used be-

Table 2–5 Average Mid-Upper
Arm Muscle Circumference
in Adults

Age (yr)	Men	Women
45–54	28.2	22.7
55–64	27.8	22.8
65–74	26.8	22.8

Source: Bishop, C.W., et al., Norms
for nutritional assessment of American adults by upper arm anthropometry, *Am. J. Clin. Nutr.* 34:2530,
1981.

cause of accessibility; however, the subscapular skinfold is less subject to error. It does not have to be measured at a precise spot because the fat layer in that area is uniform (6) (see Table 2–6).

When using standards for comparison of body measurements, it should be remembered that often the reference data have been obtained from white adults. Therefore, they may be inappropriate for use with other racial groups. In fact, absolute weight itself is not a good indication of nutritional status. More important is the person's usual weight and a history of weight change. A loss of 10 lb within 6 months, without dieting, may indicate a problem. In a survey of 4700 hospital admissions, the death rate of those over 40 was found to be 19 times higher in those who reported an involuntary 10-lb weight loss in the preceding 6

Table 2–6 Average Triceps
Skinfold Thickness
in Adults (in mm)

Age (yr)	Men	Women
35–44	12	23
45–54	11	25
55–64	11	25
65–74	11	23

Basic data on anthropometric measurements and angular measurements of the hip and knee joints for selected age groups 1–74 years of age, United States, 1971–1975 National Health Survey, Vital and Health Statistics Series No. 219, U.S. Dept. of Health and Human Services, Public Health Service, 1981.

months (7). Alternatively, significant weight gain over a short period of time may be a clue to development of edema or ascites, both of which may arise as a result of malnutrition or other medical illness.

Available standards are best used as a starting point to monitor changes in body measurements reflective of alteration in nutritional status and/or the effects of nutritional intervention (8).

LABORATORY MEASUREMENTS

A variety of laboratory measurements can be used to assess nutritional status. Norms that have been developed for these measurements are based on data from children and younger adults so that they may not be suitable for use with older persons. In addition, some test results depend on normal liver and kidney function and thus would not be appropriate for all individuals.

Depletion of body protein levels is reflected in lowered serum albumin, which takes about 2 weeks of starvation to be substantially depressed, and serum transferrin, which can be depressed in a few days. Total iron binding capacity (TIBC) may be used when serum transferrin levels are not obtainable. Multiplying TIBC by 0.8 and subtracting 43 gives the transferrin value, an approximation of the transferrin level. A transferrin level under 190 is considered low in most laboratories.

Immune function is decreased with protein malnutrition. Peripheral lymphocytes are decreased owing to deficiences in calories an precursor amino acids. Serum albumin levels less than 3.5 g/dl and total lymphocyte counts (percent lymphocytes × total white blood cells) of under 1500 mm are associated with increased mortality rates in hospitalized patients. These two parameters along with a weight loss of 10 lb, as described previously, have been suggested as a readily available indication of malnutrition (7, 9).

Skin testing to common substances people have been exposed to may be used as a measure of cellular immunity. In a malnourished person, the allergic response to allergens placed on the skin is delayed or absent. Disease, surgery, radiation, and immunosuppressant drugs can also affect the immune response (10). Skin testing is considered to be of little diagnostic value and may be misinterpreted because of age-related changes in immune function (11). Thus, skin testing is rarely used as the sole measure of nutritional adequacy.

On occasion, urinalysis may be helpful in nutritional assessment. However, some urine tests require collection of uncontaminated 24-hour urine samples, which may be difficult or even impossible for some older individuals. Twenty four-hour urine samples are used to measure creatinine, and creatinine excretion, which can be used as an indirect measure of lean body mass and degree of protein depletion. When there is protein malnutrition, creatinine excretion is lowered. Total nitrogen excretion can also be measured with a 24-hour urine sample in order to determine nitrogen balance.

CLINICAL EXAMINATION

Examination for physical signs that may indicate malnutrition is another usual method of assessment. However, commonly recognized deficiency symptoms may be misleading. In a study of 789 elderly subjects, 57 were diagnosed as having angular stomatitis, a classical sign of riboflavin (vitamin B$_2$) deficiency. In only four cases, however, could the symptoms be related to deficiency of the vitamin (12). This is true of other "deficiency symptoms" as well. There is a need for studies that separate abnormalities due to aging from those due to malnutrition. Some clinical signs of malnutrition are often considered part of normal aging, such as skin and hair changes, oral signs, missing teeth, muscle wasting, and mental confusion.

Table 2-7 lists the clinical signs of nutrient deficiencies. These should be considered only as a general guide. All signs must be evaluated on an individual basis.

DIET ASSESSMENT

A variety of methods may be used to collect dietary information from older adults. These include a diet history along with a food frequency check, food records kept for varying numbers of days, and a 24-hour recall. These methods depend on the cooperation of the clients as well as the clients' ability to accurately recall food eaten. Therefore, they are subject to errors, particularly with older adults who may have failing memories. In addition, hearing loss and poor communication skills may affect the validity and reliability of the information obtained. Often, alcohol and dietary supplements are not considered as part of the diet; they should be. In all methods of diet assessment, it must be remembered that people tend to "talk a good diet." That is, they overestimate the consumption of "good" foods while underestimating amounts of calories and other food eaten.

One of the authors remembers performing a diet study with a group of elderly individuals. They were given forms in which to keep 7-day food records. On the front of the form was an example of how the

Table 2-7 Clinical Signs of Nutrient Deficiencies

Body area	Normal appearance	Signs associated with malnutrition
Hair	Shiny; firm; not easily plucked	Lack of natural shine; hair dull and dry; thin and sparse; hair fine, silky and straight, color changes (flag sign); can be easily plucked
Face	Skin color uniform; smooth, pink, healthy appearance; not swollen	Skin color loss (depigmentation); skin dark over cheeks and under eyes (malar and supraorbital pigmentation); lumpiness or flakiness of skin of nose and mouth; swollen face; enlarged parotid glands; scaling of skin around nostrils (nasolabial seborrhea)
Eyes	Bright, clear, shiny; no sores at corners of eyelids; membranes a healthy pink and are moist; no prominent blood vessels or mound of tissue or sclera	Eye membranes are pale (pale conjunctivae); redness of membranes (conjunctival injection); Bitot's spots; redness and fissuring of eyelid corners (angular palpebritis); dryness of eye membranes (conjunctival xerosis); cornea has dull appearance (corneal xerosis); cornea is soft (keratomalacia); scar on cornea; sign of fine blood vessels around cornea (circumcorneal injection)
Lips	Smooth, not chapped or swollen	Redness and swelling of mouth or lips (cheilosis); especially at corners of mouth (angular fissures and scars)
Tongue	Deep red in appearance; not swollen or smooth	Swelling; scarlet and raw tongue; magenta (purplish color) of tongue; smooth tongue; swollen sores; hyperemic and hypertrophic papillae; atrophic papillae
Teeth	No cavities; no pain; bright	May be missing or erupting abnormally; gray or black spots (fluorosis); cavities (caries)
Gums	Healthy; red; do not bleed; not swollen	"Spongy" and bleed easily; recession of gums
Glands	Face not swollen	Thyroid enlargement (front of neck); parotid enlargement (cheeks become swollen)

Table 2-7 (Cont.) Clinical Signs of Nutrient Deficiencies

Body area	Normal appearance	Signs associated with malnutrition
Skin	No signs of rashes, swelling, dark or light spots	Dryness of skin (xerosis); sandpaper feel of skin (follicular hyperkeratosis); flakiness of skin; skin swollen and dark: red swollen pigmentation of exposed areas (pellagrous dermatosis); excessive lightness or darkness of skin (dyspigmentation); black and blue marks due to skin bleeding (petechiae); lack of fat under skin
Nails	Firm, pink	Nails are spoon-shaped (koilonychia); brittle, ridged nails
Muscular and skeletal systems	Good muscle tone; some fat under skin; can walk or run without pain	Muscles have "wasted" appearance; baby's skull bones are thin and soft (craniotabes); round swelling of front and side of head (frontal and parietal bossing); swelling of ends of bones (epiphyseal enlargement); small bumps on both sides of chest wall (on ribs)—beading of ribs; baby's soft spot on head does not harden at proper time (persistently open anterior fontanelle); knock-knees or bow legs, bleeding into muscle (musculoskeletal hemorrhages); person cannot get up or walk properly
Internal systems Cardiovascular	Normal heart rate and rhythm; no murmurs or abnormal rhythms; normal blood pressure for age	Rapid heart rate (above 100 = tachycardia); enlarged heart; abnormal rhythm; elevated blood pressure
Gastrointestinal	No palpable organs or masses (in children, however, liver edge may be palpable)	Liver enlargement; enlargement of spleen (usually indicates other associated diseases)
Nervous	Psychological stability; normal reflexes	Mental irritability and confusion; burning and tingling of hands and feet (paresthesia); loss of position and vibratory sense; weakness and tenderness of muscles (may result in inability to walk); decrease and loss of ankle and knee reflexes

Source: Nutritional Assessment in Health Programs Part I—Methodology, Clinical Assessment of Nutrition Status, *Am. J. Public Health* 63:18, Nov. 1973.

records should be kept. The example for breakfast listed orange juice, an egg, cereal, milk, and toast. Almost every participant listed exactly this breakfast on each of the 7 days.

Very often, the public health nurse, home health aide, or volunteer worker who sees the elderly on a regular basis in their homes has not had the necessary training to completely evaluate an individual's food intake. They can, however, identify potential nutritional problems and alert a nutritionist to the need for further investigation. Figure 2-1 is a checklist that may help the home visitor identify problems that might otherwise have been overlooked.

Diet History

The diet history is based on food frequency checklists. It elicits information about what a person usually eats. It is qualitative rather than quantitative and gives a picture of general food patterns for a period of time. As the nutritional state of an older person reflects previous intake as well as current practice, a diet history is helpful in filling in gaps from other methods of diet assessment and compensates for variations in daily consumption (see Figure 2-2).

Food Records

These are records of all food eaten and are recorded by the individual for periods of from 3 days to 1 week. When recorded accurately, they can give useful information about kinds and amounts of food eaten. It is time consuming, however, to keep such records, and may not be appropriate for meals eaten away from home. Also, interest may wane after keeping a detailed record for a day or two; so it is recommended that the record be limited to 3 days, only one of which is a weekend day.

Twenty-Four-Hour Recall

This is the most frequently used method of assessing current nutritional intake of older adults. A trained interviewer asks, "Tell me everything you ate in the last 24 hours beginning with the last food eaten." The reliability of the 24-hour recall is not found to be as accurate in elderly persons as in younger persons (13). Foods may be forgotten, estimates of amounts may be inaccurate, and the 24-hour period may not be representative of the person's usual diet. In Figure 2-3, Twenty-Four-Hour

Recall, there is a checklist based on the Four Food Groups developed by the U.S. Department of Agriculture. In this tool, foods are divided into four major classifications—milk, meat, fruits and vegetables, and grains. For practical purposes, using a checklist based on the four food groups will give an estimate of adequacy of food intake. It will also point out neglected food groups that need to be emphasized in counseling.

Interviewing Skills

A skilled interviewer is essential in obtaining accurate information. The following guidelines for diet assessment interviewing will help to set the stage for a productive session.

Choose a quiet, comfortable setting where there will be few interruptions.

Determine whether the person is willing and able to talk about food intake. Fatigue, anxiety, or discomfort may make it desirable to postpone the interview.

Before the interview familiarize yourself with the person's record or chart if it is available. Determine whether there are any hearing or visual problems.

If the person interviewed is ill, be sure to keep the session short, so it will not be tiring. Many older adults, because of mental and physical conditions, are unwilling and/or unable to sustain an interview for more than several minutes. When this is so, several short interviews should be planned so that as complete a diet picture as possible can be obtained.

Introduce yourself and say the person's name. Don't use the person's first name unless you are on a first-name basis.

Shake hands or use another friendly approach to help make the interviewee comfortable.

Ask open-ended questions that do not suggest answers. An interviewer should avoid using questions that suggest a correct answer or can be answered with a perfunctory "yes" or "no." It is better to say, "Tell me, what was the first thing you ate this morning?" than "Do you eat cereal for breakfast?"

Listen carefully. It is often a good idea to say little or nothing for the first few minutes, allowing the client to speak.

Do not interrupt unnecessarily. Sometimes seemingly irrelevant material may impact on nutrition. Interrupt only if the interview gets too far away from its purpose, or if a point needs clarification.

Name_____Referred by_____

Address_____Telephone_____

Date of birth_____Male_____Female_____

Marital status: Single_____ Married_____ Widowed_____ Separated_____

Race/Ethnic Background: Caucasian_____ Indian_____ Black_____ Oriental_____ Spanish_____

                    Other_____

Household composition: Live alone_____ Spouse_____ Child_____ Other_____

Local church affiliation_____

Local club affiliation_____

Have you been active in a nutrition/feeding program before?_____

What kind?_____

Emergency contact_____
                   (Name)   (Address)

_____
             (Phone)   (Relationship)

Do you have a refrigerator?_____ Stove?_____

           Kitchen?_____ Kitchen privileges?_____

Estimated yearly income_____

Are you eligible for food stamps? Yes_____ No_____

Do you use food stamps? Yes_____ No_____

Are you able to grocery shop independently? Yes_____ No_____

If not, what assistance is necessary?_____

Ambulation: Full_____ Partial_____ Wheelchair_____

           Crutches_____ Cane or walker_____ Bedfast_____

Neuromuscular problem affecting eating? Yes_____ No_____

Vision: Adequate_____ Partial_____ Blind_____

Hearing: Adequate_____ Partial_____ Hard of hearing_____

           Deaf_____

Teeth: Own in good condition_____ Dentures_____ None_____

Mental competence: Adequate_____ Inadequate_____

Comments_____

_____

Do you take medication daily? Yes_____ No_____ What kind?_____

Do you take vitamin/mineral supplements daily? Yes_____ No_____ What kind?_____

    _____ How much?_____

Are you on a special diet? Yes_____ No_____

  What kind?_____

  Who prescribed it?_____

Do you usually eat alone?_____ With someone?_____

Is mealtime pleasurable? Yes_____ No_____

Recommendations_____

_____

Figure 2–1. Assessment of need for nutritional intervention.

Name_____ Date_____

Birth date_____ Age_____

Informant_____ Telephone_____

Address_____

Race_____ Ethnic origin_____ Religion_____

Educational level_____Marital status_____

Occupation_____Hours of working day_____

Hours/week_____

Family composition

Name_____ Age_____ Sex_____

_____ _____ _____

_____ _____ _____

_____ _____ _____

Housing: Room_____ Apartment_____ Own home_____

Income: Source_____

Adequacy_____

Height_____ Weight_____

Has weight increased?_____

Has weight decreased?_____

Teeth: Good condition_____ Missing_____ No dentures_____

Dentures_____

Chewing ability: Good_____ Fair_____ Poor_____

Appetite: Good_____ Fair_____ Poor_____

Indicate any problem with the following:

Sense of taste_____

Sense of smell_____

Digestion_____

Elimination_____

Vision_____

Daily activities

Do you smoke?_____How much?_____

Do you drink beer?_____ wine?_____ alcohol?_____

How much?_____

Do you take any medication?_____ What type?_____

Who prescribed it?_____

Figure 2–2. Nutritional assessment form.

Do you take vitamin/mineral supplements?_____

What type?_____

Who prescribed it?_____

Do you take any food supplements such as rutin, bone meal, protein supplements?_____

What kind?_____Why?_____

Do you exercise?_____How often?_____

   How long?_____

Do you go outdoors?_____Daily?_____Occasionally?_____

   Hardly ever?_____

Diet information:

Have you even been on a special diet?_____ What kind?_____

Are you on one now?_____ What kind?_____

Who prescribed the diet?_____

Do you follow the diet: All the time?_____ Part of the time?_____

   Hardly ever?_____

Do you use salt? Yes_____ No_____ A small amount_____

   Salt substitute_____

Do you use low-sodium (salt) foods? Yes_____ No_____

Which one?_____

Do you use artificial sweeteners? Yes_____ No_____

Which one?_____

Are you allergic to any food?_____ Which ones?_____

Who diagnosed the allergy?_____

Do you have religious prohibitions regarding foods?_____

Which foods?_____

Are there any foods yo don't use for other reasons?_____

_____

Do you prepare all your own meals? Yes_____ No_____

Do you do your own marketing? Yes_____ No_____

Do you eat out?_____ Once a day?_____ Occasionally?_____

   Hardly ever?_____

   Where?_____

Do you eat differently on weekends?_____

How is it different?_____

How many times a day do you eat?_____

Do you eat alone?_____

Do you skip meals?_____ Which ones?_____

How often?_____

Have you increased, decreased, or eaten about the same amount of the following foods?

Food	Increased	Decreased	Same
Margarine			
"Corn-oil"			
"Diet"			
Butter			
Milk			
Skim milk (fresh)			
or Powdered milk			
Ice cream			
Cooking oil			
Solid canned fat			
Bacon			
Red meat			
Fish			
Poultry			
Eggs			
Cheese, low-fat			
Tofu			
Beans			
Peanut butter			
Whole-grain bread			
Cooked cereal			
Dry cereal			
Pasta			
Coffee			
Decaffeinated coffee			
Tea (herb or regular)			
Potatoes			
Raw vegetables			
Cooked vegetables			
Cooked fruits			
Raw fruits			
Salty snacks			
Baked goods			
Juice			
Soda			
Cocoa			
Other			

Figure 2–2 (*cont.*)   Nutritional assessment form.

There are so many "convenience foods" on the market today; do you use them?

	Yes/frequency	No/why not? (expensive, don't like them, servings too large)

Instant milk (dried)_____

TV dinners_____

Frozen main meals_____

Frozen vegetables_____

Special reinforced milks_____

Imitation sour cream_____

Special margarines_____

Nondairy cream_____

Instant breakfasts_____

Powdered orange juice_____

Instant coffee_____

Canned meats_____

Cake-muffin mixes_____

Pudding mix_____

"Boxed" main meals_____

Others_____

_____

_____

Amount and food item

Milk group
2 cups or more daily

Meat group
Eggs, meat, fish, poultry, cheese, peanut butter
2 or more servings daily

Bread and cereal group
Whole-grain, fortified, or enriched pasta noodles, rice, kasha
4 or more servings daily

Fruit and vegetable group
A variety
4 or more servings daily

Vitamin C
1 good source daily
List food

	Morning Time___ Where___	Midmorning Time___ Where___	Noon Time___ Where___	Afternoon Time___ Where___
Amount and food item				
Milk group				
Meat group				
Bread and cereal group				
Fruit and vegetable group				
Vitamin C				

Evening
Time_____
Where_____

Night
Time_____
Where_____

Is the intake of any of the following excessive?

_____ Alcohol
_____ Concentrated sweets
_____ Fats

Is this a typical day's diet?_____ If not, how does it differ?_____

Food dislikes?_____
Special food preferences?_____
Special food problems (allergies, diabetes, etc.)?_____

Evaluation: (consider consumption of alcohol, concentrated sweets, and fat)
_____

Name_____ Date_____

Address_____ Age_____ Height_____ Weight_____

Figure 2–3. 24-hour recall.

Allow sufficient time for the person to think and respond fully to each question. This is particularly important when working with the elderly.

Speak slowly, using simple, easy-to-understand language. Explain unfamiliar terms. Food models, measuring cups, and various-sized plates are useful to help determine portion size.

Do not be judgmental or express either approval or disapproval at the clients' responses. People tend to talk a good diet— underestimating calories by underreporting large quantities of food eaten and by overestimating small quantities. Your attitude should not encourage this.

If the older individual is unable to communicate adequately, diet information may be obtained from a relative or friend.

Evaluating Food Intake

The Recommended Dietary Allowances (RDA) and adaptations of them are the most commonly used standards for diet evaluation. The RDA are currently in their ninth revision and the tenth revision is expected by the end of 1985. The allowances are planned to cover the needs of 97.5% of the healthy population. In all cases, except for energy (calories), the recommendations for those over age 51 are extrapolated from the allowances for younger people because there is insufficient information on needs of the aged. Energy recommendations are more specific to the older individual (see Table 2–8).

The RDA were developed as guidelines for overall good nutrition of the population and were not intended to represent exact nutritional needs of individuals although they are often used in this way. They are even less appropriate to use for evaluating the food intake of older adults, who may not be in good health and who, because of their age, health history, food habits, and activity level, have more individualized requirements.

Nutritional assessment as discussed in this chapter should be used to screen patients at risk of nutritional depletion. These are persons who are grossly underweight or overweight; have recently lost 10% or more of body weight; are alcoholics; have been NPO (not by mouth) for more than 10 days on simple intravenous solutions; have had prolonged nutrient losses owing to draining wounds, fistulas, malabsorption, or renal dialysis; have increased metabolic needs; are on drugs that interfere with nutritional state; or have severe depression or mental incompetence.

Table 2-8 Mean Heights and Weights and Recommended Energy Intake[a]

Category	Age (years)	Weight (kg)	Weight (lb)	Height (cm)	Height (in)	Energy Needs (with range) (kcal)	Energy Needs (with range) (MJ)
Males	23–50	70	154	178	70	2700 (2300–3100)	11.3
	51–75	70	154	178	70	2400 (2000–2800)	10.1
	76+	70	154	178	70	2050 (1650–2450)	8.6
Females	23–50	55	120	163	64	2000 (1600–2400)	8.4
	51–75	55	120	163	64	1800 (1400–2200)	7.6
	76+	55	120	163	64	1600 (1200–2000)	6.7

[a]Recommended Dietary Allowances. Revised 1980. The data in this table have been assembled from men and women between the ages of 18 and 34 years as surveyed in the U.S. population (HEW/NCHS data).

The allowances for the two older groups represent mean energy needs over these age spans, allowing for a 2% decrease in basal (resting) metabolic rate per decade and a reduction in activity of 200 kcal/day for men and women between 51 and 75 years, 500 kcal for men over 75 years and 400 kcal for women over 75. The customary range of daily energy output is shown for adults in parentheses, and is based on a variation in energy needs of ± 400 kcal at any one age emphasizing the wide range of energy intakes appropriate for any group of people.

REFERENCES

1. 1983 Metropolitan Height and Weight Tables. Statistical Bulletin Metropolitan Life Insurance Co. 64(Jan-June):3, 1983.

2. Weight by height and age for adults 18–74 Years: United States, 1971–74. National Center for Health Statistics, Public Health Service, U.S. Dept. of Health, Education and Welfare.

3. Master, A.M., et al., Tables of average weight and height of Americans aged 65 to 94 years, *JAMA* 172(7):658, 1960.

4. Burke, D., et al., Copper and zinc utilization in elderly adults, *J. Gerontol.* 69(5):558, 1981.

5. Chumlea, W.C., et al., *Nutritional Assessment of the Elderly Through Anthropometry.* Ross Laboratories, March 1984.

6. Bishop, C.W., et. al., Norms for nutritional assessment of American adults by upper arm anthropometry, *Am. J. Clin. Nutr.* 35:2530, 1981.

7. Seltzer, M.H., Use of admission test data to assess nutritional status of the hospitalized patient. *Intern. Med.* 4(7):149, 1983.

8. Frisancho, A.R., New norms of upper limb fat and muscle areas for nutritional status. *Am. J. Clin. Nutr.* 34:2540, 1981.

9. Salmond, S.W., How to assess the nutritional status of acutely ill patients. *Am. J. Nurs.* May 1980, p. 922.

10. David, L.M., et al., Review of patient response to skin test antigens, *Nutr. Support Serv.* 4(3):26, 1984.

11. Wright, R.A., Heymsfield, S., *Nutritional Assessment.* Boston: Blackwell Scientific Publications, Inc., 1984.

12. Durnin, J.V., Nutrition, in: *Textbook of Geriatric Medicine and Gerontology*, J.C. Brocklehurst (ed.) New York: Churchill Livingstone, 1978.

13. Bowman, B.B., Rosenberg, I.H., Assessment of the nutritional status of the elderly, *Am. J. Clin. Nutr.* 35:1142, 1982.

Chapter 3

NUTRIENT NEEDS AS PEOPLE AGE

More than 40 different substances—carbohydrate, protein, fat, vitamins, minerals, fiber, and water—are needed for health and vigor. The amount of each of these nutrients needed depends on gender, body size, activity, and state of health as well as age. Because older adults differ so much from one another, it is difficult to generalize about their requirements. Certainly the wear and tear of living produces changes that act to individualize needs. At the present time, not a great deal is known about how nutrient requirements change with aging (1). Most recommendations currently used are based on studies of younger persons. The following sections provide an overview of nutrients along with what is known about the special requirements of older adults.

ENERGY

Food, or rather the protein, fat, and carbohydrates in food, provides energy to fuel the body. Alcohol is also a source of energy. This energy is measured as calories or, more commonly, as kilocalories (kcal). One kilocalorie is 1000 calories, the amount of heat needed to raise the temperature of 1 kilogram (kg) of water 1°C. Recently, the standard international unit kilojoules (kJ) has come into use as a unit of energy. One kilocalorie is equal to 4.184 kJ. Fat provides more energy than an equal weight of protein or carbohydrate.

Fat yields 9 kcal (38 kJ) per gram
Carbohydrate yields 4 kcal (17 kJ) per gram
Protein yields 4 kcal (17 kJ) per gram
Alcohol yields 7 kcal (30 kJ) per gram

Therefore, foods that are rich in fat (oil, butter, margarine, olives, nuts, and seeds) are higher in calories than foods that contain less fat.

As people age, there is great variation in individual energy requirements. However, in general, as people age, their energy needs are reduced. This is because, after age 21, the resting metabolic rate declines, at a rate of about 2% per decade. When this is coupled with the reduced activity common in older adults, the result is a lowered caloric need. The recommended daily caloric allowances for adults are given in three categories: those under age 52, those age 52–75, and those over age 75 (see Table 2–8, p. 41). The energy allowances for those 52–75 is 90% of that for younger adults; for those over 75, it is 75–80%.

The reduced caloric needs of the elderly require that more care be used in choosing foods so that all necessary nutrients are included. The intake of fats and sweets should be cut down as much as is practical. Older adults gain additional benefits from these reductions as a high-fat intake can cause indigestion and contribute to degenerative changes. Furthermore, the elderly often have an impaired glucose tolerance (2).

Most surveys show that average energy intakes in older adults are less than two-thirds of the RDA. However, some of the same studies show that weight increases consistently as people age (3). Reduction of caloric intake to the point where weight gain would not occur would mean a greater likelihood of inadequate nutrient intake. A better approach might be to increase activity level so that more energy is used and a more liberal diet can be eaten. Furthermore, studies show that elderly people who consume few calories often are fatigued and lack interest in their surroundings (4).

Alcohol is another source of calories that should not be overlooked. These calories may displace needed foods. In addition, alcohol, while providing little in the way of nutrients, causes nutrients to be destroyed for its metabolism. See Chapter 5 for more about the effect of alcohol intake on nutritional status.

ENERGY NUTRIENTS

Protein

About 20 different amino acids make up the protein in the body and in food. Of these 20, 9 are essential in the diet as the body cannot make them. The other amino acids can be made by the body from the nine essential amino acids, carbohydrate, and nitrogen.

All amino acids must be present in adequate amounts at the same time for the body to synthesize needed proteins. That is why older adults should be encouraged to eat foods containing all the essential amino acids at each meal or snack. A complete assortment of all amino acids is found in protein from eggs, milk, meat, fish or poultry or in mixtures of two or more incomplete protein foods such as rice, beans, cereals, seeds, or nuts. These mixtures provide inexpensive sources of protein.

Protein nutritional status can be determined by nitrogen balance. When the amount of nitrogen taken in from foods equals the amount lost in urine, feces, and through the skin, the individual is said to be in equilibrium or balance. A positive nitrogen balance exists when the body is retaining more nitrogen than it is losing. This occurs during growth, pregnancy, wound healing, and recovery from stress. A negative nitrogen balance indicates that the body is losing more nitrogen than it is taking in. This is likely to occur during injury, surgery, fever, infection, emotional stress, or metastatic disease or during a period of inadequate protein or calorie intake. The protein needs of a healthy older adult may be quite different from those of an older person who is ill. Many nitrogen balance studies do not show significant differences between young and elderly people (5). This implies that protein requirements of the elderly are no different from those of younger adults. However, there is some evidence that because of reduced bioavailability, there is increased need for certain amino acids and thus an increased need for total protein. The general consensus is that the elderly, because of their special needs, should receive 12–14% of their calories as protein instead of the RDA recommendation for adults, which is slightly more than 9% (6, 7).

Carbohydrates

Carbohydrates include sugars and starches. Sugars are often referred to as simple carbohydrates and starches as complex carbohydrates. These are a major source of calories in the diet of most older adults because they are relatively inexpensive, tasty, able to be stored for long periods without refrigeration, and easy to prepare and chew.

The elderly should be encouraged to eat about 60% of their calories as carbohydrates, mainly complex starches as in bananas, legumes, potatoes, whole grains, and enriched breads and cereals. Dry, ready-to-eat cereal can be an excellent addition to the older adult's diet. These foods are digested over a period of several hours and so satisfy hunger for a longer time than the simple sugars found in cake, cookies, and other sweets. Sugar has been shown to cause a rise in serum cholesterol and tryglycerides when it is substituted in the diet isocalorically for starch (8).

A carbohydrate intake of 100 g daily is recommended for all adults. When the amount of carbohydrate is restricted to less than 50 g, there is the danger of developing ketosis, the accumulation of ketone bodies that are formed when fat is metabolized. Without sufficient carbohydrate intake, fat cannot be completely oxidized, and ketones accumulate. Some are metabolized, but others must be eliminated from the body, which results in a loss of energy, water, and minerals. If this persists, there may be disruption of acid-base balance. Thus, it may be unsafe for older adults to follow a low-carbohydrate, weight-reducing diet such as the Atkins or the Scarsdale diet. These diets induce ketosis as a means of reducing calorie utilization and also to suppress appetite. Beside being unsafe, they are not an effective way to achieve sustained weight loss.

High-carbohydrate diets have been shown to be beneficial to elderly diabetics, reflected both in clinical condition and in laboratory tests. Furthermore, frequent consumption of carbohydrates, six or more times daily, results in reduced insulin requirements in diabetics along with lower serum cholesterol levels and greater nitrogen retention (9).

Fat

There is fat in all animal and vegetable foods. Sometimes the fat can be seen, as in meat and butter. In other foods, like milk, the fat is not visible.

It is essential to have some fat in the diet, to provide energy, carry fat-soluble vitamins, insulate and cushion the body, and make essential body compounds and structural tissue. In addition, fat in the diet provides flavor and satiety value. A small quantity of the fatty acid linoleic acid is essential in the diet as it cannot be made by the body. Other fats and fatty acids can be made from excess carbohydrate, protein, and linoleic acid.

For many older adults, it would be better to reduce the amount of fat eaten. Besides providing a concentrated source of calories, which can lead to being overweight, fat is believed to contribute to the development of cardiovascular disease and some types of cancer. Also, fat, because it takes longer to digest, may cause indigestion and reduced appetite in the older person.

A lot of effort has been expended in educating the public about the "benefit" of polyunsaturated fats and the dangers of cholesterol. It has been shown that diets restricted in cholesterol and higher in polyunsaturated versus saturated fat can lower serum cholesterol levels and therefore minimize a risk factor in cardiovascular disease (10). Such a diet may also reduce platelet adhesiveness (11). However, there is some question about the value of markedly altering the type of fats consumed after age 55 (12).

It is considered prudent to reduce one's total fat intake from the presently common level of about 43% of daily calories to a level of about 30%. That amount is more than sufficient to provide the benefit of fat and reduce the risks associated with its consumption.

FIBER

Dietary fiber refers to nondigestible material, carbohydrate and carbohydrate-related, present in plant foods. The values for crude fiber, given in food tables and on food packages, underestimate the amount of fiber because it is based on laboratory measurements of material remaining after food has been treated by strong acid and alkali. Natural digestion of food leaves a greater residue.

Fiber helps to control constipation by softening and increasing the volume of the stool. It also is helpful in treating the symptoms of diverticulosis. Some types of fiber, particularly pectins, have been shown to reduce serum cholesterol levels (13). Eating more fiber is helpful in controlling weight as its bulk satisfies hunger, displacing other higher-calorie foods and also reducing absorption of food. A diet high in complex carbohydrate and fiber from legumes and cereals has been shown to improve all aspects of diabetic control (14).

The role of fiber as a factor protecting against colon cancer and breast cancer is more controversial, and further research is needed before definite conclusions can be reached (15).

It is unwise to make drastic changes in the diet based on incomplete knowledge of the physiological function of fiber. However, in view of the fact that most Americans consume less fiber than our ancestors did, and less than many other population groups, and also that some increase in fiber might be beneficial, it seems appropriate to increase dietary intake moderately. The ideal level of dietary fiber is estimated to be between 25 and 50 g/day. This can be achieved by eating less refined foods and emphasizing unprocessed, whole-grain cereals, brown rice, unpeeled fruits and vegetables, legumes, nuts, and wheat or corn bran. Usual servings of fruits, vegetables, and whole-grain breads and cereals contain 2–3 g of dietary fiber. A level teaspoon of bran has about 2 g. Some bran-containing cereals like All Bran or Raisin Bran have more per serving (see Table 3–1). If bran is to be added, start with 1 teaspoon daily and increase up to no more than 2–3 tablespoons. Plenty of fluids must be taken along with the bran to prevent impaction and intestinal obstruction.

Excessive intake of fiber can irritate the intestinal linings and cause flatulence and interfere with mineral absorption. The latter effect can result in a deficiency of iron, calcium, or zinc if the diet, as is typical in many older adults, is marginal in these minerals (see Chapter 6, Digestive Disorders, for more information on fiber).

Table 3–1   Dietary Fiber in Foods

Food	Portion	Grams of dietary fiber
Apple, unpeeled	1 medium	5.7
Apple, peeled	1 medium	2.0
Banana	1 small	2.1
Beans, cooked		
Baked	½ cup	9.3
Kidney	½ cup	9.7
Lentils	½ cup	3.7
Limas	½ cup	8.3
Pintos	½ cup	8.9
White	½ cup	7.9
Bran	1 tbsp	1.8
Bread, white	1 slice	0.7
Bread, whole-wheat	1 slice	2.1
Broccoli, cooked	½ cup	3.2
Cabbage, cooked	½ cup	2.5
Cauliflower, cooked	½ cup	0.4
Carrots, cooked	½ cup	2.9
Cereal		
All-Bran	1 oz	9.0
Bran Buds	1 oz	8.0
Corn flakes	½ cup	1.4
Cracklin' Bran	1 oz	4.0
40% Bran Flakes	1 oz	4.0
Fruit and Fiber	½ cup	3.0
Grape Nuts	¼ cup	2.1
Mini Wheats (Frosted)	½ cup (4 biscuits)	3.0
Most	1 oz	4.0
Raisin Bran	1 oz	4.0
Special K	½ cup	0.8
Sugar Puffs	½ cup	0.9
Chestnuts	6	4.4
Corn, canned	½ cup	4.7
Fibermed	1 biscuit	5.0
Fig, dried	1	3.7

Table 3–1   (Cont.)

Food	Portion	Grams of dietary fiber
Lettuce	⅙ head	1.5
Peanut butter	1 tbsp	1.2
Peach, fresh, unpeeled	1	2.3
Pear, unpeeled	1	12.6
Peas, cooked	½ cup	6.7
Pineapple, raw	½ cup	0.8
Potato, sweet, baked	1 small	2.1
Potato, white, baked	1 small	1.9
Prunes, dried	2	2.4
Rye-krisp	3 wafers	2.3
Strawberries	1 cup	2.7
Tomato	1 medium	1.9

Adapted from: Anderson, J.W., et al., *Plant Fiber Source Book*. Lexington, Ky.: HCF Diabetes Research Foundation, 1980. *Product Information: Fibermed*. Norwalk, Ct.: The Purdue Fredricks Co. *Product Information: Kellogg's Foodservice Products Nutritive Values and Purchasing Guide*. Battle Creek, Mich.: Kellogg. Southgate, D.A.T. Dietary fiber; analysis and food sources, *Am. J. Clin. Nutr.* 31:5107, 1978.

WATER

The elderly are at greater risk of dehydration than younger adults. Fluid intake is less in older adults of both sexes, and this may explain their lower body water content (16). They may be less sensitive to the normal sensation of thirst, fluids may not be conveniently available, or they may be too debilitated to drink water when it is available. In other cases, the elderly person may restrict fluid intake so as to prevent sleep being disturbed by nocturia. In addition, some elderly persons may have conditions that increase the need for fluid such as diuretic therapy, a high-protein intake, fever, excessive sweating, vomiting, severe diarrhea, and polyuria. Water also may help to counteract constipation, and a generous intake of liquids may prevent the formation of renal or bladder stones in susceptible bed- or wheelchair-bound persons. Sufficient water must be given to comatose, tube-fed patients so that they do not develop hypernatremia.

Normally, there is a balance between water intake and output. Water intake includes that found in food and drink as well as metabolic water produced by the oxidation of food. Water is lost via urine and feces (more so with diarrhea) and through the skin and lungs. A good rule of thumb is that sufficient liquid should be taken in so that 1 qt or more of urine is produced daily. For most mature adults, 6 cups of fluid will provide for this. Studies show that the average 132 lb person, aged 65–90 needs 1.3 qt of water daily to maintain balance (17). About one-half of this can be obtained from food itself exclusive of liquids.

Dehydration may be found along with many disease states. Signs of dehydration include confusion, dry tongue, dry mouth, sunken eyes, dry loose skin, and urine output of less than 500 ml/day or a urine specific gravity greater than 1.030 (18). Daily weighing is useful to determine the extent of water loss. Treatment consists of increasing fluid intake so that it equals the amount of water lost.

VITAMINS AND MINERALS

These include a wide group of substances, organic in the case of vitamins, inorganic in the case of minerals, that are needed in the diet in small quantities.

Vitamins perform specific functions as regulators of metabolism. Minerals help control water and electrolyte balance, are activators for enzyme-catalyzed reactions, are components of body tissue and compounds, and act in muscle and nerve function. Neither is an energy source to the body, but rather catalyze energy release from carbohydrate, fat, and protein.

Vitamins are categorized as being either fat-soluble or water-soluble. The fat-soluble vitamins A, D, E, and K are found dissolved in the fat of plants and animals. They are absorbed from the gastrointestinal tract along with fat so that anything interfering with fat absorption such as the cholesterol-lowering drug *cholestyramine* (Questran), mineral oil, or the condition steatorrhea may lead to a deficiency of these vitamins. Fat-soluble vitamins are stored in the body. They are not easily excreted, and thus there is the danger of excessive accumulation when large amounts are ingested.

The water-soluble vitamins, vitamin C, thiamin, riboflavin, and the B-complex group, are not stored in the body in large amounts and are easily excreted in the urine. Because of this, toxic accumulation of water-soluble vitamins is generally not thought to be a problem. However, recently, ingestion of large quantities of these vitamins has become comonplace and reports indicate that, in excess amounts, they too may have undesirable effects. The elderly may be especially susceptible to this risk if there is reduced renal function.

Minerals are grouped according to the amount needed daily. *Macrominerals* have a daily requirement of 100 mg or more, whereas *microminerals* are required in smaller amounts. Microminerals are also referred to as trace minerals. Excessive amounts are often toxic; so it is unwise to supplement the diet to provide more than the suggested intake. Furthermore, many functions of these nutrients are interrelated and impinge on others. Excess supplementation can disrupt this balance.

Tables 3–2 and 3–3 list the vitamins and minerals known to be necessary for health along with information about functions and food sources plus additional information about each nutrient that will help in clinical practice.

USE OF NUTRIENT SUPPLEMENTATION

In 1982, 37% of American adults took vitamin supplements, spending more than 1.7 billion dollars. More women than men use them, and use is higher among those with more education and higher incomes. People in households without children are more likely to take supplements. Multivitamin products are most commonly used, followed by vitamin C, B vitamins, and vitamin E in decending order of use (19).

A high percentage of older adults take some type of supplement, and the number increases with age, income, and education (20). Studies of noninstitutionalized elderly show that up to 49% take vitamins regularly (21).

Most people decide to take supplements on the advice of family members or friends or because of the influence of advertising. Studies show that few, less than 1 out of 10, have had supplements prescribed by a physician. About 30% of users consult a physician about their supplements (22). The remainder purchase and use supplements on their own.

In view of the widespread use of supplements, particularly by older adults, a natural question is "Do they really need them?" This question has been debated by experts. The consensus of opinion seems to be that supplementation, at moderate levels, is the wisest course. Although it is true that a varied diet of 1800 to 2000 kcal can, if well chosen, provide all necessary nutrients, it has been shown in food consumption surveys that many people do not get all needed nutrients in sufficient amounts. Calcium and B vitamins are the nutrients most likely to be in short supply in diets of older adults. In addition, caloric intakes are often less than the recommended levels. Considering these along with such factors as drug use, disease, chewing difficulties, and dieting, there is less probability that older adults regularly obtain all needed nutrients from food.

A multivitamin-mineral supplement containing RDA levels or less of nutrients is a convenient, inexpensive way to ensure dietary adequacy

Table 3-2 Vitamins

Fat-soluble vitamins	Functions	Sources	Noteworthy
A (retinol) animal source; provitamin A (carotene) vegetable source	Maintains health of mucosal epithelium; maintains visual acuity in dark	Liver, egg yolk, butter, whole milk, cream, fish liver oils, fortified margarine, dark-green leafy vegetables, yellow vegetables and fruits	Vitamin A analogs are used to treat acne; vitamin A deficiency increases susceptibility to infections and to epithelial cancers; antitumor activity of pharmacological dose of vitamin A and its analogs is being studied; large amounts of retinol are toxic; severe deficiency damages eyes; mineral oil taken with meals interferes with absorption; conversion of carotene to vitamin A impaired in diabetes and hypothyroidism; excess carotene causes yellowing of skin
D (calciferol) D_2 ergocalciferol (ultraviolet radiation of plant sterol) D_3 cholecalciferol (sunlight converts 7-dehydrocholesterol in skin to this)	Regulates calcium and phosphorus absorption and mobilization and calcification of bones	Fortified milk, fish liver oils, limited amounts in butter, liver, salmon, exposure to sunlight	Large amounts are toxic causing hypercalcemia and kidney stones; deficiency causes osteomalacia in adults; D converted to active metabolite in liver and kidney; housebound or institutionalized elderly at risk of deficiency

Vitamin	Function	Sources	Comments
E (tocopherol)	Acts as an antioxidant: reduces oxidation of vitamin A, carotenes, and polyunsaturated fatty acids; protects against the peroxidation of lipid in cell membranes	Vegetable oils, wheat germ, nuts, green leafy vegetables, legumes	Related to action of mineral selenium; may be used to treat decreased blood circulation and fibrocystic disease of breast
K (naptho-quinones)	Acts in the formation of prothrombin; possible coenzyme in oxidation phosphorylation	Spinach, cabbage, broccoli, liver, egg yolk, cheese, synthesis in intestine	Large amounts are toxic; antibiotic therapy may reduce supply; some anticoagulants are K antagonists so their effectiveness can be altered if a diet high in K-rich food is consumed; some chemotherapeutic agents antagonize K
C (ascorbic acid)	Formation of collagen	Citrus fruits, tomatoes, melons, cabbage, broccoli, strawberries, potatoes, green leafy vegetables, peppers	Found concentrated in more metabolically active tissue; increased requirement in fevers, infections, stress, and for wound healing and with cigarette smoking and long-term use of aspirin
Thiamin (B_1)	Coenzyme in carbohydrate metabolism	Whole-grain or enriched bread and cereals, organ meats, pork, meat, poultry, fish, legumes, nuts, green vegetables	Deficiency causes fatigue, depression, gastrointestinal problems, cardiac problems, neurological problems, memory loss; increased need in fever, leukemia, alcoholism, hyperthyroidism and in high-carbohydrate diets and when intravenous glucose is used as sole food source; some evidence that elderly use thiamin less efficiently than younger adults

Table 3-2 (Cont.) Vitamins

Fat-soluble vitamins	Functions	Sources	Noteworthy
Riboflavin (B_2)	Coenzyme in protein metabolism	Milk, organ meats, eggs, green leafy vegetables, enriched bread and cereals	Deficiency causes sore tongue and mouth, sensitivity to light, burning itchy eyes; B_2 not effective in treating cataracts
Niacin (nicotinic acid, nicotinamide)	Coenzyme in tissue oxidation to produce energy	Meat, poultry, fish, whole-grain and enriched breads and cereals, nuts, legumes	Can be made from amino acid tryptophan; nicotinic acid is a vasodilator and, when given in large amounts therapeutically to reduce serum cholesterol (and experimentally to treat mental illness), causes burning, itching, and tingling of face; deficiency causes weakness, dermatitis, and central nervous system damage
Pyridoxine (B_6)	Coenzyme in amino acid and essential fatty acid metabolism; needed for conversion of tryptophan to niacin and glycogen to glucose	Wheat, corn, meat, poultry, fish, potatoes, sweet potatoes, vegetables	Deficiency causes anemia, nervous irritability, neuritis; D-penicillamine and isoniazid increase need for B_6; L-dopa affected by B_6, so intake must be monitored

Vitamin	Function	Sources	Deficiency / Notes
Pantothenic acid (B_3)	Coenzyme in formation of active acetate (CoA)	Meat, poultry, fish, whole-grain cereals, legumes, fruits, vegetables, milk	Deficiency found only in cases of severe B-complex deficit
Folic Acid (folate, folacin)	Coenzyme for transfer of single carbon units	Organ meats, green leafy vegetables, asparagus	Easily destroyed by heat of prolonged cooking; interrelated with vitamin B_{12}; deficiency causes macrocytic anemia; there is danger that high doses of folate could mask the diagnosis of pernicious anemia
B_{12} (cobalamin)	Coenzyme in protein synthesis	Liver, meat, milk, eggs, cheese	Deficiency causes pernicious anemia (usually due to deficiency of intrinsic factor needed for absorption of B_{12}); neuropathy of B_{12} deficiency precedes hematological changes in 25% of patients; used to treat neuritis of diabetes and alcoholism and used following gastrectomy; B_{12} is a source of mineral cobalt to body
Biotin	Coenzyme for synthesis of fatty acids, amino acids, purines	Organ meat, egg yolk, nuts, legumes	Deficiency when many raw egg whites eaten, also after prolonged use of antibiotics
Choline	Lipotropic agent; donor of methyl groups	Egg yolk, meat, fish, poultry, milk, whole grains	Not considered a true vitamin: used experimentally in the treatment of Alzheimer's disease, senile dementia, and fatty liver of alcoholics

Table 3-3 Minerals

Major minerals	Functions	Sources	Noteworthy
Calcium	Bone and teeth formation; aids blood clotting, muscle and nerve action; activates enzymes	Milk, cheese, green leafy vegetables, whole grains, shrimp, salmon, and sardines including the bones	Deficiency causes retarded bone calcification, osteomalacia, osteoporosis; absorption hindered by lack of vitamin D, excess phosphorous, antacids, tetracyclines, diuretics, fat, oxalic acid, phytic acid, and immobilization; calcium absorption decreases as age increases
Phosphorus	Bone and tooth formation; functions in metabolic processes; acts as buffer; acts in maintenance of neurological function	Milk, cheese, eggs, whole grains, legumes, nuts, meat, food additives, soft drinks	*Hypophosphatemia* found when recovering from diabetic acidosis, in malabsorption (sprue) and bone disease; excess use of aluminum hydroxide antacids can cause hypophosphotemia and may lead to osteomalacia; *hyperphosphatemia* found in renal insufficiency, hypoparathyroidism, tetany
Magnesium	Bone and tooth structure; activator and coenzyme in carbohydrate and protein metabolism; acts in nerve and muscle irritability	Whole-grain cereals, nuts, legumes, meat, milk, vegetables	Deficiency seen in alcoholism and after gastrointestinal losses; used to treat delirium tremens in alcoholism
Sulfur	Constituent of cell protein; activates enzymes; acts in detoxification reactions; makes up high-energy sulfur bonds	Meat, eggs, cheese, milk, legumes, nuts	Diet adequate in protein will meet need for sulfur

	Function	Food Sources	Comments
Sodium	Principal cation of extracellular fluid; acts in water balance, osmotic pressure, acid-base balance, cell permeability, muscle irritability and contraction, transmission of nerve impulses, in glucose transport	Table salt, milk, meat, eggs, fish, poultry, baking soda, baking powder	Diet usually provides much more than needed; may be a factor in etiology of hypertension; deficiency may occur as result of prolonged vomiting, diarrhea, profuse sweating, in chronic nephritis, or in Addison's disease
Potassium	Principal cation of intracellular fluid; acts in water balance, osmotic pressure, acid-base balance; regulates neuromuscular excitability and muscle contraction; synthesis of protein and glycogen	Whole grains, meat, legumes, fruits, vegetables	Rapid glycogen production as occurs in treatment of diabetic acidosis depletes potassium levels; deficiency can be due to starvation, adrenal tumors, use of some diuretics, prolonged vomiting or diarrhea; low potassium levels affect heart rate
Chlorine	Major extracellular fluid anion; acts in water balance, acid-base balance, and digestion because it makes up hydrochloric acid in gastric juice	Table salt	Diet usually provides more than needed
Iron	Part of hemoglobin, myoglobin, and oxidative enzymes	Organ meats, meat, poultry, egg yolk, whole grains, enriched breads and cereals, dark green leafy vegetables	Iron absorption decreases with age, marrow stores of iron in elderly are often very low; deficiency causes anemia; oral iron supplements may irritate gastric mucosa; vitamin C and meat improves absorption; antacids decrease absorption as do high-fiber diets, tea; use of iron utensils increases supply

Table 3-3 (*Cont.*) Minerals

Major minerals	Functions	Sources	Noteworthy
Copper	Aids in absorption and utilization of iron in hemoglobin synthesis; component of metalloenzymes involved in energy release; melanin synthesis	Liver, meat, seafood, whole grains, legumes, nuts, corn oil, margarine	Deficiency is rare; use of copper utensils for food increases intake as does the presence of copper water pipes; zinc antagonizes absorption of copper
Iodine	Part of thyroid hormones; regulates rate of energy metabolism	Iodized salt, seafood	Deficiency can cause goiter; at present, excess is a greater problem because iodine is often used as sanitizing agent and food additive; goitrogens are found in cabbage, cauliflower, Brussels sprouts, broccoli, kale, kohlrabi, turnips, and rutabagas and interfere with iodine uptake; excess amount may reduce effectiveness of thyroid medication
Manganese	Activates many enzymes involved in urea formation, carbohydrate oxidation, protein metabolism; bone development	Cereals, whole grains, soybeans, legumes, nuts, tea, coffee	Deficiency not described in humans; may be needed for proper utilization of thiamin

Mineral	Functions	Food Sources	Comments
Zinc	Part of many enzyme systems; combines with insulin for storage of hormone	Seafood, organ meats, fish, wheat germ, yeast, whole grains	Deficiency retards wound healing and reduces taste and smell acuity; zinc depletion may be a factor in osteoporosis; supplement of more than 15 mg/day not recommended as it may aggravate marginal copper deficiency
Fluorine	Increases resistance of teeth to decay; may protect against periodontal disease and osteoporosis	Fluoridated water, tea, seafood	Excess amounts cause fluorosis; part of tooth and bone structure
Selenium	Antioxidant (destroys peroxidases formed in cell membranes); cofactor in cell oxidation and enzyme systems	Seafood, meat, whole grains	Associated with vitamin E functions in body
Chromium	Maintains normal carbohydrate metabolism; is part of glucose tolerance factor	Liver, meat, clams, whole grains, cheese, yeast	Does not cure diabetes but may improve condition; glucose tolerance factor (GTF) sold as food supplement is ineffective in humans
Molybdenum	Constituent of metalloenzymes that are involved in purine, aldehyde, and sulfite metabolism	Organ meats, legumes, whole-grain cereals	Supplements of additional molybdenum over what is provided in the diet are not recommended; excess is associated with urinary copper loss

for these substances. However, a supplement should never be considered a substitute for a well-chosen diet. Instead, it should be used as insurance which may also provide the additional benefit of discouraging excessive use of other supplements. In no circumstances should large amounts of supplements, more than 10 times the RDA, be used without medical supervision.

Patient aid:

What Can Vitamins Do for Me Now?
A guide to vitamins for mature adults

available from:

Vitamin Nutrition Information Service
Hoffman-LaRoche Inc.
Nutley, New Jersey 07110

REFERENCES

1. Food and Nutrition Board, National Academy of Science, *Recommended Dietary Allowances*, 9th ed. Washington, D.C. 1980.

2. Bierman, E.L., Obesity, Carbohydrate and lipid interactions in the elderly, in Winick, M. (ed.). *Nutrition and Aging*, New York: John Wiley & Sons, 1976.

3. Abraham, S., *Weight by Height and Age for Adults 18–74 years, United States 1971–1974*. Hyattsville, Md: National Center for Health Statistics, 1979. Vital and Health Statistics: Series II: Data from the National Health Survey, no. 208 (DHEW Publ. no (PHS) 79–1956).

4. Guthrie, H.A., *Introductory Nutrition*, 4th ed. St. Louis: C.V. Mosby Co., 1979.

5. Cheng, A.H.R., et al., Comparative nitrogen balance study between young and aged adults. Using three levels of protein intakes from a combination wheat-soy-milk mixture, *Am. J. Clin. Nutr.* 31:12, 1978.

6. Munro, H.N., Young, V.R., Protein metabolism in the elderly, *Postgrad. Med.* 63:143, 1978.

7. Gersovitz, M., et al., Human protein requirements. Assessments of the adequacy of the current recommended dietary allowance for dietary protein in elderly men and women, *Am. J. Clin. Nutr.* 35:6, 1982.

8. Thompson, R.G., et al., Triglyceride concentrations: The disaccahride effect, *Science* 26:828, 1979.

9. Bierman, E.L., et al., Principles of nutrition and dietary recommendations for patients with diabetes mellitus, *Diabetes* 20:633, 1971.

10. Turnpeinen, O., Effect of cholesterol-lowering diet on mortality from coronary disease and other causes, *Circulation* 59:1, 1979.

11. Moncada, S., Vane, J.R., Arachidonic acid metabolism and the interactions between platelets and blood vessel walls, *N. Engl. J. Med.* 300:42, 1979.

12. Blackburn, H., How nutrition influences mass hyperlipidemia and atherosclerosis, *Geriatrics* 33:42, 1978.

13. Kelsoy, J.L., A review of research on effects of fiber intake in man, *Am. J. Clin Nutr.* 31:142, 1978.

14. Simpson, H.C.R., et al., A high carbohydrate leguminous fibre diet improves all aspects of diabetic control, *Lancet* 1:8210, 1981.

15. Vahoury, G.V., Conclusions and recommendations of the symposium on dietary fibers in health and disease, *Am. J. Clin. Nutr.* 35:152, 1982.

16. Scheller, J.G., et al., Patterns of fluid intake among U.S. adults, *Am. J. Clin. Nutr.* 34(4):692, 1984.

17. Albanese, A.O., Nutrition and health of the elderly, *Nutr. News* 39(2):5, 1976.

18. Albanese, A.A., *Nutrition for the Elderly.* New York: Alan R. Liss, 1980.

19. *The Gallup Study of Vitamin Use in the United States Survey, Survey VI, Volume I.* Princeton, N.J.: Gallup Organization, December 1982.

20. Whanger, A.D., Nutrition, diet and exercise in: *Handbook of Geriatric Psychiatry* (E.W. Busse and D.G. Bhager, eds). New York: Van Nostrand Reinhold, 1980.

21. Kellett, M., et al., Vitamin and mineral supplement usage by retired citizens, *J. Nutr. Elderly* 3(3):7, 1984.

22. Scala, J., Are food supplements necessary? *Nutr. Today* 15(9):25, 1980.

Part II

NUTRITIONAL INTERVENTION IN DISEASE

Chapter 4

COUNSELING AND COMPLIANCE

Addressing the nutritional needs of an older client is essential to total health care, and when instituted early, it is one of the most cost-effective treatments in terms of health care dollars (1). Unfortunately, it is also a well-documented fact that compliance with dietary advice and recommendations is poor (50% or less) (2,3,4).

Nutrition counseling, helping people establish and keep good nutritional habits, is a complex process. Eating, especially for the older adult, is interwoven through life's experiences, reflecting culture, religion, ethnicity, and family structure. In addition, eating will be affected by the client's physical, economic, and social situation. Chronicity of disease exacerbates the difficulty of changing lifelong eating habits (5).

There are two keys to effective nutritional counseling. One important aspect is identifiable counseling characteristics. Counselors who show empathy, sincerity, and unconditional positive regard for clients are the most effective in producing lasting change (6). Second and equally important is the element of time. Lasting nutritional changes occur when there is continuous care over an extended period (5). Compliance decreases with decreased follow-up (4). A long-held misconception in the medical community is that dietary changes require only a few, highly structured interviews where the caregiver simply instructs the patient to make prescribed dietary changes. In actuality, the best results are obtained when the patient is referred for diet instruction early in treatment and followed up regularly. Giving the patient printed diet instructions and/or providing only short-term referral for diet instructions are poor intervention techniques (5,7). One study showed that surgeons were more likely to refer patients for nutritional support than any other specialty group followed by internists and gastroenterologists (8). This might suggest which physicians would be most willing to help establish a nutrition support and referral protocol.

COUNSELING TECHNIQUES TO IMPROVE COMPLIANCE

A basic prerequisite to successful nutrition counseling is a realistic and honest understanding that the client, not the caregiver, bears the responsibility for change (6). This must be communicated to the client. To reinforce this concept, caregivers should substitute the word *adherence* for *compliance*. Adherence is less authoritative and places the decision-making responsibility on the client.

Identify the Client's Concerns and Expectations and Attempt to Meet Them

Often a client will have genuine concerns about his/her ability to initiate dietary changes. These concerns must be examined before change can be instituted. Expectations of the caregiver and client may differ. These too should be discussed. The health professional needs to understand the client's belief system so that it can be integrated into the counseling plan. Adherence to dietary regimens is poor when the caregiver does not adjust the diet prescription so that it takes into account the client's concerns and expectations (4).

Develop Communication Skills

Effective communication used both body language and verbal responses to establish an atmosphere of acceptance so that the client will feel free to discuss concerns. One can practice and become skillful at using specific types of verbal responses that can aid in successful counseling (9).

Continuing responses help to initiate a dialogue. *Content continuing responses* reflect or summarize what the counselor perceives as the client's prior statement. Client: "I love coffee with sugar and I don't want to stop drinking it that way." Counselor: "You only enjoy sweetened coffee.'' *Affective continuing responses* reflect a feeling that the client has not yet labeled. Client: ''Dieting is hard when other people are eating around you all day.'' Counselor: ''You feel deprived because you have to watch what you eat.'' These continuing responses allow the client to hear back what he/she has just said, initiating and continuing a conversation. If the counselor inaccurately interprets the client's message, the reflected response system allows for correction.

It is essential to ask questions when providing nutrition counseling. Questions that start with ''what'' or ''how'' are *open questions* that are less likely to be answered with a ''yes'' or ''no.'' Counselor: ''What did you eat this morning?'' instead of ''Did you eat this morning?'' or ''How do you enjoy eating vegetables?'' instead of ''Why don't you eat vegetables?'' Open questions are less threatening and often provide insights to the roadblocks the client may be facing.

Plan Gradual Changes in Eating Habits

Some clients may be eager to change all aspects of their eating behavior immediately; others may be overwhelmed and unable to focus on the problem. The counselor should point out that slow but steady changes in eating habits are most likely to persist over time. The client need not and indeed should not attempt to change overnight. This graduated approach to dietary change relieves the counselor from setting arbitrary goals. Each successful small change will set the stage for a subsequent additional small change resulting in an overall positive effect on eating behavior (5).

Regularly Review Goal Achievement

Reviewing and adapting the diet prescription to accommodate a client's wants or needs may reduce barriers to adherence and facilitate the achievement of long-term dietary goals. It is often hard for the counselor to accept that the success or failure of a client is not a reflection of the counselor's ability. The responsibility for change rests with the client. At times it may appear that the counseling sessions are not progressing toward a positive goal. This is the time to examine why there is a roadblock. There are four reasons why a person cannot achieve a goal: lack of skills, lack of knowledge, lack of risk taking, lack of social support (9). When the client is unable to progress, review the capabilities he/she possesses and see which one is causing the obstacle. Setting up a gradual-change approach will often help the client overcome the obstacle to goal achievement. For example, if an older diabetic woman is afraid to shop alone, the counselor can arrange for a shopping-assistance program. Once this is in progress, the counselor can once again focus on appropriate food selection and preparation to adhere to a diabetic meal plan.

Provide Positive Feedback to the Client on His/Her Progress

No matter how small the change, all clients need reinforcement so that they know they are doing well. Sometimes the only positive action the client may take is to keep his/her follow-up appointment. This, however, does evidence a desire for change; it just may take longer to accomplish. Avoid being judgmental if progress is slow. Change is threatening, especially when it involves long-standing eating habits. An explanation of the need for change with praise for the degree of change already accomplished will usually promote further adherence.

See Chapter 2 for information on nutritional assessment and guidelines for conducting a dietary interview.

AGING FACTORS THAT AFFECT COMPLIANCE

Many caregivers are not optimistic about counseling older clients. They associate aging with declining memory, slowness, and even dementia. Studies reveal, however, that most older individuals have accurate memories, keen minds, and the ability to learn and apply new concepts. Elderly participants in a government feeding program completed food frequency questionnaires with impressive accuracy. Others have shown that older clients keep accurate diet histories but have difficulty recalling information for a 24-hour food recall (10). This information is consistent with the fact that short-term memory is least effective as a person grows older (11).

Visual acuity declines with age making the perception of detail difficult. An 80-year-old needs four times as much light to perceive an image as does a younger adult. If handouts or visual materials are employed in counseling, they should be in large type and uncluttered, and the colors used should be different and distinct. Discrimination between blue, blue-green, and violet is particularly difficult (11).

Eye-to-eye contact is important in counseling as many older individuals have a hearing loss and they may partially lip-read. Older Asians, however, would find this eye contact uncomfortable because looking downward is a sign of courtesy in their culture (12). Noisy set-

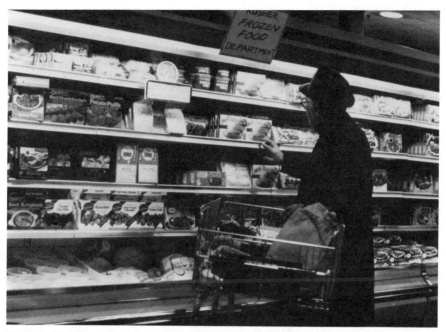

Diet modifications must be individualized, taking into account a person's belief system. Courtesy of *Progressive Grocer Magazine.*

tings, rapid speech, and the inability to clearly hear phonetically similar words may cause difficulty in following normal conversation (13).

Decreasing ability to taste food is a major factor in food acceptance. As individuals age, food flavors become more similar and less distinguishable (14). It is particularly difficult to discern the flavor of pureed items (15). Edentulous patients on soft or pureed diets often complain of lack of flavor.

Flavor depends on many senses: hearing, taste, and smell. Loss of smell begins in middle age and is progressive. Taste is more robust, but most older adults have trouble perceiving weak tastes as early as age 60 (14). An 80-year-old has 74 to 85 taste buds per papilla, of which half may be atrophic, in contrast to a young adult who has 248 functioning taste buds per papilla (16). Older adults often describe food flavors as sour, bitter, or dry. This might be explained by the increasing loss of smell as one ages. Many foods, such as green pepper, have a bitter taste but a pleasant odor. If olfactory sensitivity is markedly impaired, green peppers would simply taste bitter (15).

Loss of smell compounds the difficulty in determining food rancidity and spoilage, which increases the hazard of food-borne illness. Over 50% of those 65 and older are unable to smell domestic gas if it is escaping from an open but unlit gas jet. Studies show that over three-quarters of the deaths from domestic gas poisoning are in persons over 60 (17). An older person using a gas range should be cautioned to check the range controls several times throughout the day. Marking the *off* position with a brightly colored dot of paint will help a person visually recognize when gas may be escaping.

PHYSICAL LIMITATIONS THAT AFFECT COMPLIANCE

A person with arthritis, someone recovering from a stroke, or an older client with Parkinson's disease may be mobility-impaired and require adaptive devices for independent self-care.

Tremors, partial paralysis, impaired vision, and other physical conditions can make the activities of daily living unpleasant endurance events. If a person has a disabling physical condition, tasks must be simplified and wasted motions eliminated. Let dishes drain dry instead of wiping them; use precut onions, peppers, vegetables, and other foods to eliminate peeling, chopping, and slicing; instead of lifting, roll objects on a wheeled cart. Every task must be reduced to its essential motions.

Easy-open packages and flip-top cans are of no convenience to an arthritic person with limited strength or joint movement. The arthritic homemaker will tire easily and should plan activities in small sessions. For mixing and stirring, a large spoon held between flat palms provides a less painful, more secure grasp (18).

Stroke or surgery may result in the loss of part or all of one arm. If the cause is hemiplegia (paralysis of one side of the body), there may be an accompanying loss of perception and decreased quick mental recall. These individuals must be taught to turn their heads to compensate for visual field limitations. In food preparation, if they do not intermittently turn the head to scan the entire countertop, an ingredient can be omitted because it cannot be seen. Hemiplegia makes mealtime tasks difficult owing to the weakness on one side (19). A cutting board with two stainless steel nails hammered through it can secure food for cutting or peeling. A wet facecloth or spongecloth under a bowl can anchor it so it will not spin. Knees can hold packages as they are opened or unwrapped. Glass jars can be opened with one hand by putting the jar in a drawer, leaning a hip against the drawer to hold the jar securely, and twisting the top off with the free arm (18).

With aphasia (partial or full loss of the power of expression by speech, writing, or signs, or loss of comprehension of spoken or written language) the person must be taught to plan activities and repeat them over and over again (19). Recipes such as the example in Table 4–1 make use of a repetition of skills and can be used to help reestablish the habits of meal preparation.

An older person in a wheelchair will find the ordinary kitchen full of architectural barriers. Structural changes need to be made so this person may continue to function independently. The cost of equipment and rehabilitation is partially covered by local, state, and federal funds as homemaking is recognized as the largest single occupation among the physically handicapped (20).

Adaptive feeding aids are useful in assuring the independence of an older adult who is having trouble handling regular utensils. A built-up handle on a standard eating utensil may be all that is needed to provide a secure grasp for impaired hands. Utensils of this special type can be purchased, or a regular eating utensil can be adapted by slipping a foam rubber curler over the handle. The foam surface of the curler increases friction and aids in the maintenance of a steady grasp. These curlers are inexpensive and available in drug and variety stores. Handles may be angled or bent to compensate for limited motion, and a collar or band may be attached to the end of the handle that fits over the person's hand to help prevent the utensil from being dropped.

Plastic and metal plate guards and plates with rims enable the person to pick up his food by first pushing it against the raised edge. A suction cup or sponge cloth under the plate can keep the dish in place while the person is eating.

A spouted cup, extended straws, and pedestal cup can aid in drinking liquids. A two-handled drinking cup is especially useful for older persons with incoordination. Stretch terry cloth glass covers designed for use on cold-drink glasses provide a secure grasp when holding a glass. These are available where picnic supplies are sold or can be hand-knit or crocheted. To hold a straw steady and in place, a pen clip can be attached to a cup, and the straw threaded through where the pen was originally held. The spork, a combination of fork and spoon, often serrated down one edge, can replace three utensils for a person who has the use of only one hand.

The elderly blind can make use of many of these feeding aids. The lipped plate on which food is place in a prescribed clockwise fashion is often used to train the blind to feed themselves (18,21).

Figures 4–1 through 4–4 show a variety of these eating aids. Table 4–2 lists suppliers of adaptive eating devices for ADL-impaired individuals. It is important to remember that the ability to feed oneself is a very important factor in feeling independent. It is uncomfortable, humiliating, and embarrassing for an older person to be fed, and every effort should be made to encourage self-feeding.

Table 4-1 Repetitious Recipe to Retrain Kitchen Skills

Endless Variety Skillet Casserole

Carbohydrate	Protein	Vegetables	Liquid	Seasoning	Topping
$2/3$ C rice, uncooked	$1/2$ C cooked, cut-up chicken, or turkey, or beef, or veal or pork	$1/2$ C fresh or frozen carrots, or peas, or corn, or green beans, or chopped broccoli, or mixed vegetables	$2 1/4$ C beef or chicken broth	1 T dehydrated onion, or parsley, or chives or celery	$1/4$ C seasoned bread crumbs
1 C fine or medium noodles, uncooked	$1/2$ C flaked tuna	$1/2$ C canned vegetables (same variety as above)	$2 1/2$ C tomato sauce	$1/4$ C frozen diced green pepper or onion	$1/4$ C crushed cornflakes or other dry cereal
1 C elbow macaroni, uncooked	1 C cooked, cut-up breakfast sausage		$2 1/4$ C canned gravy	2 T diced pimento	$1/4$ C crushed potato chips or corn chips
2 C diced raw potatoes*	$1/4$ lb raw chopped meat		1 can (11-12 oz) condensed cream of mushroom, or cream of celery, or cream of		$1/4$ C grated Swiss, or cheddar, or American

⅔ C cooked or canned chick-peas

¾ C soy bean curd, diced

chicken, or cream of tomato soup (mix all of above with 1 soup can water)

1 can (11-12 oz) condensed barley-mushroom soup (mix with 1 soup can water)

cheese

1 hard-cooked egg, finely chopped

2 T wheat germ

¼ C cracker crumbs

1. In a 10-in. skillet combine 1 carbohydrate, 1 protein, 1 vegetable, 1 choice of liquid, and 2 choices of seasoning; stir to combine thoroughly.
2. Bring mixture to a boil, reduce heat to simmer, cover and continue cooking 25 to 30 minutes, stirring occasionally.
3. When casserole is done, transfer to a serving dish and sprinkle with selected topping and serve. Yield: 3 cups or two 1½ cups servings.

*When selecting potatoes as the casserole carbohydrate do not use beef or chicken broth as the liquid.

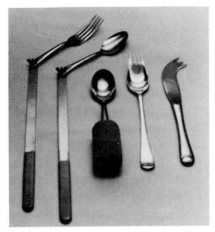

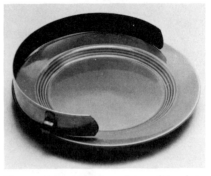

Figure 4-2 Dinner plate with plate guard. Photograph by S. Natow.

Figure 4-1 Left to right: (1) extended, angled fork and spoon; (2) regular utensil with builtup handle using a foam curler; (3) spork (spoon, fork, knife in one), one edge is serrated for cutting; (4) rocker knife/fork, for use by a person with one usable hand. Photograph by S. Natow.

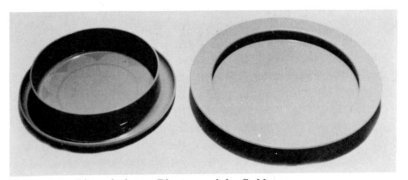

Figure 4-3 Lipped plates. Photograph by S. Natow.

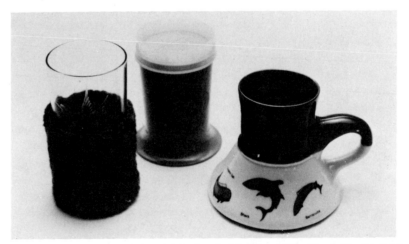

Figure 4-4 Left to right: (1) knitted drinking glass "cozy"; (2) lidded, tip-proof glass; (3) no-spill mug. Photograph by S. Natow.

Table 4–2 Suppliers of Feeding Aids

Research Products Corporation
1015 East Washington Avenue
Madison, Wisconsin 53701

Fred Sammon, Inc.
Box 321
Brookfield, Illinois
60513—0032

J.A. Preston Corporation
71 Fifth Avenue
New York, New York 10003

Cleo Living Aids
3957 Mayfield Road
Cleveland, Ohio 44121

REFERENCES

1. DRG's/A Disastrous Dilemma, *NSS Today* 1:1, Sept. 1984.

2. Gillum, R.F., Barsky, A.J., Diagnosis and management of patient non-compliance, *JAMA* 228:1563, 1974.

3. Marston, M.V., Compliance with medical regimens: A review of the literature, *Nurs. Res.* 19:312, 1970.

4. Eckerling, L., Kohrs, M.B., Research on compliance with diabetic regimens: Application to practice, *J. Am. Diet. Assoc.* 84:807, July 1984.

5. Zifferblatt, S. M., Wilbur, C.S., Dietary counseling: Some realistic expectations and guidelines, *J. Am. Diet. Assoc.* 70:591, June 1977.

6. Danish, S.J., Developing helping relationships in dietetic counseling, *J. Am. Diet. Assoc.* 67:107, Aug. 1975.

7. Ramsay, L.E., et al., Weight reduction in a blood pressure clinic, *Br. Med. J.* 2:244, 1978.

8. Mu-Chow, K.J., Baptista, R.J., Disease states and attending physicians' specialties of patients referred for formal nutrition support, *Nutr. Support Serv.* 5:56, Feb. 1985.

9. Danish, S.J., et al., The anatomy of a dietetic counseling interview, *J. Am. Diet. Assoc.* 75:626, Dec. 1979.

10. Karbeck, J.M., Assessment of nutritional status of the elderly, *Nutr. Support Serv.* 4:23, Oct. 1984.

11. Hallburg, J.C., The teaching of aged adults, *J. Gerontol. Nurs.* 2:13, 1976.

12. Spencer, H., The hidden meaning of body language, *Am. Pharm.*, NS21(7):416, July 1981.

13. Pelcovits, J., Nutrition education in group meals for the aged, *J. Nutr. Educ.* 5:118, 1973.

14. Cain, W.S., Flavoring foods for a grayer U.S., *Food Engineering* 56:103, May 1984.

15. Schiffman, S.S., Moss, J., Erickson, R.P., Thresholds of food odors in the elderly, *Exp. Aging Res.* 2:389, 1976.

16. Bayless, T.M., Malabsorption in the elderly, *Hosp. Pract.* 14:57, 1979.

17. Chalks, H.D., Dewhurst, J.R., Coal gas poisoning. Loss of sense of smell as possible contributory factor with old people. *Br. Med. J.* 2:915, 1957.

18. Klinger, J.L., *Mealtime Manual for People with Disabilities and the Aging*, Campbell Soup Company, Camden, N.J., 1978.

19. Rusk, H.A., Nutrition in the fourth phase of medical care, *Nutr. Today* 5:24, 1970.

20. Agan, T., et al., Adjusting the environment for the elderly and the handicapped, *J. Home Econ.* 69:18, 1977.

21. Rankin, G., The therapeutic value of a dining room program in a geriatric setting, *J. Gerontol. Nurs.* 1:5, 1975.

Chapter 5

ALCOHOL

Alcohol abuse, here used synonymously with alcoholism, is a serious personal, social, and health problem among older adults while remaining an elusive problem, often going undetected and untreated. Alcoholism refers to a spectrum of problems ranging from occasional excessive drinking to alcohol addiction. Often included in the phenomena associated with alcohol abuse are habitual excessive drinking in social situations, drinking to induce sleep, early-morning drinking, and "blackouts" during heavy drinking. Although none of these phenomena are necessary or sufficient to establish one as an "alcoholic," alcohol intake that routinely and repeatedly interferes with an individual's social functioning or physical health is definitely dangerous and should be considered to be alcohol abuse.

The following discussion will deal largely with the nutritional implications of chronic ingestion of alcohol. However, the reader who deals with the alcoholic individual must recognize that nutrition is only one of many aspects of the alcohol abuser's problem.

The incidence of alcohol abuse peaks in middle age, near 40, with a second peak in the 65-to-74-year-old group (1). The former group may have a history of alcohol abuse from their 20s while the latter group usually begins drinking owing to external factors associated with aging—bereavement, loneliness, depression, retirement with related boredom, loss of status, and lowered income (2,3).

The actual incidence of alcoholism in those over 55 is uncertain. Estimates suggest that from 2 to 30% of this population experience alcohol-related problems (4,5). Twenty percent of all nursing home residents have been categorized as problem drinkers, with the number increasing to 30% for Veterans Administration domiciliary residents. The National Institute on Alcohol Abuse and Alcoholism estimated that in 1980, one to three million elderly were either chronically heavy or problem drinkers (6).

Physicians and family, however, are often reluctant to suggest that the older individual is an alcoholic. The only sign of alcoholism may be the person's loss of ability to function in his environment. When this loss of function follows a major crisis—retirement, loss of spouse or home, illness—the family and physician may associate the symptoms with senility and/or depression (2). If this same patient becomes increasingly confused or suffers insomnia, gastritis, general weakness, or hyperuricemia, excessive drinking should be suspected (7).

Alcohol intoxication, alcohol withdrawal symptoms, and alcohol-drug interactions plus coexisting physical disorders such as congestive heart failure, hypertension, and emphysema can have life-threatening effects in the older adult. Early death is common among alcoholics; many die of complications of alcoholism before their sixty-fifth birthday. Some researchers suggest 50 as the age when the active drinker should be considered "elderly" (3).

The effects of alcohol intake are intensified by aging. Decreased coordination plus alcohol may result in falls or burns; decreased cognitive ability plus alcohol results in confusion; borderline hypertension plus alcohol may lead to marked hypertension; borderline diabetes and alcohol leads to overt diabetes; and mild depression plus alcohol leads to deeper depression (2).

EFFECTS OF ALCOHOL

All alcoholics are at nutritional risk, but the older alcoholic may be at particularly great risk. When alcohol is present, tissues cannot utilize or store nutrients in the normal manner. Osteoporosis, usually considered a sign of aging and seen principally in older women, is found in significant numbers of middle-aged male alcoholics (8). Because of the physiological changes in aging, mature adults are more susceptible to the toxic effects of alcohol, and adverse reactions occur with smaller doses (5,9).

Clinical observations suggest that with advancing age, many older adults decrease their drinking. These observations support the theory

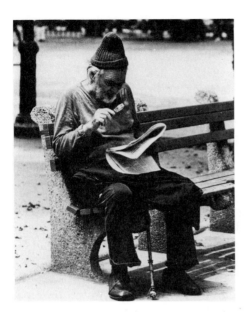

Photograph by L. Miller.

that tolerance to alcohol decreases with age, even in active drinkers. Animal studies indicate that aged organisms are more sensitive to the effects of alcohol. Aged mice become more severely intoxicated than younger mice and suffer more severe withdrawal signs after similar alcohol intakes (10,11).

Studies in older humans have yielded results similar to comparable animal studies. For a given height and weight, the older individual will demonstrate an increased blood alcohol concentration after a measured dose as compared to a younger person. This higher peak blood alcohol level is probably due to the combined reductions in body water and lean body mass that occur in aging. Consequently, older individuals may experience intensified reactions to alcohol such as greater depression of motor skills, impaired cognition, and sleep disturbances (5,9). Though these problems would be most evident in heavy drinkers, the reactions also occur in light to moderate drinkers. Chronic use of alcohol, even in relatively small amounts, may mimic or magnify changes in the nervous system associated with normal aging. The confused, disoriented older patient may not be demented but intoxicated (5). It is important in a clinical assessment to determine not only whether the person drinks but when and how much. Drinking small amounts throughout the day may lead to symptoms that could easily be misdiagnosed as dementia.

Studies show that the metabolic clearance of alcohol is not altered with age. Liver disease, illness, and malnutrition, however, can decrease the metabolic clearance in the older adult as they would in the young (5,9). This would prolong the amount of time alcohol circulates, potentiating its toxic effects. The synergistic effect of poor nutrition and the hepatotoxicity of alcohol may initiate organ damage and cause abnormal changes in body functions (9,12).

Alcoholic beverages contain calories and a few nutrients. One gram of alcohol yields 7.1 kcal but does not behave as other kilocalorie equivalents since the oxidation of alcohol in the liver is an energy-wasting process. As the older individual takes in more alcohol, weight gain often does not occur because the net increase in calories is less than would be expected, and as alcohol calories increase, food intake usually decreases. Weight loss may be seen in some alcoholics owing to irregular eating or total abstinence from food during, or immediately after, a drinking episode. Alcohol-induced anorexia is common and complex in origin. Contributing factors in addition to inebriation may be depression, heavy cigarette smoking, gastrointestinal disturbances, chronic pancreatitis, and liver disease (13).

Ethyl alcohol, or ethanol, is completely miscible in water, requires no digestion, and is inherently toxic to living tissues. Consequently, every cell in the body is liable to damage or destruction. Alcohol will damage the gastrointestinal tract and impair absorption of nutrients (9). In the esophagus, stomach, and small intestine alcohol irritates the mucosa, leading to ulceration and hemorrhage. Alcohol may increase pancreatic secretion while at the same time obstructing release of the enzymes, causing damage to pancreatic cells. Pancreatitis, associated with abdominal tenderness, distention, and vomiting, may become chronic and will be triggered by binge drinking. Concomitant with these symptoms is the malabsorption of amino acids and fat caused by maldigestion resulting from a decreased availability of pancreatic enzymes.

Alcohol affects intestinal motility and contributes to diarrhea. Chronic or even intermittent diarrhea poses the possible complication of dehydration for the older drinker.

Alcohol ingestion interferes with the metabolism of minerals. Zinc absorption is decreased while excretion is increased, depressing wound healing. Magnesium is also excreted in larger-than-normal amounts, potentiating the cardiac effects of thiamin deficiency. Hypokalemia is common in chronic drinkers and may be the cause of arrhythmias associated with alcoholic heart disease (13). In wine, 80% of the available iron is in the physiologically active ferrous form (14). Wine drinkers, therefore, may ingest excess amounts of iron. In addition, iron absorption is enhanced, in part, by increased gastric acidity and folic acid deficiency. This excess iron absorption and subsequent storage may result in hepatic damage. Hemochromatosis (iron-overload disease) has been clinically observed among middle-aged alcoholic men (13). For this reason, routine iron supplements are contraindicated for older alcoholics.

Vitamin deficiency in the chronic drinker has multiple causes—low dietary intake, intestinal malabsorption, hyperexcretion, and impaired synthesis to the active or coenzyme forms. Utilization of vitamins by alcohol-damaged tissues is impaired while this same damage increases the need for vitamins by the tissues. Vitamin needs of the alcoholic exceed those of the nonalcoholic.

Deficiences of folic acid, thiamin (B_1), pyridoxine (B_6), pantothenic acid, and cobalamin (B_{12}) have been documented among groups of alcoholics (9,13). Vitamin D metabolism may also be disturbed, contributing to an increase in fractures owing to poor calcium utilization(8). Wernicke's disease and Korsakoff's psychosis are disorders of the central nervous system seen in the elderly with a long history of alcohol abuse and poor diet. The specific lack of thiamin (B_1) is the main nutritional problem in these disorders, and supplementation can reverse many of the symptoms (13). The incidence of Wernicke-Korsakoff's syndrome is high in elderly female alcoholics. No evidence suggests a gender relationship. A more likely explanation is that older women outlive men, and the number of older women alcoholics may be underestimated (5). It is important to realize that the early symptoms may be misinterpreted as being due to aging (unsteady gait, double vision, confused agitation, and hallucinations) and may thus be allowed to progress to an irreversible chronic brain syndrome characterized by memory loss and inability to function independently (13).

Even though chronic drinkers suffer multiple nutrient deficiencies, clinicians must be aware that alcoholics are heavy users and abusers of over-the-counter vitamin preparations and tonics. Physicians, particularly psychiatrists, often prescribe vitamins as a prophylaxis and to prevent organic brain syndrome. However, because of liver damage, elderly alcoholics may be more susceptible to vitamin toxicity. Hypervitaminosis A and niacin "intoxication" have been reported (13).

Although the liver is the primary site for the detoxification of alcohol, the cells and function of this organ can be damaged by alcohol and its metabolites (9). Alcohol replaces fat as the preferred energy source of the liver. Oxidation of fat thus ceases, and lipid accumulates in the liver, depressing hepatic function and leading to progressive liver disease (15). Damage to the liver adversely affects all parts of the body. Alcohol alters amino acid metabolism in the hepatic cells causing certain amino acids to accumulate in the liver. The synthesis of other proteins, such as albumin and transferrin, is inhibited.

Alcohol also interferes with gluconeogenesis. This may lead to a hypoglycemic reaction—weakness, irritability, incoordination, trembling, perspiration, rapid heartbeat, nausea, vomiting, and confusion. This reaction could be misread as signs of intoxication. An alcoholic coma may in fact be a hypoglycemic coma (16). If a glucose infusion is delayed, death or brain damage may result.

With excessive alcohol ingestion, large amounts of lactate are produced. The lactate is excreted readily by the body and in preference to the excretion of uric acid. As a result, uric acid levels in alcoholics are increased. Male patients with serum uric acid levels of 9.0 mg/dl or more should be questioned about alcohol use. In one study of admissions to a general hospital, male patients with these uric acid levels had a 30% likelihood of being alcoholic (7).

Liver Disease

The major effect of alcohol ingestion is on lipid metabolism resulting in hypertriglyceridemia and fatty liver (15). Fatty liver develops when alcohol replaces fat as the preferred energy source for the liver. Combustion of fat ceases and lipid accumulates in the liver. The older drinker may have varying degrees of liver involvement from fatty liver to alcoholic hepatitis to irreversible cirrhosis. Nutritional support is a cornerstone in the treatment of these hepatic problems.

In addition to the obvious need for abstinence from alcohol and the treatment of withdrawal symptoms, a major aspect of medical care of the alcoholic is the correction of nutritional deficiencies. Patients with alcoholic hepatitis usually exhibit signs of chronic malnutrition with resultant immunosuppression and increased susceptibility to infections. A diet with adequate (but not excessive) protein (60–100 g/day) and supplemental vitamins and minerals is recommended. A low fat intake is warranted especially when jaundice or steatorrhea is evident. A useful way to supply fat to bile-deficient patients is by using medium-chain triglyceride (MCT) oil. MCT oil does not facilitate the absorption of fat-soluble vitamins nor does it provide essential fatty acids (EFA). Supplementary EFA must be supplied. Oral administration of safflower or sunflower oil can be used. The cirrhotic patient also requires high protein, low fat, adequate calories, and vitamin/mineral supplementation. However, if hepatic encephalopathy is present, protein restriction must be imposed. If ascites is present, salt is restricted to 2 g/day and fluid intake to 1500 ml/day. Use of potassium chloride salt substitutes is contraindicated as many patients with ascites are treated with potassium-conserving diuretics. Supplementary potassium could cause hyperkalemia, cardiac arrhythmias, and death (12,17). See Chapter 6 for further discussion of nutrition in liver disease.

ALCOHOL AND DRUGS

Alcohol interacts with more than 150 commonly prescribed drugs. A drug-alcohol interaction is predictable, but the intensity or duration of the reaction may vary markedly from one individual to another and from one occasion to another depending on the casual or chronic nature of a person's alcohol consumption. The acute effect of alcohol is to impair liver metabolism, prolonging the half-life and potentiating the drug's effect. In addition, there is the possibility of additive effects of the drug and alcohol. Chronic alcohol ingestion enhances the metabolism of certain drugs, necessitating increased doses for effectiveness (5).

Alcohol's effect in modifying the action of drugs is important for many older adults who may be on multiple-drug regimens both prescription and nonprescription. Aspirin, commonly used for arthritic pain, irritates the mucosa of the stomach and interferes with certain clotting functions. Taking aspirin regularly along with the chronic use of alcohol will result in an additive effect that could lead to serious gastric hemorrhage (18). This additive effect is even more lethal in combination with barbiturates. Six hundred milligrams of Seconal (secobarbital) taken with alcohol can result in death. An elderly patient with decreased hepatic reserve is at risk for a barbituate overdose unless he is cautioned to avoid alcohol completely (5). The solvent action of alcohol may hasten the absorption of medication. Alcohol increases the absorption of nitroglycerin, leading to hypotension (18). Alcohol potentiates the effect of tranquilizers and sedatives. This interaction is more pronounced for older individuals who are taking drugs like Librium (chlordiazepoxide) resulting in side effects such as hypotension, sedation, confusion, and central nervous system depression (5).

The caregiver should question the older client about his use of alcohol and give specific instructions as to its interaction with medications. Table 17–8 (p. 261) gives numerous alcohol/drug interactions to aid the caregiver in detailing medication instructions.

ALCOHOL IN PHARMACEUTICAL PRODUCTS

More than 500 pharmaceuticals are aqueous-alcohol mixtures. Most are vitamin tonics or antitussive-decongestant liquids, which are frequently used by older adults. Thirty milliliters (2 tablespoons) of a cough/cold preparation containing 25% alcohol (i.e., NyQuil), can cause a disul-firamlike reaction in an elderly diabetic taking Diabinese (chlorpro-pamide). Gastric acid is stimulated by solutions with a 10% alcohol content, and erosive gastritis may be provoked with solutions in excess of 20% alcohol with concomitant inhibition of gastric activity leading to digestive distress.

Aqueous-alcohol preparations combined with sedatives, antianx-iety agents, or mild tranquilizers may enhance their depressant effects on the central nervous system and can compromise the person's safety by interfering with balance, judgement, and coordination.

Elderly persons taking prescription drugs must be counseled to seek advice when selecting cough/cold preparations or vitamin tonics to be sure that the self-medication is not contraindicated by the medication that is prescribed (19). Furthermore, the caregiver must determine *when* and *how much* of the aqueous-alcohol mixture is used. Often these sub-stances are taken in the evening or right before bed, and "just a little ex-tra" is added to the suggested dose. One tablespoon of a cold remedy that is 20% alcohol (40 proof) has the equivalent alcohol content of 1 oz of wine. Some elderly persons may be using these medications for their sed-ative effect or as a camouflaged and acceptable way to ingest additional alcohol. Table 17–7 (p. 259) is a list of the alcohol concentrations of vari-ous prescription and nonprescription pharmaceuticals.

ALCOHOL IN LONG-TERM CARE

The use of beer, wine, or a cocktail is gaining acceptance in long-term care. Studies suggest many beneficial effects including improved sleep, morale, appetite, alertness, friendliness, and social interaction (9,20).

Clinical and laboratory studies have confirmed that alcohol can stimulate appetite. Only small or moderate doses of alcohol are needed to enhance appetite and enjoyment of meals. This effect is most useful among those elderly who show a lack of interest in eating.

Even with the benefits noted, alcohol use in long-term care must be handled judiciously; a substantial percentage of residents may already be alcohol abusers. Although their intake may have been moderated by institutionalization, access to alcohol might initiate chronic drinking once again. Because of decreased physiological function, the elderly are more susceptible to the effects of alcohol, and these effects may last longer owing to decreased elimination. Falls, fractures, and aggressive and violent behavior have been precipitated by drinking. If alcohol is used for its sedative/euphoric effect, patient-management problems may develop when increasingly large amounts are denied to those who have developed a tolerance (1,18). Nursing home supervisors report on many ingenious ways that the elderly manage to secure the extra alcohol they desire. Even over-the-counter aqueous-alcohol solutions have been used to supplement therapeutically prescribed amounts.

ALCOHOL USE IN THERAPEUTIC DIETS

Low-Sodium Diets

One or two drinks a day (1½ oz of distilled liquor, 12 oz of beer, or 5 oz of table wine is equal to one drink) have been associated with a decreased risk of coronary death. The effect is apparent only in light drinkers. Among heavy drinkers, high blood pressure, abnormal heart rhythms, and cardiomyopathy are common (13).

Several studies have suggested that regular consumption of alcohol is associated with hypertension (21,22). Other studies have disputed this finding (9,21). Chronic alcohol consumption, coupled with age-related physiological changes in which the mechanism of blood pressure control becomes compromised, can cause a rise in blood pressure. Hypertension due to alcohol abuse appears to be reversible (21). Therefore, moderation of alcohol intake is an important nonpharmacological intervention for the control of hypertension. Alcohol abuse is also prevalent in stroke victims under age 50 and may precipitate cerebrovascular accidents in those over 60 (21,23).

In small amounts, alcohol can enhance the flavor of food. However, it would be prudent to counsel older clients on low-sodium diets to keep alcohol consumption minimal. Most wines contain less than 20 mg of sodium in a 5-oz glass. Wineries can supply sodium values for a given brand. Only those wineries that use iron-exchange resins to stabilize and clarify white wines will produce wines containing more sodium. The potassium content of wine is generally high, resulting in a favorable potassium-to-sodium ratio, an important consideration on a low-sodium diet.

Eighty percent of the sodium content of beer comes from the water in the area of the brewery. Manufacturers can supply exact amounts of sodium for their specific brand. An average 12-oz can of beer contains a range of sodium from 25 to 198 mg. Those brands that fall at the lower end of the range would be useful on a low-sodium diet. Distilled spirits (such as gin, scotch, and vodka) have virtually no sodium or potassium.

Mixers, however, may contain substantial amounts of both and need to be selected judiciously (20).

Remember that alcohol is contraindicated when a person is taking a diuretic or an antihypertensive agent or has a history of alcohol abuse.

Diabetic Diets

Alcohol contributes to energy intake as does the beverages in which it is mixed; consequently, chronic alcohol use may interfere with weight management in some older diabetics. For insulin-treated diabetes, large amounts of alcohol are hazardous, potentiating the hypoglycemic action of insulin (16). In well-controlled, mild diabetics moderate alcohol ingestion produces no impairment of diabetic control. Wine in amounts of 4–6 oz showed no significant effect on blood glucose (20). A 4-oz serving of dry red wine or dry white wine contains 0.2–0.5 g carbohydrate; dry rosé and dry champagne, 1.3–1.8 g; dry sherry, 2.4 g. Sweet dessert wines should not be used.

Beer and "light" beer have more carbohydrate and need to be used with care. A 12-oz glass of ale has 12.0 g of carbohydrate; beer, 15.8 g; light beer, 5.5 g. Distilled spirits contain no carbohydrate; it has all been fermented to alcohol. But mixers may add carbohydrates when the alcohol is served as a cocktail. Cordials such as fruit brandy and crème de menthe will provide an average of 6.0 g of carbohydrate per 1½-oz serving (14). Mixers that may be used in any amount are mineral water, Perrier water, club soda, diet soda, and sugar-free tonic. All older diabetics should be counseled to keep alcohol intake low and not to take alcohol on an empty stomach but rather at, or shortly after, a meal. The older diabetic treated with oral hypoglycemic agents is at risk for an alcohol-drug interaction (see Table 17–1, p. 252).

Weight Control

Some research shows that a glass of wine may reduce the tension associated with eating and aid in weight control programs. For those with reduced tastes, a small amount of alcohol may stimulate appetite (14).

Recommending alcohol indiscriminately to older patients is imprudent considering the physiological changes that occur in the aging process, the potential for alcohol-drug interaction, and the possibility of underlying alcohol abuse. If, however, an older person is functioning well and consuming small amounts of alcohol, this practice should not be discouraged as it may benefit health and the enjoyment of life. In addition, active treatment for elderly alcohol abusers has a high success rate as their drinking problems usually result from the psychosocial stresses of aging (3,9). Once the social problems are addressed, older alcoholics respond more positively to behavioral treatment for alcohol abuse than do younger alcoholics (1,24,25).

Professional resource:

The Unseen Alcoholics—The Elderly

available from:

Public Affairs Committee, Inc.
381 Park Avenue South
New York, N.Y. 10016

REFERENCES

1. Zimberg, S., The elderly alcoholic, *Gerontologist* 14:221, June 1974.
2. Pattee, J.J., Uncovering the elderly "hidden" alcoholic, *Geriatrics* 37:145, 1982.
3. Blum, L., Rosener, F., Alcoholism in the elderly: An analysis of 50 patients, *J. Natl Med. Assoc.* 75(5):489, 1983.
4. Zimering, S., Domeischel, J.R., Is alcoholism a problem of the elderly? *J. Drug Educ.* 12(2):103, 1982.
5. Hartford, J.T., Samorajski, T., Alcoholism in the geriatric population, *J. Am. Geriatr. Soc.* 30(1):18, 1982.
6. Williams, M., Alcohol and the elderly: An overview, *Alcohol Health Res. World* 8(3):3, Spring 1984.
7. Drum, D.F., Elevation of serum uric acid as a clue to alcohol abuse, *Arch. Intern. Med.* 141:477, March 1981.
8. Bone loss associated with alcoholism, *Alcohol Health Res. World* 8(3):22, Spring 1984.
9. West. L.J., Alcoholism, *Ann. Intern. Med.* 100(3):405, March 1984.
10. Gomberg, E.L., Patterns of alcohol use and abuse among the elderly, in: National Institute on Alcohol Abuse and Alcoholism. *Special Population*

Issues, Alcohol and Health Monograph No. 4. Rockville, MD: NIAAA, 1982, pp. 263–290.

11. Responses to alcohol differ for elderly vs. young, *Alcohol Health Res. World*, 8(3):20, Spring 1984.

12. Sherlock, S., Nutrition in the alcoholic, *Lancet* 1:489, March 3, 1984.

13. Roe, D., Nutritional concerns of the alcoholic, *J. Am. Diet. Assoc.* 78:17, 1981.

14. McDonald, J., Mixing alcohol with nutrition, *Professional Nutritionist* 3:1, Summer 1981.

15. Isselbocher, K.J., Metabolic and hepatic effects of alcohol, *N. Engl. J. Med.* 296(11):612, March 17, 1977.

16. Eisenstein, A.B., Nutritional and metabolic effects of alcohol, *J. Am. Diet. Assoc.* 81:247, Sept. 1982.

17. Gitlin, N., Heyman, M.B., Nutritional support in liver disease, *Nutr. Support Serv.* 4(6):14, June 1984.

18. Seixas, F.A., Drug/alcohol interactions: Avert potential dangers, *Geriatrics* 34:89, Oct. 1979.

19. Dukes, G.E., Kuhn, J.G., Evens, R.P., Alcohol in pharmeceutical products, *Am. Fam. Physician* 16:97, Sept. 1977.

20. McDonald, J., Moderate amounts of alcoholic beverages and clinical nutrition, *J. Nutr. Educ.* 14(2):58, 1982.

21. Clark, L.T., Alcohol use and hypertension, *Postgrad. Med.* 75(8):273, June 1984.

22. Ueshima, H., Asakura, D., Alcohol and hypertension, *J. Chronic Dis.* 37(7):597, 1984.

23. Taylor, J.R., Alcohol and strokes (letter), *N. Engl. J. Med.* 306:1111, May 6, 1982.

24. "Sunset" shines light on alcohol abuse, *Geriatrics* 37(3):35, March 1982.

25. Dupree, L.W., Broskowski, H., Schonfeld, L., The gerontology alcohol project: A behavioral treatment program for elderly alcohol abusers, *Gerontologist* 24(5):510, 1984.

Chapter 6

DIGESTIVE DISORDERS

Indigestion, abdominal pain, heartburn, gas, constipation, and the other gastrointestinal complaints collectively referred to as dyspepsia are very common in older adults. Seven percent of people over 45 experience acute gastrointestinal problems each year (1). It is all too easy to blame these ills on aging. However, the lessened sense of taste and smell, decreased secretion of saliva, hydrochloric acid, mucous, intrinsic factor, and digestive enzymes that are characteristic of aging and occur to varying degrees in most elderly persons usually do not significantly affect digestion. This is because the enormous reserve capacity of the gastrointestinal tract is able to minimize the effect of these changes (2).

It appears that the increasingly common practices of overeating, use of highly processed foods, alcohol, smoking, sedentary life-style, and polypharmacy are major causes or contributing factors to the digestive complaints of the elderly. Drugs such as aspirin, nonsteroidal antiinflammatory agents, steroids, erythromycin, digoxin, and theophylline often cause indigestion. Diets low in fiber and lack of physical activity have been linked to constipation. Furthermore, many of the other health problems of the elderly, and their treatment, may lead to digestive disorders.

It should not be overlooked that emotional upset, such as grief, anxiety, or loneliness may result in digestive aberrations. One of the cardinal signs of depression is loss of appetite. A very common cause of diarrhea, flatulence, or abdominal pain is anxiety. In addition, anxiety can result in increased or decreased appetite.

Tooth loss may predispose to digestive problems. The loss of many or most teeth has been accepted as part of normal aging, but this need not be. "Older people lose teeth because they have dental disease, not because they are old" (3). Seventy percent of all nursing home residents and 45% of adults over age 65 have lost all their teeth (4). However, these numbers represent a decline since the early 1960s (5). With widespread fluoridation of water supplies and improved dental care, many more adults will retain their natural teeth throughout life.

CONDITIONS OF THE GASTROINTESTINAL TRACT

Food Obstructions

Bezoars are tightly packed masses of hair, fruit, or vegetable matter that form and may become lodged in the gastrointestinal tract causing pain, fullness, nausea, vomiting, and acute constipation. Although bezoars develop in people of all ages, they are more often found in persons over age 60 (6). Chewing problems due to tooth loss and ill-fitting dentures and conditions that delay gastric emptying are predisposing factors. These masses are usually composed of pulp, seeds, husks, and skins of fruit and vegetables, often oranges, persimmons, potato skins, or even unshelled pumpkin seeds (7).

Liquid and low-fiber diets have been used to treat bezoars. Enzyme preparations are given to dissolve them. As these remedies are not always helpful, it is better to prevent bezoar formation. Precautions should be taken with persons at risk of developing them such as those with delayed gastric emptying or who have had gastric surgery. They should not eat large amounts of high-fiber foods. Others, taking medications like cholestyramine or aluminum hydroxide gels, should be instructed to drink plenty of liquids.

Pureeing fiberous fruits and vegetables may be necessary for persons who cannot chew normally so that they do not swallow large amounts of unchewed cellulose (6).

Malabsorption

Weight loss, diarrhea, and reduced blood levels of albumin, cholesterol, calcium, iron, vitamin B_{12}, and folic acid are often signs of malabsorption but may be due to other problems. Weight loss may be caused by depression, carcinoma, heart failure, pulmonary disease, or diabetes, while diarrhea may be due to functional bowel syndrome, infection, or carcinoma. Steatorrhea with bulky, light-colored, foul-smelling stools is a positive sign that there is a significant abnormality of digestion, absorption, or bile secretion (8).

Hydrochloric acid secretion by the stomach gradually diminishes with age. This reduction in acid reduces the absorption of iron and calcium and also can permit the proliferation of bacteria in the stomach as maintenance of a pH less than 4 is necessary for gastric secretions to have bactericidal effects.

Pancreatic insufficiency, caused by chronic pancreatitis, cancer, or resection of the pancreas, requires oral replacement of enzymes. Most commonly, an enzyme supplement such as Viokase is usually given before each meal, along with an antacid (so that the enzymes are not destroyed by gastric acid). Using such a preparation will allow nearly normal absorption of all nutrients.

Biliary obstruction due to stones, strictures, or tumors will reduce the absorption of calcium and vitamin A, D, E, and K. This interference with vitamin K is of particular importance for patients who are on anticoagulant therapy. Medium-chain triglycerides (MCT), composed of fatty acids with 6 to 10 carbons, are frequently administered to patients with biliary obstruction or any of a number of other malabsorption problems. About one-third of the MCT oil can be absorbed without the presence of bile salts. Supplements of fat-soluble vitamins A, D, E, and K may also be needed.

Persons with gluten-sensitive enteropathy (celiac sprue) frequently have folic-acid- or vitamin-B_{12}-deficiency anemia as well as hypocalcemia. Their intestinal epithelial cells can be damaged by as little as 3 g of gliadin (a component of gluten) daily. A carefully followed gluten-restricted diet is needed. Gluten is found mainly in wheat and rye and in lesser amounts in oats and barley. Rice, corn, and soy are allowed.

Bacterial overgrowth in portions of the small intestine is caused mainly by stasis—the slowing or stopping of the movement of intestinal contents down the gastrointestinal tract. This is particularly common after certain surgical procedures in which the intestine is diverted and new conduits and blind loops are formed. This bacterial overgrowth causes bile salt deconjugation and mucosal cell damage interfering with the absorption of fat, iron, vitamin B_{12}, vitamin D, and niacin. Antibiotics are useful to combat the overgrowth, and nutrient supplements are used to overcome deficiencies (9).

Acute bacterial or viral infection can cause transient but severe malabsorption as does parasitic infestation such as amebiasis and giardiasis. Giardiasis is not uncommon in older adults. Immunodeficiency syndromes and achlorhydria may be reasons for the increased incidence in elderly compared with younger adults (10). The *Giardia* organisms, found in travelers and in institutionalized persons, interfere with absorption and cause mild diarrhea. For more information on infectious disease, see Chapter 14.

Disaccharidase deficiency, the most common of which is lactase deficiency, is another cause of malabsorption. Only small amounts of lactose, milk sugar, can be tolerated without the symptoms of pain, gas, and diarrhea. As an alternative to milk, yogurt may be tolerated well (11). See the section on lactose intolerance.

Surgical alterations of the gastrointestinal tract will affect digestion and absorption. A total gastrectomy results in poor digestion of fat and protein as the digestive juices of the stomach are no longer secreted into the gastrointestinal tract. The lack of intrinsic factor needed for the absorption of vitamin B_{12} necessitates parenteral administration of the vitamin. Iron and calcium are not well absorbed after gastrectomy, so that supplements may be needed.

The dumping syndrome, with its symptoms of flushing, sweating, and lightheadedness, results from rapid entry of the gastric contents into the jejunum of the small intestine. This may occur after certain surgical procedures for duodenal ulcer. Dietary treatment of this problem is given in Table 6–1.

Alcohol and drug use contribute to digestive problems and malabsorption. Alcohol alters mucosa, fluid and electrolyte transport, and vitamin and mineral absorption. Excessive use of cathartics and mineral oil can result in more rapid transit through the intestine and impaired absorption of fat and fat-soluble vitamins. Neomycin binds fatty and bile acids and injures intestinal mucosa causing loss of electrolytes and fats. Colchicine may cause fat malabsorption and diarrhea and also decreases absorption of bile acids, carotene, and vitamin B_{12}. Cholestyramine binds bile salts and fat-soluble vitamins. Phenytoin lessens absorption of folic acid and vitamin B_{12}. Paraaminosalicylic acid causes diarrhea. See Chapter 17, on drugs, for further discussion of some of these areas.

Table 6–1   Dietary Treatment for Dumping Syndrome

Small, frequent meals: 5 or 6 daily
Relatively low carbohydrate content with little simple sugars
Relatively high in fat and high in protein content
No milk, alcohol, or regular sweetened soft drinks
Liquids 30 to 60 minutes after meals
Relatively low fiber
Avoid very hot or very cold food
Rest after eating

Obstruction of the intestinal lymphatics due to fibrosis, tumor, lymphoma, or even severe congestive heart failure causes regurgitation of lipid and protein back into the lumen of the gut. This results in impaired fat absorption and may even cause a net loss of protein, referred to as protein-losing enteropathy. If the lymphatic obstruction cannot be relieved, strict fat restriction should be imposed in order to minimize lymph flow and consequent protein loss (8).

Esophagitis (Gastroesophageal Reflux)

The lower esophageal sphincter is believed to become weakened with aging, allowing reflux of gastric acid into the esophagus, which, in turn, causes esophagitis. Persons with this problem have low sphincter pressures. Recent studies suggest that it is the episodes of reflux that lead to the lowered pressure of the esophageal sphincter. Thus, a cyclic process is set up that allows perpetuation of reflux esophagitis once it has begun (12).

Esophagitis is commonly referred to as heartburn. It is usually worse at night and when reclining after a big meal. The acid, pepsin, and bile that reflux up from the stomach may irritate the esophagus, and chronic esophagitis may lead to permanent damage to the esophagus.

Obesity, especially extra fat on the abdomen, increases the chance of food refluxing back into the esophagus. A large meal also predisposes to reflux, so it is best for the obese client with reflux to eat smaller amounts more often. Three small meals with a midmorning and midafternoon snack are suggested. No food should be eaten later than 2 hours before bedtime, since a reclining position further increases the chance of reflux.

Fats, chocolate, alcohol, peppermint, and spearmint should be avoided as they impair lower esophagael sphincter function. Cigarette smoking does too. Tomato products and citrus juices are known to aggravate heartburn apparently because, although they do not affect sphincter function, they have a direct (pH-independent) irritant effect on the inflamed esophageal mucosa (13). One study has shown that coffee actually reduces gastric acid secretion in susceptible persons who have heartburn after drinking coffee. In these persons, the pressure of the lower esphogeal sphincter is also reduced. This supports the idea that heartburn is often due to an abnormality in sphincter function (14). Substituting decaffeinated coffee for regular coffee does not help as the acid secretion responses are higher for the decaffeinated than other coffee (15).

Antacids are used to treat heartburn both for their acid-neutralizing effect and also because they increase lower-esophogeal-sphincter pressure and thus decrease reflux. However, there have been no controlled clinical trials to support their use (12). Moreover, excessive use of antacids may be harmful because aluminum-containing antacids cause constipation and can block the absorption of phosphates by bone so that prolonged or excessive use can cause osteomalacia (16). Magnesium-containing antacids can cause diarrhea and also are not appropriate for use by persons with renal disease. Calcium-containing antacids cause rebound hyperacidity and also hypercalcemia (17). Many commonly used antacids contain considerable amounts of sodium (see Table 6–2). Antacid therapy is planned such that something is in the stomach at all times to neutralize acid. Older adults are frequently advised to take antacid or eat food every 2 hours when awake and to take an additional dose of antacid at bedtime. This number of doses may result in a high sodium intake that might be ill-advised for many persons with heart or kidney disease.

Table 6–2   Sodium Content of Antacids

Antacid	Size	Milligrams of sodium
Alka-Seltzer	1 tablet	276.0
Amphojel	0.3-g tablet	1.4
	5 ml	6.9
Gavison	1 tablet	18.4
	5 ml	26.8
Maalox	1 #1 tablet	0.84
	1 #2 tablet	1.80
	5 ml	2.5
Maalox Plus	1 tablet	1.4
Milk of magnesia	100 ml	10.0
Mylanta	1 tablet	5.0
	5 ml	5.0
Riopan	1 tablet	3.0
	5 ml	3.0
Riopan Plus	1 tablet	3.0
	5 ml	3.0
Rolaids	1 tablet	53.0
Sal Hepatica	1 dose	1000.0
Sodium bicarbonate	1 dose	89.0
Tums	1 tablet	3.0

Bicarbonate of soda is often used as an antacid by older adults. Because it is frequently found on the pantry shelf it is considered safe, but it may not always be. A recent report described an adult whose stomach ruptured spontaneously shortly after he took ½ teaspoon of bicarbonate of soda in a glass of water (18).

Body position is another factor in treatment of heartburn. The recommendation is to elevate head and shoulders 30 degrees when in bed. This can be accomplished by placing blocks under the legs at the head of the bed. Extra pillows actually make reflux worse by increasing intraabdominal pressure. Tight clothing, belts, and girdles should not be worn.

Hiatus Hernia

Hiatus hernia is a common problem in which the stomach protrudes upward into the chest through the esophageal opening of the diaphragm. The incidence increases with aging and is found in 40–60% of those who are middle aged and 90% of those over 70. It affects more women than men. Causes include obesity, pregnancy, severe coughing, straining at stool, vomiting, wearing clothes that are tight around the waist, and even weight lifting. In short, hiatus hernia can be caused by any condition that causes increased intraabdominal pressure. Many people have this condition and are unaware of it. In others, bleeding and ulceration of the esophagus occur. Treatment is similar to that for esophageal reflux.

Another unusual source of abdominal pain has been reported. Bay leaves used as flavoring may become lodged in the gastrointestinal tract, causing pain. Because these leaves are not broken down in the gut, they should be removed from food before it is served (19,20).

Patient aid:

Person to Person About Acid Reflux and Hiatal Hernia

available from:

American Digestive Disease Society
7720 Wisconsin Avenue
Bethesda, Maryland 20814

Diverticulosis

Diverticulosis refers to a condition in which small distended sacs form in the colon. These sacs are found in 40% of those over age 70 (21). They usually cause no symptoms but may become inflamed or infected. This condition, called diverticulitis, can cause nausea, vomiting, fever, gas, and pain. It is treated by bed rest, liquid diet, antibiotics, antispasmodics, and sedatives. After the inflammation is controlled, moderate amounts of fiber are added to the diet (22).

Consumption of a low-fiber diet of largely refined and processed foods is believed to predispose to the formation of diverticula. High-fiber diets have been proposed as a possible preventive measure and as useful after the inflammation is controlled to help prevent recurrence. Ample fiber will prevent constipation and help to move the stool through the bowel quickly. This puts less strain on the intestinal wall and reduces the chance of residue being caught in the diverticula.

Lactose Intolerance

Lactose is the principal sugar in milk. The intestinal enzyme lactase is needed to break it down into simple sugars that can be absorbed. The normal state of human beings, except those from Northern and Western Europe, is to become lactase deficient by the first or second decade of life. This deficiency is not influenced by dietary lactose (23). When there is not enough lactase to hydrolyze the lactose in the milk and milk products eaten, the unabsorbed sugar remains in the lumen of the intestine and acts osmotically to retain water. This effect and the subsequent fermentation of lactose by intestinal bacteria cause cramping, diarrhea, bloating, and gas. There may be a loss of other nutrients owing to these gastrointestinal disturbances.

The range of tolerance for lactose is wide. Studies show that the number of persons who can tolerate the lactose in one glass of milk (12 g) ranges from 0 to 75%. It is believed that most people who are intolerant of milk learn to recognize the amount they are able to drink without developing symptoms.

Recent studies show that lactose in yogurt can be digested by persons who are deficient in lactase. It appears that lactase is released from the microorganisms in the yogurt (24). This is true only of yogurt that is not pasteurized after culture. Not all fermented dairy products have this feature as buttermilk, pasteurized yogurt, and sweet acidophilus milk are not tolerated well by persons who are lactase deficient (25).

Small amounts of milk, up to one cup, may be well tolerated by some, especially when taken with meals. Others may wish to try Lact-Aid, a preparation containing an enzyme from yeast (*Saccharomyces lactis lactase*) that can digest the lactose in milk. It is available in drugstores. A few drops are added to milk the night before it is to be used. By the next morning, there is little lactose left in the milk. In some areas of the country, Lact-Aid fluid milk is available in supermarkets as is Lact-Aid-treated cottage cheese. Other such treated products including American cheese and ice cream will soon be available. Regular hard cheese is well tolerated by most people with lactose intolerance as it contains little if any milk sugar. Most lactase-deficient persons can tolerate small amounts of lactose without symptoms, but those who cannot should be cautioned to avoid any products, food, or drugs listing whey or lactose or dry milk powder among their ingredients.

Lactose is a basic ingredient in many varieties of tube feedings. Common side effects of these feedings are abdominal distention, cramping, and diarrhea. It has been shown that even individuals with normal lactose tests may exhibit these symptoms when large amounts of lactose are ingested. Caseinate and soy isolate base formulas such as Sustacal, Portagen powder, or Ensure can be used (26).

Recently there have been reports suggesting a connection between senile cataracts and high lactose consumers who also have high lactase activity as adults. The glactose that is produced when lactose is digested has been found to induce cataracts in animals when fed at high levels. A study of adults in Italy suggests that those who are able to absorb galactose from a lactose-rich diet may be especially susceptible to developing senile or presenile cataracts (27).

The clinician should be aware that diarrhea does not necessarily indicate lactose intolerance. A dietary cause of diarrhea can be excessive coffee consumption, that is, over 10 cups a day. Fructose, which is sometimes considered a more healthful form of sugar, and sorbitol, often used in diabetic products, can cause diarrhea too. Sorbitol, used in sugarless gum, candy, and mints and as vehicle for certain drugs, can cause diarrhea when over 50 g a day is consumed. One piece of sugarless gum contains from 1.2 to 4.4 g sorbitol. Persons with chronic diarrhea should be questioned about their intake of milk, milk products, coffee, fructose, and sorbitol (28).

Intestinal Gas

A common complaint of many older adults is that they have too much gas. Symptoms of this may be repeated eructation (belching), bloating and abdominal pain, and excessive passing of flatus.

Occasional belching after eating or drinking is a normal result of the air swallowed in the act of eating or the air contained in the food. Whipped cream is an obvious example of air in food, but there are other less obvious examples. An apple is said to contain 20% air (29). Persons who belch very frequently are bringing up air they have swallowed as a nervous habit.

Abdominal pain and bloating that the patient believes to be due to too much gas may actually represent only a greater sensitivity to distention of the intestines (30). This has been termed spastic or irritable bowel.

Excessive passage of flatus is caused by excessive gas production in the intestines. Diet influences this production as some foods contain gas or provide a substrate for bacteria that, then ferment them, producing gas. Gas is produced from foods that are not absorbed completely and that remain in the intestine and are fermented by bacteria. These are mainly carbohydrate foods and small amounts of protein (see Table 6–3). Milk can be a problem for those who are deficient in lactase. Dried peas and beans and wheat flour may also cause gas. Relief from the gas can be obtained by eliminating milk sugar (lactose), wheat, and legumes, the main offenders (31). Because of the popularity of adding bran and other high-fiber foods to the diet, many people are noticing more gas than usual. Usually, gas from a change in the diet moderates in a few weeks.

The most effective way for the individual to eliminate intestinal gas is to selectively remove foods from the diet in order to determine which foods are most gassy for that person. The client should then avoid these

Table 6–3   Gas-Producing Foods

Main offenders	Minor offenders
Milk sugar (lactose)	Potatoes
Wheat	Eggplant
Legumes	Citrus fruits
Onions	Apples
Celery	Bread
Carrots	Pastries
Raisins	Bran
Bananas	
Apricots	
Prune juice	
Pretzels	
Bagels	
Wheat germ	
Brussels sprouts	

foods and substitute nutritionally equivalent choices. If no offensive foods are found, then the client should reduce the fat in meals, eliminate foods with a high gas content like soda and whipped cream, eat and drink more slowly, and chew with the mouth closed. In addition, one should not talk while chewing, and not chew gum or use a straw to drink liquids.

Ulcers

Peptic ulcers affect 10% of the elderly, the same percent as in younger adults. However, older adults have a greater proportion of peptic ulcers in the stomach, rather than in the duodenum as is the case in younger people. This is believed to be due to reduced production of protective gastric mucus in older individuals. More men than women have ulcers.

Diet therapy of ulcers includes frequent, small meals eaten slowly and calmly, and antacids given 1 hour after each meal and at bedtime. Foods can be eaten as tolerated with the exception of alcohol, coffee (both regular and decaffeinated), meat extracts like bouillon, gravy, and broth, cola drinks, and black pepper. Smoking and the use of aspirin should be avoided also.

Gone are the days of drinking heavy cream to soothe the ulcer, eating pureed fruits and vegetables, and avoiding "gassy" food. Each person reacts differently to food. What causes discomfort for one may not for another (32).

Gallbladder Disease

The incidence of gallstones increases with age, 10% for men and 20% for women aged 55–64, and by age 60–90, at least 60% of the women and 30–50% of men have them (33). As many as 90% of gallstones are composed mainly of cholesterol. These are commonly associated with obesity. Refined carbohydrates are considered a major contributing factor owing to their lack of fiber and tendency to cause overweight. It is recommended that susceptible individuals avoid refined carbohydrate foods and replace them with whole-grain products, fruits, and vegetables to reduce the risk of cholesterol gallstone formation (34).

The most frequent disorder caused by gallstones is acute cholecystitis, which may occur when the stones become impacted in the cystic duct. Pain results from the gallbladder contracting against this obstruction. Inflammation of the gallbladder and surrounding tissue occurs.

The traditional dietary treatment of cholecystitis is a low-fat diet to decrease secretion of the hormone cholecystokinin, which causes contractions of the gallbladder. This may not stop the pain as dietary protein also stimulates the release of cholescystakinin (35).

Chenodeoxycholic acid has been used to dissolve gallstones and is effective in select cases but can cause liver abnormalities and increased low-density-lipoprotein (LDL) cholesterol. Other treatments are being tested.

Constipation

Constipation is a common problem among older adults, the major consumers of laxatives. Frequent complaints are that defecation is less frequent, the amount of stool passed is less, and bowel movements are either painful or difficult to initiate.

There is no evidence that aging causes constipation. Persons over 60 have as many bowel movements as do younger adults, ranging from three a day to one every three days for 98% of all adults. About 70% have a daily movement (36).

Many older adults were taught that a daily bowel movement was necessary to prevent accumulation of "poisons" in the body. Although that is no longer accepted, preliminary studies link chronic constipation to both breast dysplasia and lower-bowel carcinoma (36). Chronic retention can lead to fecal incontinence. Because of the variability in frequency of defecation, the term "constipation" should be reserved for prolonged retention of feces with infrequent and difficult passage of dry, hard stools.

Constipation can be caused by a variety of factors including inadequate food, fiber, and fluid intake, immobility, decreased intestinal muscle tone, ignoring of the normal urge to defecate, laxative abuse, medical problems such as tumors or spasms, and some medications (see Table 6–4).

Laxative use is widespread in older adults but may cause problems. Magnesium salts can be dangerous if kidney function is not normal as excessive amounts of magnesium may be absorbed and retained. Overuse of castor oil can cause dehydration and loss of electrolytes. Mineral oil interferes with the absorption of vitamins A, D, E, and K. Chronic use of laxatives fosters dependency on them.

Increased fiber intake can help constipation. Fiber absorbs many times its weight in water, softening the stool and also increasing the propulsive action of the colon, leading to decreased transit time. Many older adults eat a lot of highly processed foods that contain little fiber.

Table 6–4 Drugs That Can Cause Constipation

Aluminum-containing antacids, e.g., Maalox
Bismuth, e.g., Pepto-Bismol
Calcium
Iron
Codeine
Diphenoxylate
Dicodid (Hydrocodone)
Ephedrine, e.g., Tedral
Isoproterenol (Isuprel)
Phenylephine, e.g., Neosynephrine, Dimetapp
Phenylpropanolamine, e.g., Dimetapp, Ornade, Sine-Aid, Dexatrim
Pseudoephedrine, e.g., Actifed
Terbutaline, e.g., Brethine
Disopyramide (Norpace)
Nifedipine (Procardia)
Verapamil (Calon, Isoptin)
Amitriptyline, e.g., Elavil
Doxepin (Adapin, Sinequan)
Imipramine, e.g., Tofranil
Diuretics, e.g., Lasix
Antihistamines, e.g., Benadryl, Chlortrimeton

Adapted from Sparberg, M., Practical pointers for treating constipation, *Drug Ther.* p. 68, May 1984.

Thirty-five to forty grams of dietary fiber daily is recommended to maintain normal bowel movements. Minimally processed cereals are the richest source of fiber, followed by dried peas and beans, then root vegetables, and finally fruits and leafy vegetables containing the least amount of fiber because they are over 90% water (see Table 3–1, p. 48). Bran is about 44% fiber and is a helpful supplement to the diet when used in moderate amounts—that is, no more than 3 tablespoons a day along with generous fluid intake. It can be sprinkled on or cooked in cereals, added to casseroles and hamburgers, and used as breading. Moderation is important as bran itself can cause an impaction. In addition, too much fiber can interfere with the absorption of calcium, magnesium, iron, zinc, and other minerals and also increase the amount of intestinal gas produced.

Adding two bran biscuits (Fibermed*), containing 7.5 g bran each, daily to the diets of elderly subjects with an average age of 80 proved useful. There was increased stool weight, a reduction in the number of stool-free days, and fewer laxatives prescribed (37).

*Purdue Fredrick, Co., Norwalk, Connecticut 06856.

The first step in restoring normal bowel function in severe constipation is to eliminate all laxatives. Initially, enemas may be used to induce bowel evacuation until responsiveness of the rectum is reestablished. Then, a regular time each day for a bowel movement should be set, allowing 5–10 minutes for this, usually after breakfast or dinner. A hearty breakfast, which includes foods high in fiber like whole-grain bread or cereal plus a hot drink, should be served.

Six or more glasses of liquid daily will help keep the feces from becoming hard and dry. A glass of prune juice, which has laxative effects, may make up part of this intake. Some older adults drink a glass of warm water and lemon juice upon arising each day and find this helpful. Exercise is important for regular bowel movements. Walking and/or an appropriate exercise program should be part of an older adult's daily routine.

LIVER DISEASE

The liver has many vital functions. It serves to synthesize many necessary proteins, inactivate toxins, and store nutrients. When the liver is diseased, these functions are no longer maintained. As liver failure reaches the end stages, and the liver's functional reserve is exhausted, the patient may develop ascites, endocrine disturbances, renal failure, bleeding, and hepatic encephalopathy. Excessive alcohol consumption, viral hepatitis, and other liver diseases can progress to cirrhosis and liver failure.

Appropriate nutrition is extremely important in the management of the patient with cirrhosis (38). Modest restriction of sodium and water is important, as these individuals are prone to develop salt and fluid overload. Reduction of dietary protein is also important, particularly for the patient with hepatic encephalopathy.

Restricting the daily protein intake to 30–40 g can greatly improve the mental status of the patient with hepatic encephalopathy. Of course, in patients with hepatic coma, all dietary protein must be withheld. With improvement in mental state, the protein intake can be increased by 10–20 g/day every 3–5 days, watching closely for any deterioration in mental state.

In addition to decreasing the quantity of ingested protein, it is important to modify the type of ingested protein. There is some evidence that vegetable protein is tolerated better than animal protein (38). This may be due to the differences in the content of nitrogen and aromatic compounds (tyrosine, phenylalanine, tryptophan) in animal versus vegetable proteins.

Finally, endogenous protein degradation must be prevented. This can be accomplished by ensuring that the patient obtains at least 1600 calories/day in the form of glucose. In addition, adequate vitamin intake, especially folic acid and vitamin K, is important in patients with liver disease.

REFERENCES

1. Morgan, W., et al., Gastrointestinal system, in: *Nursing and the Aged.* Irene Mortenson Burnside, ed. New York: McGraw Hill, 1981.
2. Bayless, T.M., Malabsorption in the elderly, *Hosp. Pract.* 14(8):57, 1979.
3. Niessen, L.C., Jones, J.A., Oral health changes in the elderly, *Oral Health* 75(5):231, 1984.
4. Craig, A., *Oral Health for Long-Term Care Patients.* Chicago: American Society for Geriatric Dentistry.
5. U.S. National Center for Health Statistics, Edentulous Persons in the U.S. *Vital Health Statistics* 10:89, 1974.
6. Goldstein, S.S., Lewis, J.H., Bezoars: Clinical recognition and management in the geriatric patient, *Geriatr. Med. Today* 3(11):58, 1984.
7. Chandrasekhara, K.L., Pumpkin seed impaction (letter), *Ann. Intern. Med.* 98(5):675, 1983.
8. Gebhard, R.L., Malabsorption—A cause of geriatric nutritional failure, *Geriatrics* 38(1):97, 1983.
9. Heyman, M.B., Nutritional management of intestinal bacterial overgrowth, *Nutr. Support Serv.* 4(4):61, 1984.
10. Maasdam, C.F., Anuras, S., Are you overlooking G.I. infections in your elderly patients? *Geriatrics* 36(2):127, 1981.
11. Savaiano, D.A., et al., Lactose malabsorption from yogurt, pasteurized yogurt, sweet acidophilus milk and cultured milk in lactose-deficient individuals, *Am. J. Clin. Nutr.* 40(6):1219, 1984.
12. Richter, J.E., Castell, D.O., Gastroesophageal reflux, *Ann. Intern. Med.* 97:93, 1982.
13. Price, S.F., et al., Food sensitivity in reflux esophagitis, *Gastroenterology* 75:240, 1978.
14. Cohen, S., Pathogenesis of coffee-induced gastrointestinal symptoms, *N. Engl. J. Med.* 303(3):122, 1980.
15. Cohen, S., Booth G.H., Gastric acid secretion and lower esophageal sphincter pressure in response to coffee and caffeine, *N. Engl. J. Med.* 293:897, 1975.
16. Antacid osteomalacia, *Nutr. & M.D.* 7:5, 1981.
17. Port, J.H., et al., Antacid therapy for peptic ulcer disease. Questions and answers, *JAMA* 248:2045, 1982.

18. Mastrangelo, M.R., Moore, E.W., Spontaneous rupture of the stomach in a healthy adult man after sodium bicarbonate ingestion, *Ann. Intern. Med.* 101:649, 1984.

19. Brokaw, S.A., Wonnell, D.M., Complications of bay leaf ingestion (letter), *JAMA* 250(6):729, 1983.

20. Palin, W.E., Richardson, J.D., Complications from bay leaf ingestion, *JAMA* 249(6):729, 1983.

21. Berman, P.M., The aging gut. II. Diseases of the colon, pancreas, liver and gallbladder, functional bowel disease and iatrogenic disease, *Geriatrics* 27(4):117, 1972.

22. Plumley, P.F., Francis, B., Dietary management of diverticular disease, *J. Am. Diet. Assoc.* 63:527, 1973.

23. Newcomer, A.D., McGill, D.B., Clinical importance of lactose deficiency, *N. Engl. J. Med.* 310(1):42, 1984.

24. Kolars, J.C., et al., Yogurt—An autodigesting source of lactose, *N. Engl. J. Med.* 310(1):1, 1984.

25. Savaiano, D.A., Nutrition and therapeutic aspects of fermented dairy products, *Contemp. Nutr.* 9(6):1, 1984.

26. Ross, G., Geriatric enteral hyperalimentation. Part I, *Nutr. Support Serv.* 1(6):29, 1981.

27. Rinaldi, E., et al., High frequency of lactose absorbers among adults with idiopathic senile and presenile cataracts in a population with a high prevalence of primary adult lactose malabsorption, *Lancet* 1:355, 1984.

28. Babb, R.R., Coffee, sugars, and chronic diarrhea, *Postgrad. Med.* 75(8):82, 1984.

29. Levitt, M.D., Gastrointestinal gas and abdominal symptoms. Part 1, *Practical Gastroenterol.* 7(6):6, 1983.

30. Levitt, M.D., Gastrointestinal gas and abdominal symptoms. Part 2, *Practical Gastroenterol.* 8(1):6, 1983.

31. Levitt, M.D., Foods that produce gas, *Nutr. & M.D.* 8(4):1, 1982.

32. American Dietetic Association: Position paper on bland diet in the treatment of chronic duodenal ulcer disease, *J. Am. Diet. Assoc.* 59:244, 1971.

33. Friedman, G.D., et al., The epidemiology of gallbladder disease. Observations in the Framingham study, *J. Chronic Dis.* 19:273, 1966.

34. Thornton, J.R., et al., Diet and gallstones. Effects of refined and unrefined carbohydrate diets on bile cholesterol saturation and bile acid metabolism, *Gut* 24(1):2, 1983.

35. Hanson, R.F., Gallstones—The case for medical management, *Geriatrics* 37(7):72, 1982.

36. The ins and outs of constipation, *Transition* 1(8):20, 1983.

37. Pringle, R., et al., Bran and bowel function in the elderly, *Age and Aging* 13(3):175, 1984.

38. Hoyumpa, A.M., et al., Hepatic encephalopathy, *Gastroenterology* 76:184, 1979.

Chapter 7

RENAL DISEASE

The kidneys perform three major functions in the body: excretion of excess fluid and wastes, regulation of the body's internal chemistry, and production of two hormones: erythropoietin (an important regulator of blood production) and the most active metabolite of vitamin D (1).

Most people have three or four meals each day, and so the body receives several large doses of water, protein, minerals, and toxins. These would disrupt the body's chemistry if the kidneys were not doing their job properly. The normal kidneys can sense changes in blood chemistry on a minute-to-minute basis and can excrete or conserve large amounts of water, sodium, potassium, ammonia, urea, phosphorus, calcium, and other substances. In addition, the kidneys can sense the amount of blood that is circulating and can produce more or less erythropoietin, depending on the body's need for blood. Also, depending on the body's need for calcium, the kidneys can produce more dihydroxyvitamin D, which is the most potent form of this vitamin.

AGING AND THE KIDNEY

After age 40, virtually all people have a slow, progressive decline in all aspects of renal function (2). By age 80, it has been shown that renal blood flow decreases by 55% (3). Consequently, the kidneys are slower to respond to changes in blood chemistry, and they can adequately compensate only for changes in blood chemistry over a narrower range. An elderly person's kidney has a decreased ability to concentrate urine—a water-conserving measure; therefore, the *minimum* amount of fluid that an elderly person must take in daily is higher than that of a younger person whose kidney function is better. Similarly, the ability of an elderly person's kidney to excrete excess water (as dilute urine) is decreased, so the *maximum* amount of fluid that an elderly person may drink in a day is less than that of a younger person. The same situations hold for essentially all the other functions of the kidney. Most elderly persons without renal disease continue to have normal body chemistry, even though they are more prone to disturbances if they take in relatively large or relatively small quantities of food or liquid.

The exact cause of the progressive decline in renal function seen with aging is not known, but it has been recently proposed that at least one important factor may be excessive dietary protein intake (4). There is a great deal of experimental data in animals to support this idea. It has also been proposed that dietary protein has an important role in initiating and causing progression of many types of chronic renal disease (5).

CHRONIC RENAL DISEASE

Chronic renal disease is the irreversible loss of normal kidney function from any of a number of different causes: diabetes, hypertension, kidney stones, exposure to toxins, drug reactions, and perhaps recurrent kidney infections. Regardless of the original cause, chronic renal disease always progresses with slow, continued, predictable loss of kidney function. In the early stages, nutritional intervention is important because this may slow or even prevent progression to later stages (6). In the later stages, nutritional intervention is essential for survival.

The signs and symptoms that occur with chronic renal disease depend on the stage of the disease. In the early stages, there may be occasional swelling (edema) of the legs and mild hypertension. As renal function worsens, edema may be seen more often and may even involve the face, especially the area around the eyes. There may be shortness of breath from fluid buildup in the lungs. In later stages, anorexia, altered taste sensation, and anemia (from decreased production or erythropoietin and gastrointestinal bleeding) may occur. There may also be cardiac arrhythmias from electrolyte imbalances, easy bruisability from abnormal blood clotting, joint pains from calcium deposits, and a wide range of neurological symptoms.

The two blood tests most commonly used to evaluate kidney function are the creatinine and BUN (blood–urea–nitrogen). As kidney disease progresses, both these levels increase. This is because these substances are normally excreted by the kidney, and as kidney function worsens, they are not excreted as efficiently and their levels increase (7).

Reduced Renal Reserve

In this, the earliest, stage of chronic renal disease, kidney function is decreased but is still greater than 50% of normal. The only detectable abnormalities may be occasional slight elevations of the BUN and creatinine. In this situation, most of the time, the client functions normally. However, the kidneys cannot retain or excrete large quantities of water or electrolytes. Therefore, it is important to make sure to counsel the client not to take in very large or very small amounts of salt and water or else fluid overload or dehydration may occur (7). (See Table 7–1.)

Mild to Moderate Renal Insufficiency and Renal Failure

In these stages, kidney function is between 20 and 50% of normal. With mild to moderate renal insufficiency, the BUN is elevated at all times, and there is mild anemia. The kidneys cannot make a normally concen-

Table 7–1   Key Points for Nutritional Intervention in Different Stages of Chronic Renal Disease

Reduced renal reserve
   Avoid extremes of fluid intake

Mild to moderate renal insufficiency
   Avoid dehydration
   Watch for iron deficiency anemia

Renal failure
   Avoid dehydration and fluid overload
   Avoid excess potassium intake
   Watch for iron deficiency anemia
   Use oral phosphorus binders to keep phosphorus level in normal range
   Use vitamin supplements as needed
   Give low protein intake

ESRD (end state renal disease)
   Maintain protein and calorie balance
   Maintain sodium and potassium levels
   Prevent fluid overload and dehydration
   Maintain normal phosphorus and calcium levels

trated urine, and so dehydration can be a problem. Nocturia occurs, because with decreased urine concentration, a greater amount of urine is formed.

With deterioration of kidney function to approximately one-third of normal, there is a loss of other regulatory processes in the kidney. The ability to produce a dilute or concentrated urine is also impaired, thereby predisposing to fluid overload or dehydration. Phosphorus and calcium balance become abnormal, and so calcium phosphate salts can be deposited under the skin, in blood vessels, and in joints. At a further reduction in renal function, potassium excretion is reduced, and potassium overload may occur (7).

In these stages of kidney disease, modification of the diet is important to prevent changes in blood chemistry. Diet intervention may also help to slow down or prevent further deterioration of the kidneys (8).

Fluid intake should be monitored and adjusted so that the client's weight is stable. For most people, daily fluid intake will be approximately 1.1–1.5 liters. The client should be weighed at least three times a week. Any weight change of 1 lb or more should be first considered as due to fluid, and the client's intake should be adjusted accordingly.

Serum potassium levels should be checked at least every 3–4 months, and foods that are rich in potassium should be eaten sparingly or avoided altogether. Foods rich in potassium include oranges, grapefruit, tomatoes, bananas, strawberries, raisins, grapes, nuts, and salt substitutes. If these foods are avoided, the client may need additional vitamin supplementation (9).

The anemia associated with renal failure is usually due to low production of erythropoietin by the kidney. However, persons with chronic renal disease are prone to gastrointestinal bleeding, and so blood studies to check for possible iron deficiency anemia should always be done. If iron deficiency is found, then iron supplements should be given. It is important to remember, however, that clients with renal disease may not absorb iron normally, and parenteral supplementation may be necessary (7).

In renal failure, phosphorus levels in the blood increase, and calcium levels decrease. This may lead to calcium deposits in the skin and other organs and also may led to weakening and destruction of the bones, because of calcium loss from them. As a first measure, to counteract elevated phosphorus levels, it is important for the client to take phosphorus binders at mealtime. The most commonly used binders are aluminum antacids such as Amphogel. If calcium levels remain low after phosphorus levels have been reduced, then calcium or vitamin D supplements may be given, but only very cautiously, and with close monitoring of serum calcium (10).

Recommendations about the optimum amount of dietary protein for a client with chronic renal failure are rapidly changing (11,12,13). Until recently, it was believed that once the creatinine rose to approximately 4 mg/dl, chronic renal failure then progressed irreversibly to end-stage renal disease, and dialysis would be required. Now, however, it has been shown that dietary intervention, particularly drastic reductions in protein intake, may slow down or block this progression (13).

Both excess and inadequate intake of protein may be a problem for the renal client at different times. Most clients find the restrictive renal diet unpalatable and do not follow it carefully. In addition, total food intake may be reduced because of anorexia due to renal disease. A good rule to determine the maximum protein intake for a client with renal failure is one that keeps the BUN no higher than approximately 10 times the creatinine. However, diets that provide less than 0.75 g/kg/day of protein may be inadequate to prevent the breakdown of muscle protein, regardless of the level of the BUN. With protein intakes below 1 g/kg/day, it is important to ensure that at least 35 kcal/kg of additional calories as carbohydrate and fat is provided to prevent tissue breakdown. If there is a large amount of protein in the urine, dietary protein intake must be supplemented (11).

Further research is necessary before more specific recommendations can be made about the optimum amount of protein in the diet that will slow the progression of chronic renal disease. However, if it can be tolerated by the client, a diet that is more restricted in protein should be encouraged over one that is more liberal.

End-Stage Renal Disease and Dialysis

When the kidney's function has declined to less than 20% of normal, the client has end-stage renal disease (ESRD), and progressive renal disease necessitating dialysis is unavoidable. A hemodialysis machine is used to take over the role of the kidneys. The client's blood travels through the dialysis machine, which removes excess fluid, electrolytes, and nitrogenous wastes. Treatments are usually done three times a week for 4 hr at a time. At present over 55,000 persons receive hemodialysis in the United States.

In ESRD, the client has little or no ability to excrete excess fluid, electrolytes, and wastes; therefore, diet modification is essential to prevent life-threatening fluid or electrolyte imbalances (1).

The objectives of the diet in ESRD are to maintain protein and calorie balance, maintain sodium and potassium levels, prevent fluid overload and dehydration, maintain calcium and phosphorus levels, and prevent destruction of the bones. Although the client has a machine to do the work of his kidneys, the dialysis diet is more restrictive than the previously mentioned diets because the clients needing dialysis have much worse kidney function than clients with earlier stages of chronic renal disease. However, dietary protein intake can be liberalized once dialysis is initiated (1).

Protein intake for clients on dialysis should be 1-1.5 g/kg/day. If the protein intake is higher than this, nausea, vomiting, weakness, and other neurological disturbances may appear. If too little protein is eaten, serum albumin levels will decrease, and there will be muscle wasting. (See Table 7–2.)

Carbohydrates and fats are metabolized to products that do not need kidney function for excretion. Therefore, they can be eaten more liberally than protein. It is generally recommended that 40–50 kcal/kg/day and certainly no less than 30–35 kcal/kg/day be eaten, with 50% of the daily calories coming from carbohydrates, 35% from fat, and the rest from protein.

The most immediate threat to life in a client with ESRD is electrolyte imbalance leading to cardiac arrhythmia. Since the client has basically no ability to excrete sodium or potassium between dialysis sessions, the dietary intake of these must be limited. Sodium and potassium intakes should be limited to 1.5–2 g each per day, though this limit can be relaxed somewhat during the meal just prior to dialysis (14).

Guidelines for fluid intake in ESRD must be based on the amount of urine that the client is able to produce. Usually, fluid intake can safely be 500 ml more than the volume of urine made. As mentioned previously, excess fluid intake will be easily detected by weighing the client (15).

Calcium and phosphorus balance must be closely monitored in ESRD. Phosphorus binders, such as Amphogel, should always be taken at mealtime. As mentioned previously, calcium and vitamin D supplements should be given very cautiously, while following serum calcium levels, and only after phosphorus levels have come down to normal. Otherwise, calcium phosphate salts can be deposited in the skin, blood vessels, and vital organs (10).

Recently, researchers have shown that vitamin B_6 (pyridoxine) supplements may be very helpful in decreasing the number of infections in dialysis patients (16).

Based on the above, a typical dialysis diet might be: 2500 kcal, 65 g protein, 2 g sodium, 1.5 g potassium, 1500 ml fluid. Often fat modification is called for, substituting polyunsaturated fatty acids (PUFA) for saturated fat because of the greater potential for atherosclerosis. This is obviously a very restricted diet, especially when the potassium-rich foods and most dairy products (which are rich in sodium, potassium,

Table 7–2   Sources of Low-Protein Foods

One of the special concerns of those caring for patients with severe kidney disease is planning and preparing meals that meet the protein restrictions often prescribed for such patients. This can be less of a problem with the use of low-protein food products that are available from several companies. Some of these include:

Anglo-Dietetics Ltd.
P.O. Box 333
Wilton, CT 06897
203/762-2504

Henkel Corporation
4620 West 77th Street
Minneapolis, MN 55435
612/828-8000

Dietary Specialties
P.O. Box 227
Rochester, NY 14601
716/263-2787

Kingsmill Foods Co., Ltd.
1399 Kennedy Road, Unit 17
Scarborough, Ontario M1P 2L6
416/755-1124

Ener-G Foods, Inc.
P.O. Box 24723
Seattle, WA 98124
206/767-6660

Source: *Nutrition & M.D.* 10(9):5, Sept. 1984.

and phosphorus) are eliminated. Phosphorus binders and vitamin supplements must also be taken in addition to any other medications that the client may need. The 12 or more hours each week spent attached to the dialysis machine is a tremendous disruption to the client with ESRD. However, unless a renal transplant becomes available, all of this is necessary for the client to stay alive.

Peritoneal Dialysis

In some situations, persons with ESRD may not be able to have hemodialysis, but instead have a different type of dialysis procedure. This involves inserting a catheter into the abdominal cavity and running solutions in and out, so that excess wastes, fluid, and electrolytes are carried away. This procedure causes more protein and electrolyte loss than hemodialysis, so clients having peritoneal dialysis need a different diet. For peritoneal dialysis, the protein intake must be 1–1.5 g/kg/day, or higher. Sodium intake can be 2–3 g/day; potassium intake, 3–3.5 g/day. At least 2 g of calcium must also be given daily (17).

KIDNEY STONES

It has been estimated that 12–14% of males and 5% of females will have at least one episode of symptomatic renal stones by age 70 (18).

Once formed, there is a tendency for kidney stones to recur. In healthy persons, diet may have little or no role in the formation of stones. In susceptible persons, however, diet can play a role in their formation and treatment.

Calcium-containing stones are the most common type. Most often, persons who form calcium stones have high concentrations of calcium in their urine. It is assumed that this high concentration is related to the process of stone formation, though this has not been proven. Decreasing the amount of dietary calcium in a stone former *does not* decrease the incidence of stone formation. This is because, in part, when calcium intake is decreased, there is more absorption of oxalate from the intestine, and thus there is formation of calcium oxalate stones. Calcium and oxalate are absorbed from the intestine by the same process, so if there is an increase in calcium in the intestine, then less oxalate can be absorbed. If less calcium is in the intestine, then more oxalate is absorbed.

It is important for a calcium-stone-former to drink large quantities of water, approximately 3–4 qt daily. This will decrease the concentra-

Table 7–3 Foods with High Oxalate Content

Vegetables	*Fruits*
Beet	Cranberry juice
Carrot	Currants
Celery	Figs
Chives	Gooseberries
Green beans	Grapefruit
Okra	Grape juice
Parsley	Orange
Sweet potato	Plum
Tomato	Prune
Greens:	Raspberries
Beet	Rhubarb
Collard	Tangerine
Dandelion	
Kale	*Miscellaneous*
Mustard	Beer
Spinach	Chocolate
Turnip	Cola drinks
Sorrel	Gelatin
	Marmalade
	Nuts
	Ovaltine
	Peanut butter
	Tea
	Wheat germ

tion of calcium in the urine and may help prevent the formation of stones. This quantity of fluid intake is safe for the older person so long as congestive heart failure is not a problem.

It has recently been suggested that a decrease in dietary protein may also be useful to decrease the incidence of calcium-containing kidney stones (19). This is because it has been conclusively shown that decreasing the amount of protein in the diet will decrease the concentration of calcium in the urine. Exactly how this happens is unknown, but this effect has been shown in persons with and without kidney stones. Until now, however, no one has shown that decreasing dietary protein will decrease the frequency of kidney stone formation.

The concentration of oxalate in the urine is more important than the concentration of calcium for the formation of calcium oxalate stones. Many people with calcium oxalate kidney stones absorb more oxalate than normal from the intestine. This may be due to malabsorption of fat. Fat that remains in the intestine is able to bind to calcium, so oxalate is free to be absorbed. In this situation, placing the client on a low-fat diet may decrease the amount of oxalate that is absorbed and may then decrease the frequency of stone formation. Also, giving calcium supplements (up to 2 g/day) to a calcium oxalate stone former will provide more calcium to the intestine, which will then lead to decreased absorption of oxalate from the intestine, and may decrease the incidence of stone formation. Drinking large amounts of water will decrease the incidence of stones. Finally, decreasing the amount of oxalates in the diet may have a role in preventing oxalate stones (20). (See Table 7–3.)

Patient aid:

The Low Oxalate Diet Book: For the Prevention of Oxalate Kidney Stones

available from:

General Clinical Research Center
The University of California
San Diego Medical Center
University Hospital
225 Dickenson Street
San Diego, California 92103

REFERENCES

1. Luke, B., Nutrition in renal disease: The adult on dialysis, *Am. J. Nurs.* 79:2155, 1979.

2. Lindeman, R.D., Changes in kidney function with age, *Geriatr. Med. Today* 13(5):41, 1984.

3. Parsons, V., What decreasing renal function means to geriatric patients, *J. Geriatr.* 32:93, 1977.

4. Breener, B.M., Meyer, T.W., Hotstetter, T.H., Dietary protein intake and the progressive nature of kidney disease: The role of hemodynamically mediated glomerular injury in the pathogenesis of progressive glomerular sclerosis in aging, renal ablation, and intrinsic renal disease, *N. Engl. J. Med.* 307:652, 1982.

5. Jamison, R.L., Dietary protein, glomerular hyperemia and progressive renal failure, *Ann. Intern. Med.* 99:849, 1983.

6. Low protein diet can slow renal function deterioration, *Intern. Med. News* 17(10):40, 1984.

7. Oestrich, S.K., Rational nursing care in chronic renal disease, *Am. J. Nurs.* 79:1096, 1979.

8. Steffee, W.P., Anderson, C.F., Enteral nutrition and renal disease, in: J.L. Rombeau, M.D. Caldwell, eds., *Enteral and Tube Feeding*. Philadelphia: W.B. Saunders Co., 1984.

9. Holliday, M.A., Nutritional aspects of renal disease in children and adults, *Hosp. Pract.*, p. 179, March 1983.

10. Goolkasian, D., Nutritional implications of drugs used in end-stage renal disease *R.D.* 4(2):3, 1984.

11. Burton, B.T., Hirshman, G.H., Current concepts of nutritional therapy in chronic renal failure, *J. Am. Diet. Assoc.* 82:359, 1983.

12. Maroni, B.J., Steinman, T.I., Mitch, W.E., Nutritional therapy of chronic renal failure, *Drug Ther.* 9(9):43, 1984.

13. Mitch W.E., et al., The effect of a ketoacid-amino acid supplement to a restricted diet on the progression of chronic renal failure, *N. Engl. J. Med.* 311:623, 1984.

14. Matthews, L., Care of the dialysis patient in the long term care setting, *J. Nutr. Elderly* 14:41, 1984.

15. Chambers, J.K., Assessing the dialysis patient at home, *Am. J. Nurs.* 81:750, 1981.

16. Casciato, D.A., et al., Immunologic abnormalities in hemodialysis patients: Improvement after pyridoxine therapy, *Nephron* 38:9, 1984.

17. Blumenkrantz, M.J., et al., Nutritional management of the adult patient undergoing peritoneal dialysis, *J. Am. Diet. Assoc.* 73:251, 1978.

18. Diet and urolithiasis, *Dairy Council Dig.* 54(5), 1983.

19. Urinary calcium and dietary protein, *Nutr. Rev.* 38:9, 1980.

20. Wilson, D.M., Medical treatment of urolithiasis, *Geriatrics* 34:65, Aug. 1979.

Chapter 8

DIABETES MELLITUS

Diabetes mellitus is a heterogenous disease in which there is an abnormally high plasma glucose concentration. The two major classifications of diabetes are Type I, insulin-dependent diabetes mellitus (IDDM), and Type II, non-insulin-dependent diabetes mellitus (NIDDM). Type I accounts for only about 10 % of the cases of diabetes in older adults.

Approximately 10 million adults in the United States have diabetes, and half of them are not aware of it (1). The prevalance increases with age. It is estimated that 16.5% of those aged 65 and 26% of 85-year-olds are affected. Impaired glucose tolerance with aging is associated with poor diet, decreased physical activity, decreases in lean body mass in which to store excess carbohydrate, decreased insulin secretion, and insulin resistance (2).

Standards for determining when the glucose intolerance seen in normal aging constitutes the abnormality diabetes are not agreed on by all diabetologists. The National Diabetes Data Group of the National Institutes of Health proposed diagnostic criteria for nonpregnant adults that include a 2-hour blood glucose value of greater than 140 mg/dl as indicating "impaired glucose tolerance" and a 2-hour reading greater than 200 mg/dl as diagnostic for diabetes. These are in addition to the criterion of a fasting blood glucose level of 140 mg/dl or greater on more than one occasion (3). Because carbohydrate intolerance increases with aging, many experts feel that the limit of abnormality should be raised approximately 10 mg/dl/decade after age 60 (4).

Many elderly persons fall into the group that would be labeled impaired glucose tolerant. Calorie restriction and weight loss may improve their glucose tolerance, but there is no evidence that treatment with diet, insulin, or oral agents has any benefit (5). These persons should be watched closely for possible future development of overt diabetes.

The usual clinical symptoms of diabetes—polyuria, polydipsia, polyphagia, and weight loss—are not common in older adults. The disease is usually discovered during an examination for some other medical problem such as cholecystitis, infection, vascular disorders, or neuropathy, which often are complications of diabetes. Slow-healing, frequent skin infections, numbness of legs, feet or fingers, blurred vision, or any change in sight is often a sign of NIDDM.

Type II, formerly called maturity-onset diabetes, usually occurs after age 40, with the peak age of onset between 45 and 50. It affects mainly obese persons, and the complication of ketoacidosis usually does not occur. However, in stress situations, such as with infections, ketosis may develop. Unlike Type I patients, those with Type II diabetes may have more than enough circulating insulin, but the insulin is not utilized normally. In Type II diabetes, the patient is insulin-resistant.

The term "non-insulin-dependent-diabetes" should not imply that the patient is non-insulin-requiring or non-insulin-treated. Insulin may be required temporarily when there is medical or surgical stress, or it may be needed for long-term therapy in patients who are unable to control their diet or cannot tolerate oral agents. Approximately 15 to 30% of all persons with NIDDM eventually need insulin (4,5). An evaluation of a group of diabetic patients over the age of 60 showed that 30% received insulin (4). Thus, it appears that aging increases the numbers needing insulin.

COMPLICATIONS

The incidence of complications is very high in patients with diabetes and older adults are at particular risk. It has been established that the prevalence and incidence of neuropathy, retinopathy, and nephropathy are strongly correlated with the degree and duration of hyperglycemia (6). Many older adults have had hyperglycemia for many years before diagnosis. In addition, usual degenerative changes in aging increase the probability and extent of the complications. The major causes of death from these complications, in order of importance, are myocardial infarction, renal failure, cerebrovascular disease, ischemic heart disease, and infections (7).

Atherosclerosis in diabetics is commonly found beginning at an earlier than usual age and progressing at a faster rate. It does not correlate with the severity of diabetes or its control. The risk of death from cardiovascular disease is twice and four times as great, respectively, in diabetic men and women compared with nondiabetics (8). Diet modifications to control this additional risk by reducing the amount of fat and cholesterol and modifying the type of fat eaten are less important than weight loss to control hyperglycemia (see Diet Considerations). It is believed that excess morbidity and mortality from atherosclerosis found in obese NIDDM persons is best treated by control of hyperglycemia through limiting calorie intake. The composition of the diet appears to be less important (9). Hypertension is another risk factor for cardiovascular disease. It is found in 8 of 10 persons with NIDDM.

Renal complications are common and often call for dietary modifications in protein and mineral intake. Nine of ten persons who have had diabetes for 10 years or longer suffer some degree of renal impairment from glomerulosclerosis.

Both cataracts and glaucoma are more prevalent in the adult with diabetes. These disorders, along with diabetic retinopathy, account for the fact that diabetes is the main cause of blindness among the elderly (5). Gangrene, often an initial sign of undetected diabetes, is responsible for five of every six amputations. These amputations plus vision loss have considerable direct and indirect impact on the nutritional status of the adult diabetic.

As all the long-term complications of diabetes seem to be linked to the metabolic abnormalities of the disease, they may be prevented or ameliorated by adequate control (10).

MANAGEMENT

Persons with NIDDM may be controlled by weight loss and diet alone, diet plus insulin, or diet plus sulfonylurea therapy. Older diabetics with nearly normal fasting and postprandial blood glucose (less than 150 mg/dl and 200 mg/dl, respectively) can be expected to achieve good control with diet, exercise, and glucose monitoring (11). Elderly patients with elevations of fasting blood glucose of more than 200 mg/dl and 2-hour postprandial glucose levels of greater than 350 mg/dl usually are treated with insulin and dietary control. Patients with blood glucose levels between these figures should be started on diet alone. If this is found to be inadequate, after about 6 weeks, sulfonylureas can be tried (11).

Diet Considerations

Obesity is commonly seen in over 80% of persons with NIDDM although it is not necessarily extreme, as only about one-half of these overweight individuals weight 20% more than their desirable weight. Weight loss is the main objective in this situation. Caloric restriction causes a reduction in blood glucose even before a significant weight loss occurs. Hyperinsulinemia and reduced sensitivity of tissues to insulin are reversed by weight loss. Weight reduction alone can often control the diabetes, even reversing it in some who have had the condition for only a few years. Weight loss has the further benefit of reducing blood lipid levels and blood pressure and normalizing clotting factors (12).

Weight reduction is difficult to achieve and much more difficult to maintain. The frightening diagnosis of diabetes may be a powerful motivating force, encouraging the patient to follow a program of reduced calorie intake and increased exercise. The motivational impact can be enhanced when the benefits of weight loss on diabetes control or even reversal of the disease are explained. (See Table 8-1.)

In the minority of persons with NIDDM who are at optimum weight, further loss of weight is not helpful. In this situation, diet considerations focus on changes in the composition, size, and spacing of meals. Also, regular exercise is recommended (13).

It is obvious that diabetes is heterogenous, as are the persons who have the disease. That is why it is vital that nutritional care of the patient be individualized. This is particularly important when working with older adults, whose food habits have become ingrained and who may require diet therapy for other conditions in addition to diabetes. Factors that must be taken into consideration are appropriateness of weight level, physical activity, physiological state, and the cultural, social, and economic background of the patient. In addition, the methods of instruction will depend on the patient's educational background and sensory adequacy. That is why it is best not to prescribe a diet in the usual manner by distributing preprinted diet sheets, but rather to elicit the food intake pattern of the individual and modify it step by step (14). Greater cooperation and compliance will be the inevitable result.

Diet Composition

The exact carbohydrate, protein, and fat content of the diet for the obese person with NIDDM is less critical than for the person with IDDM. The diet must be planned, however, in order to provide adequate nutrients. The need for vitamins and minerals is similar to that of

Table 8-1   Behavioral and Eating Changes to Help Achieve Weight Loss

How to Eat

- Eat only when you are hungry.
- Stop eating when you can still eat a little more.
- When you are home, eat at one place only.
- Never eat when you are standing.
- Eat as slowly as you can, a meal should take at least 20 minutes; a snack, 10 minutes.
- Don't read or watch TV when eating.
- Use a smaller-sized plate (salad or luncheon plate), so that usual portions of food appear generous.
- Don't leave snack food around in inviting dishes throughout your home. Keep all foods in one room out of sight.
- Practice leaving a little food on your plate.
- Always eat three meals a day. Don't skip a meal because you want to "splurge" later; just eat a little less. Never skip breakfast.

What to Eat

- Eat whole-grain breads and cereals and brown rice.
- Eat oranges, grapefruit, tomatoes, apples, prunes, and other fruits and vegetables instead of drinking their juices.
- If you must use a spread on bread, use a half teaspoon of jelly or honey for a slice of bread.
- Reduce the amount of butter, margarine, or sour cream you use on mashed or baked potatoes.
- Choose foods that require a lot of chewing—apples, shredded wheat, raw vegetables, dried fruits—because they not only slow down eating, the chewing itself is satisfying.
- Eat foods that require effort and slow down eating—nuts and seeds in the shell, unpeeled shrimp, artichokes, half melons, soup.
- Avoid fried foods because they are very high in calories. Eat baked, broiled, poached, and steamed foods.

other adults. Therefore, when calories are reduced to less than 1200 kcal daily for weight loss, multivitamin/mineral supplements may be needed.

For the adult who controls diabetes by diet alone, each day's calories should be divided fairly evenly among the main meals, so that no one meal raises the blood sugar level too high. It is best to wait 4-5 hours between meals to allow enough time for the blood glucose level to return to normal (15).

Adults with diabetes who take insulin or an oral agent, and some patients on diet therapy alone, need to maintain consistency in the time, number, and composition of meals from day to day. A rigidly structured diet based on the diabetic exchange lists (see Appendix B, p. 287) is not essential for most older persons (16). However, these exchange lists, which group foods according to their carbohydrate, protein, and fat content are useful for planning a variety of meals without needing to count calories. The lists also help patients to modify the fat content of their diet.

Carbohydrate restriction, long the cornerstone of diabetic diets, is being reconsidered and abandoned by many diabetologists (17). The dietary recommendations of the American Diabetes Association emphasize increased complex carbohydrates, which have been shown to improve glucose tolerance in most people with diabetes. They recommend also a reduction in dietary fat to reduce the risk of vascular disease and increased fiber intake as a means of reducing postprandial blood glucose elevations (18).

Anderson and Sieling advocate high-carbohydrate, high-fiber diets for treating diabetes and have reported success in reducing insulin doses and fasting blood glucose levels (19). The diets are recommended for outpatient use and provide

55–60% of calories as carbohydrate
20% of calories as protein
20–25% of calories as fat

Anderson and his co-workers believe that this diet is best suited for persons with Type II diabetes as it serves to increase the number of insulin receptors on target tissues and also increases the activity of glucose metabolism enzymes. This type of diet also delays gastric emptying thus slowing down carbohydrate absorption.

Eliminating simple sugars from the diabetic diet and eating carbohydrates principally in the complex form so as to have less effect on blood glucose is another long-held tenet that may now be subject to revision. It has been shown that not all complex carbohydrates have similar effects on blood glucose levels. The form of the food, ground or whole, and whether or not it is cooked will influence its effect on blood glucose. Also, simple sugars, which usually are proscribed in diabetes, do not always produce high blood glucose values (20).

A glycemic index has been calculated by Jenkins that shows the difference in glucose responses to various foods. The greatest increase in blood glucose levels occurs after eating root vegetables like carrots and parsnips, potatoes, breads, and cereals. Lesser increases follow eating fruit and dairy products, including ice cream. Peas, dried beans, and lentils have the least effect on blood glucose levels (21). The Canadian and British Diabetic Associations advise increased consumption of legumes by diabetics because of their low glycemic index (22).

Sugar, when consumed in controlled amounts in nutritionally balanced meals also containing protein and fat, does not increase blood

Table 8–2 Diet Guidelines for Persons with NIDDM

- A good diet for a person with diabetes is also a good diet for persons who do not have diabetes.
- Special foods such as those labeled ''dietetic'' or ''diabetic'' are not needed.
- All regular foods can be used.
- Emphasize foods with a low glycemic index: peas, dried beans, lentils.
- Concentrated sweets such as regular soda, candy, cake, pie, and cookies can be used occasionally in small amounts.
- Artificial sweeteners may be used in moderate amounts.
- Use of alcoholic beverages should be decided on an individual basis.
- Restriction and/or modification of sodium, fat, and cholesterol may be recommended.
- *If overweight, reduce to ideal weight.**

*Consult Table 2–1, page 20.

glucose significantly more than other carbohydrates such as wheat flour or potato starch (23). There seems to be no reason to deny the older diabetic person the pleasure of a small amount of added sugar in the diet, if he wants it (24). Amounts used should be moderate so that weight is not increased and other nutritious foods are not displaced.

Recent research concluded that the glycemic index of foods will be a useful guide in planning diet therapy for those with NIDDM (25). It may be more useful than diabetic exchanges and is especially useful for nonobese diabetics who do not need to pay careful attention to calorie intake. For others, an exchange system based on the glycemic index may be more useful than the current exchanges. Table 8–2 provides dietary guidelines for persons with NIDDM.

DIABETIC DIET IN LONG-TERM CARE FACILITIES

It is reported that as many as 27% of the residents in long-term care facilities have diabetes (26, 27). The diet orders for these residents are varied, ranging from strict traditional diets based on the diabetic exchange lists (usually 1500 or 1800 kcal) to more liberal regimens where the diet is simply the regular or house diet with no concentrated sweets. Diets are rarely individualized. In addition, availability of foods as gifts and from vending machines increases dietary noncompliance.

It would seem more practical and appropriate in light of current understanding of dietary management of NIDDM to liberalize the diet emphasizing foods low in fat and with a low glycemic index while controlling calories to achieve or maintain optimum body weight. Diets such as these are well accepted and followed and result in better control of the diabetes (28, 29).

DIABETIC FOODS

Sweeteners

Sweets are enjoyed by most people but traditionally have not been recommended for diabetics. This thinking is changing. Alternative sweeteners are frequently used by diabetics, and caregivers may be asked questions about their safety and efficacy.

Fructose, called fruit sugar, or levulose, is slowly absorbed by facilitated diffusion from the gastrointestinal tract. The initial steps of fructose metabolism are *insulin independent*, and for this reason it has been suggested as a sweetener for diabetics. Well-controlled NIDDM seem to react normally to fructose with little rise in plasma glucose concentrations, whereas persons with IDDM show a rise in blood sugar levels after fructose ingestion. The long-term influence of fructose, ingested in substantial amounts by diabetics, has yet to be evaluated (30).

Saccharin, an alternate nonnutritive sweetener has been in use for over 80 years. Currently, its carcinogenic potential is being evaluated. Preliminary results suggest that its potential as a carcinogen is weak, but sufficient data have not been collected for a final determination. When ingested by humans, it is readily absorbed, not metabolized, and rapidly excreted by the kidneys, essentially unchanged. The American Diabetes Association supports its use in limited amounts by diabetics (31).

Sugar alcohols, sorbitol and mannitol, are sometimes used as sugar substitutes. They are absorbed very slowly from the digestive tract and can easily promote diarrhea (32). Label warnings state this potential laxative effect, but too frequently they are ignored by the consumer. The yellowing of the lens of the eye has also been attributed to sorbitol (8). Therefore, the older diabetic should be counseled to use limited amounts of sorbitol- and mannitol-sweetened foods.

Aspartame, a dipeptide synthesized by coupling two amino acids, is sold as an alternate sweetener under the trade name Equal or Nutra-Sweet. It is intensely sweet, blends well with food flavors, and is free of the bitter or metallic aftertaste associated with saccharin. It is metabolized in the body via the metabolic pathways for amino acid breakdown, yielding a small but insignificant amount of calories (33). At present, there is no recommendation for a daily intake though some side effects, such as headache, nausea, diarrhea, rashes, hives, and menstrual disorders, have been reported (34,35). The powdered, table-use form is packaged with a lactose buffer, which may be troublesome to older individuals with sensitivity to lactose.

Polydextrose, approved for use by the Food and Drug Administration in 1981, is a 1-kcal/g bulking agent that will be used to replace sucrose or fats in foods expanding the development of many reduced-calorie foods. This reduced-calorie bulking agent should provide variety in low-calorie meal planning (33).

With the proliferation of products on the market making nutritional claims of "lite" and "sugar-free," the older consumer may find it difficult to make appropriate selections. The following list of terms that appear on food labels may be useful in counseling the diabetics.

Diabetic foods must state on the label, "Diabetics: This product may be useful in your diet on the advice of a physician." If the food is not low-calorie, the label must also state, "This food is not a reduced-calorie food." The names of these foods may not include terms like "diabetic" or "for diabetics" and may not claim to be useful in the diabetic diet simply because they are low-calorie or reduced-calorie foods.

Low-calorie foods can claim to be "low-calorie" only if a serving has no more than 40 kcal. These foods also must have no more than 0.4 kcal/g (except for sugar substitutes). The principal display panel, which almost always bears the product's trademark or trade name, must also bear the words "low-calorie," "low in calories," or "a low-calorie food." A food that is naturally low in calories, such as celery, may claim only that it is a "low-calorie food."

Reduced-calorie foods contain at least one-third fewer calories than an equivalent serving of the food for which they substitute. The label must list the caloric content of a serving of the "reduced-calorie" food and the caloric content of a serving of the food for which it substitutes. This information must appear on the same panel with nutrition and ingredient information. Also, reduced-calorie food must be similar in all sensory properties (taste, smell, mouth feel) to the food for which it substitutes and must not be nutritionally inferior.

Sugar-free or sugarless foods may be labeled "low-calorie" or "reduced-calorie" (if they meet the requirements for those foods). If not low in calories, they must be accompanied by a phrase such as "not a low [or reduced] calorie food," or a more specific statement of non-diet function such as "only helps avoid tooth decay." Sugar-free foods may contain sugar alcohols (e.g., sorbitol, xylitol, mannitol) which have the same calories as sugar (4 kcal/g), but may not cause a rapid rise in blood sugar; these foods must state that the product is not for weight control. Foods that contain apparent substantial inherent sugar content, such as juices, may contain a factual statement that the food is unsweetened or contains no added sugar.

Light ("lite") foods contain less of such substances as fat, sugar, or alcohol (in the case of beer or wine), and they are usually lower in calories. When "light" represents a claim for weight control, these foods are expected to conform with regulations for low- or reduced-calorie foods.

Foods useful in weight control that contain a nonnutritive sweetener (e.g., saccharin) must declare that fact and the percentage by weight of the nonnutritive ingredient on the label. The Food and Drug Administration considers aspartame to be a nutritive sweetener; so it is not subject to these labeling regulations.

ALCOHOL

Although in the past, it was recommended that alcohol be avoided by all diabetics, at the present time it is accepted that alcohol in moderate amounts is probably no worse for diabetics than for others. However, if the patient is overweight, it must be remembered that alcoholic drinks are often high in calories. Some persons who have high triglyceride levels in their blood respond to alcohol ingestion by forming even higher levels of triglycerides.

Alcohol should be taken with food, not on an empty stomach; or hypoglycemia can result, especially in persons who are controlled with insulin. Others who are treated with sulfonylureas may have a disulfiram (Antabuse-like) reaction, with palpitations and flushing when they drink alcohol (13). See Chapter 5 and Table 17–7, p. 259, for more information on alcohol.

DRUGS THAT AFFECT DIABETES MANAGEMENT

Older adults often take a large number of drugs. Some drugs are known to affect blood sugar levels whereas others may interfere with accuracy of urine testing for glucose levels. (See Tables 8–3 and 8–4.)

Drugs are not usually considered when one is thinking about dietary sources of sugar, but they should be. Neither sugar nor saccharin

Table 8–3   Drugs That Affect Blood Sugar Level

Raise	Lower
Thyroid preparations	Salicylates (large amounts)
Glucocorticoids	Monoamine oxidase inhibitors
Diuretics	Propranolol
Estrogens	
Nicotinic acid	
Diazoxide	
Adrenaline	
Lithium carbonate	

Note: Starvation also increases the blood sugar level as do aspirin and caffeine and vitamin C in large amounts.

Table 8–4 Drugs That Interfere with Urine Glucose Tests

	Clinitest	**Tes-Tape**
Cephalosporins	False positive	No effect
Vitamin C*	False positive	False negative
Aspirin*	False positive	False negative
Aldomet	False positive	False negative
Benemid	False positive	No effect
Achromycin†	False positive	False negative
Pyridium	No effect	False positive and false negative
Chloromycetin	False positive	No effect
Levodopa*	False positive	False negative

*Large amounts.
†Injected only.
Adapted from Grant, J. P., *Handbook of Total Parenteral Nutrition*. Philadelphia: W. B. Saunders, 1980.

need be listed on labels of nonprescription medications because they are considered to be inactive ingredients. Sugar added to medications for flavor can add a significant number of calories to daily intake particularly in the case of antacids, which may be used in fairly large amounts for prolonged periods. For example, Mylanta contains almost 0.5 teaspoon of sugar in each tablespoon (36). See Table 17–9, p. 263, for a listing of nonprescription medications with little or no sugar content.

Patient aid:

Managing Type II Diabetes

available from:

Nassau Hospital
Diabetes Education Center
259 First Street
Mineola, New York 11501

REFERENCES

1. *1984 Fact Sheet on Diabetes*. New York: American Diabetes Association.
2. Horowitz, D.L., Diabetes and aging, *Am. J. Clin. Nutr.* 36:803, 1982.
3. National Diabetes Data Group, Classification and diagnosis of diabetes

mellitus and other categories of glucose intolerance, *Diabetes* 28:1039, 1979.

4. Shuman, C.R., Optimum insulin use in older diabetics, *Geriatrics* 39(10): 71, 1984.

5. Ellenberg, M., The diagnosis of diabetes in the geriatric patient, *Geriatr. Med. Today* 3(1):43, 1984.

6. Zimmerman, B.R., A survey of lipid anomalies in NIDDM written by the head of the Mayo Clinic's Diabetes Core Group, *Transition* 2(6):31, 1984.

7. Miles, J.M., An overview of the pathophysiology of NIDDM written especially for the primary care physician, *Transition* 2(6):49, 1984.

8. Hayter, J., Diabetes and the older person. *Geriatr. Nurs.* 2(1):32, 1981.

9. Wood, F.C., Bierman, E.L., New concepts in diabetic dietetics, *Nutr. Today* 3:4, 1972.

10. Popkin, L.E., Diabetes that first occurs in older people, *Nutr. Today* 17(5):4, 1982.

11. Skillman, T.G., Oral hypoglycemic agents for treatment of NIDDM, *Geratrics* 39(9):77, 1984.

12. Arky, R., et al., Examination of current dietary recommendations for individuals with diabetes mellitus, *Diabetes Care* 5(1):59, 1982.

13. Crapo, P.A., *Diet and Nutrition in Diabetes*, National Diabetes Information—Clearinghouse, National Institute of Arthritis, Diabetes and Digestive and Kidney Diseases, U.S. Dept. of Health and Human Services, July 1983.

14. Wahlquist, M.L., Recent revisions in dietary recommendations to diabetic patients, *Pract. Cardiol.* 10(6):95, 1984.

15. Rifkin, H., Type II diabetes—The state of the art, *Diabetes Forecast* 37(4):30, 1984.

16. Committees of the American Diabetes Association, Inc., and the American Dietetic Association, *Exchange Lists for Meal Planning*. Chicago: The American Dietetic Association and the American Diabetic Association in cooperation with the National Institute of Arthritis, Metabolism and Digestive Diseases and the National Heart, Lung and Blood Institute, Public Health Service, U.S. Dept. of Health, Education and Welfare, 1976.

17. Diabetes: How effective are the new diets? *Data Centrum* 1(3):21, 1984.

18. American Diabetes Association: Principles of nutrition and dietary recommendations for individuals with diabetes mellitus, *Diabetes* 28:1027, 1979.

19. Anderson, J.W., Sieling, B., High-fiber diets for diabetics: Unconventional but effective, *Geriatrics* 36:64, 1981.

20. Diabetes Care and Education Practice Group, The American Dietetic Association, *Diabetes Mellitus and Glycemic Responses to Different Foods: A Summary and Annotated Bibliography*, Chicago: The American Dietetic Association, 1983.

21. Jenkins, D.J.A., et al., Glycemic index of foods: A physiological basis for carbohydrate exchange, *Am. J. Clin. Nutr.* 34:362, 1981.

22. Jenkins, D.J.A., et al., The glycemic response to carbohydrate foods, *Lancet* 2:388, 1984.

23. Bantle, J.P., et al., Postprandial glucose and insulin responses to meals containing different carbohydrates in normal and diabetic subjects, *N. Eng. J. Med.* 309:7, 1983.

24. Nuttall, F.Q., Diet and the diabetic patient, *Diabetes Care* 6(2):197, 1983.

25. Jenkins, D.J.A., et al., Glycemic responses to foods; Possible differences between insulin-dependent and noninsulin-dependent diabetics, *Am. J. Clin. Nutr.* 40:971, 1984.

26. Zimmer, J.G., Williams, T. F., Spectrum of severity and control of diabetes mellitus in skilled nursing facilities, *J. Am. Geriatr. Soc.* 26(10):44, Oct. 1978.

27. Matthews, L.E., Feeding the diabetic resident, *J. Nutr. Elderly*, 3(2):45, Winter 1983.

28. Barnard, J., et al., Long-term use of a high-complex-carbohydrate, high-fiber, low-fat diet and exercise in the treatment of NIDDM patient, *Diabetes Care*, 6(3):268, May-June 1983.

29. Simpson, H.C.R., et al., A high carbohydrate leguminous fibre diet improves all aspects of diabetic control, *Lancet* l:8210, 1981.

30. Crapo, P.A., Fructose's sweet future, *Professional Nutr.* 13(2):4, 1981.

31. Souney, P.F., et al., Sugar content of selected pharmaceuticals, *Diabetes Care* 6(3):231, 1983.

32. Ravry, M.J.R., Dietetic food diarrhea, *JAMA* 244(3):270, 1980.

33. American Dietetic Association: *Handbook of Clinical Dietetics*, New Haven: Yale University Press, 1981.

34. O'Brien, L., Gelardi,A., Alternative sweeteners, *Chemtech* 11:274, 1981.

35. Morris, D.H., Aspartame (letter), *JAMA* 252(15):2068, 1984.

36. Campbell, R.K., Hansten, P.D., Use with caution, *Diabetes Forecast* 35(4):27, 1982.

Chapter 9

CANCER

The total number of cancer patients will increase over the next decade. The reasons for this are twofold: (1) the population is aging, and the most conspicuous feature of most forms of cancer is that the incidence increases sharply with age; (2) at the same time, the death rate from cardiovascular disease is declining. Each person now has a slightly higher chance of dying from cancer than his parents did. The annual death rate from cancer more than doubles as one goes from 50 to 60 years old. By age 80 there is a one in four chance of developing cancer within the next 5 years; cancer is the leading cause of death in oldest age groups.

The time course of cancer and its relation to aging have not as yet been clearly defined. Perhaps with aging comes a lessened resistance to carcinogenesis. Or perhaps, and more likely, the disease process is multistep. As aging progresses, there is a higher probability of having many cells that have gone through all the preliminary stages of the carcinogenic process. Studies of experimental cancers show a multistep origin with different initiating factors causing the early- and late-stage event. Early initiating factors appear to damage DNA. Learning to prevent these initiating events will change the incidence of certain cancers 50 years in the future. Late-stage, promoting factors appear to affect cell proliferation and differentiation. Experimental carcinogenesis and epidemiologic observations have put forth some strong evidence linking late-stage carcinogenic factors to controllable environmental variables including smoking and diet (1). The practical message is that, at any age, preventive measures may prove worthwhile in reducing the risk for cancer.

DIET AND CANCER RISK

Many dietary factors have been examined for their potential to promote or protect against cancer (2,3,4,5,6,7). Currently, it is not possible, and it may never be possible, to specify diet changes that would protect everyone against all forms of cancer. Knowledgeable experts cannot agree on what advice the public should be given regarding diet, nutrition, and cancer. Most believe that diet, in combination with other life style factors, plays an important role in determining whether a person will eventually get cancer. The process of carcinogenesis, however, is so complex, interplaying with each individual's personal environment and genetic make-up that specific dietary recommendations for the entire population may not exist (8). Nevertheless, in 1984, the American Cancer Society proposed dietary guidelines that are consistent with good nutrition and may help reduce the chance of getting cancer (see Table 9–1). How much cancer will be prevented if these guidelines are applied is impossible to speculate. The guidelines are appropriate to the extent that they will aid lay people in selecting a well-balanced diet and eating in moderation.

AGING AND CANCER RISK

Management of cancer in older adults has, to date, not been studied to the same extent that it has in younger adults. Arbitrary age limitations that have excluded older patients from clinical studies are partly responsible for the lack of information about cancer management in the

Table 9–1   American Cancer Society Nutrition Guidelines to Help Reduce the Chance of Getting Cancer (1984)

1. Avoid obesity	5. Include cruciferous vegetables such as cabbage, broccoli, Brussels sprouts, kohlrabi, and cauliflower in the diet
2. Cut down on total fat intake	
3. Eat more high-fiber foods, such as fruits, vegetables, and whole-grain cereals	
	6. Be moderate in consumption of alcoholic beverages
4. Include foods rich in vitamins A and C in the daily diet	7. Be moderate in consumption of salt-cured, smoked, and nitrite-cured foods

elderly (9). In addition, it is commonplace for the older adult to have many chronic illnesses, of which cancer is but one. Thus, research protocols in chemotherapeutics have tended to exclude older patients. These factors have led to the probably incorrect clinical impression that older patients do not tolerate chemotherapy as well as younger patients (10).

For the older adult, cancer must be viewed as an increasingly protracted disease. With each passing year, it is diagnosed earlier and treated more aggressively and more successfully. Many patients will experience a prolonged survival even if their disease is in an advanced state.

Cancer of the colon and rectum is the second most common form of cancer for both sexes. Routine screening, after age 40, could, through early detection, reduce the risk of having advanced colorectal cancer. Most older patients, however, are diagnosed in the late phase of the disease, compromising survival.

Stomach, colon, rectum and prostate cancer in men, and breast cancer in women, make up 50% of all the cancer seen in patients over 60. One-half of all breast cancer patients are over 65 (9). In one study of patients over 70 who had breast cancer surgery, the survival rates at 5 and 10 years did not differ from those of younger individuals. This once again reinforces the idea that conventional treatment should not be withheld solely on the basis of age (11). Approximately 40% of acute nonlymphocytic leukemia occurs in people over 60. Recently, more aggressive treatment has been given to older patients, and the subsequent remission rate is comparable to that of similarly treated younger patients (9). Palliative surgery, radiotherapy, and judiciously used chemotherapy will afford the older patient the possibility of long-term alleviation and/or relief from symptoms. Both will add to the quality of life and, in many cases, will extend it as well.

Those who work with older oncology patients feel that they should be told openly about diagnosis and prognosis (12, 13). Children and spouses frequently request that the patient not be told. This deception, in light of a deteriorating physical condition, leads to bouts of depression, anxiety and loneliness, all of which can compromise treatment and survival (12). At the least, this deception, by its very nature, curtails communication between the patient and his family and physician in the terminal period. This lack of interaction removes family and physician support and interferes with patient comfort, peace of mind, and freedom from pain since a frank discussion of treatment approaches is impossible (14).

Most older patients can accept their condition if they feel they can retain some control over decisions and that their wishes will be respected. Though the majority of caregivers feel that cancer patients need the most support coping with their emotions, patients themselves rank emotional needs far below their need to understand and cope with their treatment and its side effects (15).

NUTRITIONAL SUPPORT

Nutritional support cannot cure a patient of cancer. However, nutrition plays a vital role in cancer care: it can shorten a patient's hospital stay, increase the effectiveness of cancer therapy, increase the length of a patient's life, and enhance the quality of the time that remains.

Cancer may adversely affect the patient's nutritional status in three ways: (1) through the systemic effects of the cancer itself, (2) through the local effect of malignant cell growth, and (3) through the effects of cancer treatment (surgery, radiation, and chemotherapy) (16).

Systemic Effects

Active neoplastic disease causes a marked loss of appetite in a significant number of patients. Although not fully understood, this phenomenon leads to anorexia (sustained lack of appetite) and may contribute to cancer cachexia (a progressive syndrome characterized by loss of appetite, weight loss leading to emaciation, and alterations in vital functions). If anorexia is allowed to proceed unchecked, the patient becomes progressively more severely malnourished. Malnutrition accentuates the anorexia leading to abnormalities in the intestinal mucosa. Patients often have increased epithelial cell loss and decreased lactose utilization. This further depresses nutrient absorption and may predispose the patient to diarrhea (16).

Localized Effects

Tumor growth in any part of the gastrointestinal tract, resulting in partial or complete obstruction, will interfere with food intake and nutrient absorption. Tumors of the pancreas, pancreatic duct, or common bile duct lead to impaired digestion and absorption of fats and fat-soluble vitamins. The decrease in fat absorption leads to increased excretion of calcium and magnesium in the feces. Interference with normal pancreatic function causes inefficient protein utilization. Tube feeding into a site beyond the obstruction or intravenous alimentation may sustain patients until normal feeding can be reinstituted (16).

Treatment Effects

Radiation therapy may induce a variety of serious, acute and chronic effects on the nutritional status of the older patient. The epithelium of the small bowel is second only to the bone marrow in its sensitivity to radiation. Radiation damage may lead to diarrhea, nausea, chronic malabsorption, stricture, and fistula formation (17). Acute effects usually disappear shortly after therapy is stopped. Chronic or "late" radiation changes are more difficult to manage, and the patient will need careful follow-up and attention to nutritional needs (16). See Table 9–2 for the nutritional side effects of radiation therapy.

More than half of all cancer patients receive radiation therapy during the course of treatment (18). When the head and neck are irradiated, a number of oral complications may arise that exacerbate problems of eating and nutrition. Xerostomia (decreased salivary flow) affects taste perception, chewing, swallowing, and speech. A dry mouth is more susceptible to infection from bacterial, fungal, or vial agents (19). Patients frequently use hard candies, sour balls, or mints throughout the day to stimulate salivary flow. This palliative measure can cause accelerated dental decay by providing cariogenic oral bacteria with a continuous source of sugar. In a radiation-compromised patient, tooth decay may occur within weeks of treatment initiation. The combination of diminished resistance, dry mouth, and ill-fitting dentures can lead to progressive dental infection that may involve the jaw, causing osteonecrosis (bone death) (20). An anticipatory oral health evaluation and instruc-

Table 9–2 Nutritional Side Effects of Cancer Treatment

Affected area	Radiation side effects	Surgery side effects
Head and upper neck	Dysgeusia "Mouth blindness," loss of taste sensation Xerostomia—dry mouth Odynophagia—painful swallowing	Difficulty chewing and swallowing Inability to swallow causing need for prolonged tube feeding in some cases

Table 9–2   (Cont.) Nutritional Side Effects of Cancer Treatment

Affected area	Radiation side effects	Surgery side effects
	Food aversions and complaints of a "tinny" or unpleasant taste	
	Stomatitis—dry, friable, inflamed oral mucosa	
	Osteoradionecrosis—"bone death" due to radiation trauma and bacterial infiltration, exacerbated by ill-fitting dentures	
	Dental decay—may occur as early as several weeks after initial treatment	
	Infection	
Lower neck and midchest area	Dysphagia—difficulty swallowing	Diarrhea
	Esophagitis—painful inflammation of esophagus	Delayed gastric function
		Steatorrhea—fatty stools
	Fibrosis with esophageal stricture	
Abdominal and pelvic area	Altered intestinal function	Dumping syndrome—accelerated flow into jejunum with flushing, dizziness, and general malaise
	Diarrhea	
	Nausea	
	Chronic or "late" changes—flattening and alteration of mucosa	Achlorhydria—decreased HCl production
	Telangiectasis (dilatation of capillary vessels and minute arteries), fibrosis	Lack of intrinsic factor to facilitate B_{12} absorption
		Hypoglycemia
	Stenosis (narrowing or stricture) of the bowel	Diarrhea
	Obstruction or fistula	Loss of bile salts
		Steatorrhea
		Moderate to severe malabsorption
		Diabetes mellitus as a result of pancreatectomy
		Disruption of water and electrolyte balance

tion in hygiene coupled with nutritional support can optimize tissue resistance and minimize oral problems (19, 20).

The use of most chemotherapeutic drugs is disruptive to the maintenance of good nutritional status. The majority of these drugs are effective because they interfere with one or more key phases in the metabolism of cells—normal as well as neoplastic. The epithelial cells of the small intestine have a rapid turnover rate; consequently chemotherapeutic agents adversely affect intestinal function. The epithelium of the mouth and large bowel is also affected. Newer treatment programs, which are increasingly effective, stress the use of multicombination, high-dose cyclical chemotherapy resulting in prolonged periods of anorexia and nausea (16). Table 9–3 lists the side effects that can be expected when these drugs are used.

Surgery to remove a malignant growth may remove part of the gastrointestinal tract or render sections of it unusable (see Table 9–2). Extensive resection of the head and neck, total gastrectomy, and colostomy are common to patients with cancer (16). Esophageal cancer is most common in men 70–80 years old (18). Radical surgery in the head and neck area leads to difficulty in chewing and swallowing. Prolonged use of a puréed diet or tube feeding may be necessary. See Chapter 12 for additional information to help manage these patients. Massive small-bowel resection, especially in older patients, presents serious, long-range problems in maintaining adequate nutrition and electrolyte and water balance (16).

Over half of all cases of colorectal carcinoma occur in those over 60 (18). The incidence of this type of cancer peaks between ages 75 and 80 with risk increase beginning at 40 (21). Surgery is frequently indicated and an ileostomy or colostomy performed. This new anatomic condition is often difficult to accept and older patients need a great deal of help and support.

Colonic surgery, by itself, does not cause significant nutrition problems. Nutrition counseling, however, can allay some of the patient's fear and help the patient deal with any problems that arise. The patient should be encouraged to eat normally once healing has occurred. The postoperative diet minimizes residue so as not to irritate the stoma. Progressively and slowly the patient should introduce additional foods according to individual preference. Any food that causes discomfort should be removed from the diet. It should, however, be tried once again, in a month to 6 weeks, when healing is more complete.

No specific dietary rules can be set down but the following suggestions may be helpful in handling common problems.

Table 9–3 Reactions Caused by Chemotherapeutic Agents

Chemotherapy agents	Possible nutrition side effects
Adriamycin	Nausea, vomiting, stomatitis, anorexia
Asparaginase	Nausea, vomiting, anorexia
BCNU	Nausea, vomiting, anorexia
Bleomycin (Blenoxane)	Stomatitis, nausea, vomiting
Busulfan (Myleran)	Nausea, vomiting, glossitis
Chlorambucil (Leukeran)	Nausea, vomiting, diarrhea (at low-level toxicity), GI discomfort, stomatitis, sore throat
Cisplatin (Platinol)	Anorexia, nausea, vomiting
Cyclophosphamide (Cytoxan)	Nausea, vomiting, abdominal pain, anorexia, oral ulcerations
Cytarabine (Ara-C)	Nausea, vomiting, diarrhea, oral and intestinal ulcerations
Dactinomycin (Actinomycin-D)	Nausea, vomiting, abdominal pain, enteritis, mucositis, anorexia, diarrhea
Daunorubicin (Cerubidine)	Nausea, vomiting, stomatitis, anorexia
5-Fluorouracil	Severe nausea, vomiting, alters taste, anorexia, stomatitis, diarrhea
Hydroxyurea	Anorexia, nausea, stomatitis, diarrhea, vomiting
Melphalan (Alkeran)	Nausea, vomiting
Mercaptopurine	Abdominal pain, nausea, vomiting, diarrhea
Methotrexate	Anorexia, nausea, vomiting, diarrhea, intestinal pain and intestinal ulcerations, gingivitis, stomatitis
Mithramycin (Mithracin)	Nausea, vomiting, gastrointestinal toxicity, diarrhea, anorexia
Prednisone	Fluid retention, muscle wasting, hypertension
Procarbazine (Matulene)	Nausea, vomiting, anorexia, intestinal ulceration, stomatitis, sore throat, dry mouth
Vinblastine (Velban)	Nausea, vomiting, stomatitis, constipation, abdominal pain, glossitis
Vincristine (Oncovin)	Muscle pain, constipation, nausea, vomiting, abdominal pain

Problem	*Possible causes*
Odorous discharge	Onions, green peppers, turnips, cabbage, beets, antibiotics, vitamin-mineral supplements
Gas	Alcoholic beverages, especially beer; any food listed under odorous discharge, but this varies greatly from person to person
Blockage of food bolus	Avoidance of very fibrous vegetables (i.e., bran, corn, celery, coconuts); all may be tolerated in small amounts
Loose stools or watery discharge	Alcohol, raw vegetables and fruits, highly spiced foods

Vitamin B_{12} is absorbed in the terminal ileum. If a large portion has been removed in surgery, parenteral B_{12} must be given so macrocytic anemia does not develop. Fluids need to be increased daily by 1 to 2 qt since the water-absorbing capacity of the body has been decreased surgically. Some patients reduce fluids hoping to control diarrhea or watery stools, but this will not help the problem. Additional dietary sodium may be necessary in some cases since sodium resorption has been altered and excretion is abnormal (22).

NUTRITIONAL ASSESSMENT IN CANCER CARE

Malnutrition is not an obligatory consequence of cancer, yet there is a definite interplay between nutritional status and disease (15). The altered host metabolism associated with cancer and the side effects of therapy commonly lead to protein-calorie malnutrition. Malnutrition, left unchecked initiates a downward spiral of apathy, anorexia, and further malnutrition. This compromises the effectiveness of oncological treatment. Equally important is the deterioration of the patient's quality of life. Among geriatric patients with metastatic cancer receiving palliative therapy, adequate nutrition greatly improves the quality of life. The improvement achieved in general health frequently is what allows the patient at least a short-term release from the hospital back to the home environment for interaction with family and friends (23).

Cancer patients 60 and older show the same nutritional deficits as younger patients and require the same nutritional intervention but need more careful monitoring and encouragement (24). Figure 9–1 is a example of a checksheet for use in determining which cancer patients are at

Figure 9–1. Checklist for identifying cancer patients at risk of developing malnutrition.

Name_____ Current weight_____

Age_____ Ideal or standard weight_____

Sex_____ % of standard weight_____

	Yes	No
1. Has the patient had a recent loss of 10% or more of usual weight?	_____	_____
2. Has the patient recently had surgery?	_____	_____
3. Is the patient currently receiving chemotherapy or radiotherapy?	_____	_____
4. Has the patient been maintained for more than a week during the previous month on a liquid or full-fluid diet?	_____	_____
5. Has the patient been maintained for more than 7 days during the last month on intravenous fluids?	_____	_____
6. Will the patient's anticipated therapy render him unable to eat (i.e., surgery of head or neck)?	_____	_____
7. Does the patient's diet history indicate nutritional inadequacy (i.e., history of meal skipping, monotonous food selections, or unorthodox diet)?	_____	_____
8. Has the patient experienced recurrent episodes of:		
nausea	_____	_____
vomiting	_____	_____
diarrhea	_____	_____
9. Does the patient have a mechanical interference to self-feeding (i.e., dentures, armboard, tremors)?	_____	_____
10. Does the patient have:		
stomatitis	_____	_____
glossitis	_____	_____
gingivitis	_____	_____
esophagitis	_____	_____
xerostomia	_____	_____
11. Has the patient complained of:		
bloating	_____	_____
"mouth blindness" (loss of taste)	_____	_____
smell alterations	_____	_____
food aversions	_____	_____

Figure 9–1.   (*Continued*)

	Yes	No
12. Is there evidence of increased metabolic requirements due to:		
fever	_____	_____
infection	_____	_____
bedsores	_____	_____
draining fistulas	_____	_____
wound healing	_____	_____
13. Is the patient's mental attitude positive?	_____	_____
14. Does the patient have a history of:		
liver abnormalities	_____	_____
impaired kidney function	_____	_____
diabetes	_____	_____
heart disease	_____	_____
alcohol abuse	_____	_____

Any **yes** answer indicates a potential for the patient to be at nutritional risk. Any **yes** answer in combination with a weight loss of 10 per cent or greater classifies the patient at nutritional risk and in need of nutrition intervention. If five or more **yes** answers are given, aggressive nutrition support is necessary.

Adapted from: A Tool for Assessing the Nutritional Status of Cancer by Jane H. Butler, R.N., M.N., UCLA Center for the Health Sciences.

nutritional risk (25). A combination of regular food supplemented with low-residue liquid feedings, providing 2000 to 3000 kcal/day has been shown to maintain nutritional status (24). Parenteral nutrition is expensive and more dangerous for an older patient and is reserved for special circumstances or critical phases in patient care. Most older patients will continue to have a positive outlook if they continue to eat conventional foods in a conventional manner (25). Body weight, levels of serum albumin, serum fatty acids, and plasma amino acids, and the 24-hour urinary excretion of creatinine and urea nitrogen may be used as a gauge of the efficacy of nutritional support.

Over 25% of all patients admitted for cancer care have depressed serum albumin levels. This does not appear to be a function of age but is due instead to the metastatic stage of the tumor. In a study of older patients, analysis of serum albumin values lower than 3.5 g/dl showed that only 20% were attributed to the terminal state of the patient (24). Therefore, the majority of older patients with depressed serum albumin levels would be responsive to nutritional support adjunctive to conventional therapy. Protein requirements for cancer patients have been suggested to be 1.5 to 2.5 times greater than normal requirements. This would approximate 84–140 g protein/day for older males and 66–110 g protein/day for females. Protein intake should be adjusted and monitored by interpreting serum albumin and serum transferrin concentrations (17). Low serum transferrin levels alone are not a reliable parameter of nutritional status since anemia may be precipitated by neoplastic disease and/or the use of some chemotherapeutic agents, and this may alter transferrin levels.

In one study, low serum albumin and transferrin were found in a significant number of patients who had poor immune competence and subsequently died (17). The patient's loss of immunocompetence is known to be compounded by protein depletion and poor nutritional status. Loss of immune competence can be solely due to malnutrition. The proper or improper function of the immune system is felt to be significant in the disease process of cancer. Depressed immunocompetence correlates with the presence of cancer, recurrence of tumor growth, poor response and intolerance to therapy, and increased mortality (26). Well-nourished cancer patients display the same immunocompetence as controls without neoplastic disease. However, cancer patients over 70 may show a depressed immune response regardless of nutritional support (27). This suggests that aging, by itself, may be an important factor in the loss of immunocompetence in older cancer patients.

The caregiver needs a simple tool for a quick determination of nutritional status. Patients' weight and deviations in weight can serve as a quick and available barometer of nutritional well-being (13, 26, 28). Patients should be weighed without shoes, with minimal or no clothing. Weight and percent of standard weight should be recorded and reevaluated at least twice weekly. Table 9–4 provides guidelines for using

Table 9–4 Weight as an Indication of Nutritional Status and Response to Cancer Treatment

% of standard weight	Nutritional status	Response to treatment
95–100%	Well nourished	Can tolerate chemotherapy and radiation; good risk for surgery
90%	Slightly undernourished	Less tolerance to radiation and unable to tolerate chemotherapy; guarded risk for surgery
80%	Moderately undernourished	Unable to tolerate radiation or chemotherapy; severe risk for surgery
70% and below	Severely undernourished	No oncological treatment possible

weight as a rough indicator of nutritional status and response to treatment (25).

The progressive syndrome of undernutrition is often accompanied by personality changes. Outgoing, even-tempered patients become increasingly apathetic, withdrawn, whiny, and self-centered. The hospitalization, life-threatening illness, or pain may be possible explanations for the behavior change. It has long been known, however, that the stress of semistarvation results in emotional instability with protracted periods of depression. Therefore, the behavioral changes seen in cancer patients may be due to the decline in nutritional status rather than to general psychological effects of coping with disease.

FEEDING THE CANCER PATIENT

Response to oncological treatment and the tolerance of that treatment depend, to a great degree, on the nutritional status of the patient. Nutrition therapy can be divided into (1) supportive, (2) adjunctive, or (3) definitive. Supportive nutrition therapy is designed to maintain or improve the patient's nutritional state prior to more definitive therapy such as surgery. Adjunctive nutrition therapy is based on the concept that improving nutritional status will contribute to the efficacy of the primary modality of treatment. For example, a well-nourished patient can tolerate higher doses of radiation or chemotherapeutic agents. When definitive nutrition therapy is used, it is the primary cancer treatment and essential to the survival of the patient. A severely undernourished patient would require definitive therapy before any additional treatment was attempted (16).

Nourishing the cancer patient is a difficult and challenging task. Many physiological and psychological problems may develop. Abnormalities appear in the intestinal mucosa, depressing nutrient absorption and predisposing the patient to diarrhea. Personality changes occur, resulting in emotional instability with protracted periods of depression. Food aversions, taste and odor alterations, the side effects of treatment, and the isolation of hospitalization adversely affect the patient's nutritional status (25).

The nutritional needs of the oncology patient are unique. Cancer often increases the demand for nutrients while at the same time the disease and the treatment diminish the patient's ability to eat. Pain, difficulty swallowing, early satiety, nausea, vomiting, obstruction of the gastrointestinal tract, taste and smell alterations, loss of saliva, malabsorption, and anorexia all interfere with eating (17).

Cancer patients need to select foods with a maximum nutrient return. Eating needs to be considered as part of treatment. For those in bed, a liquid nourishment in an ice bath should be left at the bedside. Even a few sips an hour adds to the calories and nutrients for the day. Suggest eating often, sometimes making an effort to eat a small snack every hour when meals are not well received. A plate waste study confirmed that standard hospital portions are too large for most cancer patients and may discourage intake. Patients attribute their anorexia to the hospital environment, scheduling of treatments, and timing of meals (17).

Anorexia

A significant number of cancer patients have a marked loss of appetite, which can lead to body wasting. Many explanations for this have been suggested: altered metabolism, derangement in the central nervous system, increased levels of free fatty acids, hyperglycemia and elevated lactic acid levels, and changes in taste and smell (13, 29).

Anorexia is most common in patients with cancer of the gastrointestinal tract, liver, or pancreas and in those in whom cancer is widespread throughout the body. The depressed appetite will lead to marked weight loss and progressive malnutrition, initiating changes in the gastrointestinal tract that further decrease absorption and utilization of nutrients. The anorexia and malnutrition may be accentuated by an emotional response to the diagnosis (13, 17). Though anorexia with concommitant malnutrition is difficult to manage, it is rare to find a cancer patient who cannot either be maintained in good nutrition or improved from a malnourished state.

It is well known that breakfast is the most popular meal for cancer patients, although there is no data on why this is true. Nonetheless, breakfast and breakfast foods, offered as snacks, should be emphasized (13). Dairy foods and eggs are frequently more desirable to cancer patients than meals or combination entrees (17). These foods provide good protein sources as well as calories. For patients experiencing early satiety, small, frequent meals featuring bread, breakfast cereals, rice, yogurt, milk, and eggs are usually well tolerated (13). Zinc sulfide supplements have also stimulated the appetites of patients on chemotherapeutic or radiation therapy. It is important to appreciate that a patient suffering from anorexia cannot realistically be expected to order food for the following day. A protocol should be established to allow an anorectic patient to order and change food requests spontaneously (13). This can be accomplished easily by the availability of various, appealing nourishments.

When it becomes apparent that the patient cannot maintain nutritional adequacy, the feeding program should be modified. Enteral nutrition by nasoduodenal tube is preferred as this method increases the likelihood of maintaining proper tube placement despite nausea or vomiting and decreases the likelihood of aspiration (17). When tube feeding is used, regardless of the method of administration, residual stomach contents must be checked before successive feedings. An older, debilitated patient is at great risk of regurgitation and aspiration (13).

Cachexia

Cancer-induced cachexia, the weight loss and wasting seen in many cancer patients, is not the same as simple starvation. It is the result of a complicated pathophysiological state the clinical signs of which include early satiety, anorexia, weight loss, anemia, muscle weakness, and easy fatigability (30). Left unchecked, it will result in extreme malnutrition resulting in accelerated death. Cachexia, commonplace in patients with advanced metastatic malignant disease, may also be seen in patients with localized disease. The cachectic state itself may result in slower tumor growth; therefore, it is inappropriate to aggressively nourish the patient without simultaneously treating the underlying cancer (13). The current consensus is that advanced cancer patients should receive anticancer therapy in conjunction with nutritional support (31).

Feeding Problems

Table 9–5 provides nutrition hints and suggestions for dealing with the most common side effects of cancer treatment.

For the patient with stomatitis, rinsing the mouth several times a day and before meals with an analgesic solution makes eating more tolerable. Many commercial solutions are available. Following are two homemade preparations that may be used (32).

Solution 1: 2 tablespoons sodium bicarbonate (baking soda)
        1 teaspoon salt
        Dissolve in 1 quart water
        Use 1/4 cup to rinse mouth
Solution 2: 1 tablespoon plain yogurt
        1 tablespoon liquid Tylenol
        Mix together and use to rinse mouth

Commercial mouthwashes should not be used as they tend to dry out the mouth lining; adding to discomfort and proliferation of bacteria (33).

Table 9–5   Nutritional Suggestions for Dealing with the Discomforts of Cancer Treatment

Discomfort	Feeding suggestions	Foods to try
Mouth blindness (dysgeusia)	Use odor, texture, and eye appeal to encourage eating Acidic drinks may stimulate taste Select strongly flavored foods	Wine Lemonade Lemon/lime soda Barbecue sauce Steak sauce Teriyaki sauce Smoked meats Pizza Catsup Milkshakes flavored with coffee or mint Cheese chips Herb breads
Sore mouth (stomatitis) and esophagus (esophagitis)	Avoid rough, raw, acid, and spicy foods Eat soft, bland foods Gargle before meals with an analgesic solution (see p. 143) Puréed diet or full fluid diet may be needed for a few days during peak irritation Cool and room-temperature food is most tolerable	Watermelon Honeydew Applesauce Cold liquids Cooked cereals Strained cream soup Mashed potatoes or squash Popsicles Casseroles Custard Soft-cooked eggs Plain ice cream Jello Pudding Sherbet Pumpkin and squash soup
Thick, sticky saliva	Make first meal of day liquid Have a light breakfast Milk products are not well tolerated; use soybean milk To break morning mucus try hot tea with lemon or suck on sour-lemon drops	Soups Drinks Pureed vegetables Pureed fruits Soft cooked chicken or fish Sugar-free sour candies Nondairy creamer
Dry mouth (xerostomia)	Serve foods with sauces, gravies, or in broth Serve plenty of liquid along with food	Soft-cooked chicken or fish Casseroles Milk, milkshakes, and malts

Table 9–5 (Cont.)

Discomfort	Feeding suggestions	Foods to try
	Increase saliva flow by using sugarless lemon drops or gum, lemon tea, lemonade, or sports gum (i.e., Gatorade Gum) just before or with meal	Eggnogs Cooked cereal Dry cereal soaked in milk Vegetables with sauces Melons Peaches Canned fruits Fruit juices and nectars Sherbet
	Try an artificial saliva substitute	
	"Dunk" breads and crackers in a beverage	
Nausea and vomiting	Do not eat for several hours before treatment	Plain meat, fish, and poultry Low-fat milk Saltines or salted crackers Toast Cold cereal Baked potatoes Juices Cold drinks Sherbert Gatorade Popsicles
	Salty foods or ice-cold drinks help control nausea and vomiting	
	Do not mix hot and cold foods at a meal	
	Do not eat overly sweet or greasy foods	
	Eat slowly	
	Do not drink rapidly	
	Eat small frequent meals	
	Lie down or rest after eating	
	For morning nausea use techniques for "morning sickness" during pregnancy*	
	Odorous foods aggravate nausea	
Diarrhea	Drink ample liquids	Water Fruit ades Low-acid fruit Juice (i.e., apricot, peach, pear) Lact-Aid†-treated milk Refined cereals, breads, and pasta White rice Cooked fruits and vegetables without skins and seeds Bananas
	Eat food low in fiber	
	Use soybean milk if regular milk causes discomfort	
	Eat foods high in potassium (see p. 177)	

Table 9-5 *(Cont.)* Nutritional Suggestions for Dealing with the Discomforts of Cancer Treatment

Discomfort	Feeding suggestions	Foods to try
Constipation	Eat high-fiber foods if chewing and swallowing are not a problem Add bran to cooked foods Drink prune juice Drink 8 or more glasses of liquid a day Get regular daily exercise	Whole-grain breads, cereals, and pasta Brown rice Raw fruits and vegetables with skins Fruit juices Dried fruit

*To treat morning sickness place dry toast or plain cracker at the bedside before retiring; upon awakening do not raise head off pillow, eat toast slowly, and rest a full 5 min before getting up; eat solid foods before taking any liquids.

†Lact-Aid available from Sugar Lo Company, P.O. Box 1017, Atlantic City, New Jersey 08404.

During peak irritation, a full fluid or pureed diet may be needed. The intense soreness in the mouth will persist longer if recovery is slowed by poor nutrition; with proper refeeding, the condition should clear up in a few days. It is important for the patient or caregiver to be inventive. Vegetable and pasta cooking water can be saved to add nutrients and enhance the flavor of blenderized items. Cooked cereals, especially farina and cornmeal, can be used as thickening agents. Stirring either into a soup will turn it into a gravy that can be combined with rice or small, shaped pasta. Blenderized creamed vegetables or canned peas function as an appetizing sauce over flaked fish or poached shredded poultry. Canned Chinese foods are already soft but, if needed, they can be pureed easily. Frozen fish entrees blend nicely and can be used over rice, pasta, and mashed potatoes or thinned and served as a pureed fish chowder topped with soft bread cubes. Attractive meal service will add to the acceptance of a pureed diet. Serving such a meal in many colorful Chinese bowls on an attractive tray may provide the motivation a patient needs to eat.

Nausea and vomiting are the most common side effects of chemotherapy. Some patients experience anticipatory nausea and vomiting as a learned response to treatment. Behavioral intervention and relaxation techniques substantially reduce the frequency, severity, and duration of the anticipatory side effects (33).

Many accounts of food aversions have been reported among cancer patients. These aversions are to specific foods or groups of foods and not a generalized response to all foods as in anorexia (29). Over one-third of all patients will experience an aversion to one or more foods. The following is a list of foods reported by cancer patients to have a perceived odor or taste change.

Coffee
Chocolate
Sweets
High-protein foods (red meat, meat, fish, poultry, especially fried chicken, and pork hocks)
Cereal products (except for rice and hot cereal)
Salty meats (ham, bacon, pork, breakfast meats)

If a person is given a food for which he has a known food aversion, the sight or smell of the food may cause the ''gag'' response and initiate nausea and vomiting (34). The cause of food aversions in cancer patients is speculative. The aversion may be a learned response to sickness, sickness produced by foods, or a physiological and psychological response to the disease. Certain foods, such as meats, are more likely to become aversive, and odors play a role in their unfavorable acceptance. Possibly, the aversive foods have similar odor components (35,36). Meat, casseroles, ground beef, and egg aversions have been reported in patients receiving 5-fluorouracil, while others feel chemotherapeutic agents are not related to food rejections (37). Whatever the mechanism involved, patients reporting food aversions must have their diet individualized to omit these offending foods.

Taste Alterations

While the range of taste and odor abnormalities varies greatly from patient to patient, these changes in perception contribute to anorexia and malnutrition in cancer patients (13, 37). Although the response is highly individual, it is worth noting some observations and trends from interviews with cancer patients and caregivers.

The bitter sensation may be magnified, and many cancer patients become acutely sensitive to the bitter aftertaste of amino acids in meats (17, 35, 37). This taste alteration may pose a problem when encouraging patients to eat approximately 100 g of protein a day. Nonmeat protein sources such as eggs, cheese, and milk may be better accepted (17, 37). Poultry and fish are often less offensive than red meat, though some patients rate them unacceptable as well (35). There are a number of cancer patients who, despite treatment, still enjoy meat, so it should never be assumed that meats will be universally disliked (38). Cold proteins, including meats, are often better received. Thoroughly chilling the plate before service will help to keep the protein cold for a prolonged period. This is especially helpful when there is a time lapse between service and delivery.

Soy sauce, salt, and wine sauce will make items more palatable. Fruit sauces are also well received. These can be made quickly and in small amounts by pureeing and then heating canned fruits such as peaches, plums, apples, or pineapple. Strained commercial baby food fruits also work well. Older patients react negatively to the thought of eating baby food. Therefore, these items should never be given to the patient in their original jar but rather placed in a dish or small serving pitcher. Any sauces served should be given on the side so patients can flavor to their preference. Some patients may drown meats in soy sauce, but if this increases consumption one should not be judgmental about the preference.

Alteration of patients' perception of sweet foods varies greatly. Many find chocolate unpleasant (29, 39). In some anorectic patients and some patients on chemotherapy, the sweet stimulus is altered, so that they reduce their intake of extremely sweet foods (29, 38). Many feel the unpleasantness associated with sweets stems from the consistent encouragement to eat sweet foods and drink high-calorie sweet-flavored supplements (37). Other patients readily accept sweetened foods but within a narrow range of sweetness. For example, a patient who normally puts 1 teaspoon of sugar on breakfast cereal may now request 5 teaspoons. If 6 teaspoons are accidentally used, the patient may find the cereal intolerable and nauseating (36). These varied reactions reinforce the precept that patients should be allowed to sweeten to taste and additional sweetness should be made available to them. Some may find that sprinkling brown sugar on vegetables or potatoes provides a more acceptable taste.

Conversely, some patients may request that sweetness be reduced. Serving additional milk to dilute custard or pudding, a lemon wedge to squeeze over plain cake, or plain yogurt topping on pie may encourage eating. Avoid the use of artificial sweeteners since they are sweeter than sugar, yield no calories and leave an unpleasant, bitter aftertaste for many patients during treatment. Calorie-containing salty snacks such as peanuts, peanut butter, crackers, and pretzels may be offered. These foods stimulate fluid intake, and if calories are added to fluids, the daily intake can be increased and appetite stimulated.

Some patients report that certain sour foods, like dill pickles, taste bitter while they are receiving radiation treatments. In these instances, salty and sour sensations have been dulled by treatment while the bitter sensation remains at normal intensity (39). This once again reinforces that the caregiver must focus on the individual food preferences of the patient, using known generalizations only as guideposts to potential food acceptability.

A significant proportion of cancer patients report smell alterations strong enough to trigger nausea and rejection of food (37). Meats have been reported as smelling rancid (36). Cold foods are less odorous, so cold proteins are a better choice.

At home, suggest that the patient eat in a room other than the kitchen. In a hospital, uncover the patient's tray outside the room so odors have a chance to dissipate (36). Offensive liquids should be frozen to a slush to reduce odor. These liquids and soups can be served in covered glasses or mugs and sipped through a spouted lid or a straw.

NUTRITION MISINTERPRETATION

The fear of a potential diagnosis of cancer and the devastation felt when this fear becomes an actuality can lead very rational people to irrational acts. Self-medication for prevention or treatment of cancer is common among older adults. When a patient feels he is actively contributing to his treatment and care, his response will be more positive. Therefore, the caregiver must be careful not to dispel hope by denouncing the self-help regimen proposed by the patient. Many of these suggested treatments are harmless, and a possible placebo effect cannot be overlooked. When the potential for harm exists, the decision to use a nonconventional treatment belongs to the patient, but he should be informed about the probable ineffectiveness, dangers inherent in use, and contraindications to current treatment. Table 9-6 offers the caregiver some additional advice.

Laetrile, a cyanogenic glycoside also known as amygdalin, is found in peach, apricot, apple, plum and bitter almond pits. It has been added to herbal medicines for almost 2000 years. In 1920, Ernest Krebs rediscovered amygdalin, claiming it had antineoplastic properties. He had patients eat ground apricot pits, but so many of those treated had toxic reactions that Krebs abandoned his work. In 1952, Ernest Krebs, Jr., registered amygdalin with the U.S. Patent Office under the trade name *Laetrile*. It has been touted as a miracle cure for cancer in recent years.

The physical reaction to Laetrile can be mild to severe. Often this depends on the method of administration. Oral Laetrile is far more toxic than a parenteral dose. Given parenterally, the substance is never metabolized and is eliminated unchanged in the urine. When taken

Table 9–6   How to Counteract Cancer Quackery*

1. Listen to the patients needs and fears. Offer assistance, support, dignity, and hope.
2. Learn what the current myths are so you can provide the patient with correct information.
3. Cultivate an open, accepting, and sensitive attitude so the patient will feel comfortable discussing a "miracle" cure.
4. Sensitively correct misconceptions and guide the patient to appropriate self-help techniques.
5. Report unproven methods of "cure" to the health department, consumer protection office, local medical society, or American Cancer Society.

*Adapted from Burkhalter, P.K. Cancer Quackery, *Am. J. Nurs.* 77(3):451, March 1977.

orally, Laetrile reacts with beta-glucosidase, an enzyme found in recently ingested raw foods or endogenous to the gastrointestinal tract, forming hydrocyanic acid. This acid, a cyanide, incapacitates a respiratory enzyme system, preventing energy exchange at the cellular level. Acute cyanide poisoning can occur within 30 minutes of taking laetrile and quickly progress to internal asphyxiation. Some patients suffer chronic Laetrile poisoning, developing neuropathies with ataxia and blindness, inattention, and incoordination. The skin, mucous membranes, and auditory nerves may also be affected (40). Although much publicity surrounds this controversial compound, a clinical trial reported Laetrile had no substantial benefit in terms of cure, improvement, or stabilization of human cancer. A substantial number of patients given laetrile therapy in this study showed signs of cyanide toxicity (41).

Colonic irrigations are a suggested naturopathic therapy for cancer. Some of the regimens include coffee enemas administered as often as every 2 hours. These invasive colonic irrigations force huge amounts of fluid into the large intestine, disrupt fluid and electrolyte balance, and have caused death in a number of cases. They are an unproven method of cancer care and may be life-threatening, especially to an older patient (42).

Vitamin deficiences have been suggested as an initiating event in some cancers. Several epidemiological studies have shown an inverse association between the intake of vitamin-A-rich food and the risk of lung cancer. These studies suggest that a plant source of vitamin A, beta-carotene, is the protective factor (3). Other studies suggest beta-carotene is not protective (43). This discrepancy can be explained by the simple fact that beta-carotene is probably not equally protective for all types of cancer.

Taking large amounts of beta-carotene over prolonged periods does not induce toxicity. Excess carotene will accumulate in the tissues and cause yellowed skin, but this is not harmful as far as is known. Animal sources and supplemental vitamin A are found in the retinol form. Excess retinol, 30,000 to 50,000 IU daily (6,000 to 10,000 RE) taken for prolonged periods can be toxic, leading to hair loss, dry itching skin, joint swelling, and an enlarged liver (3). Elderly persons are more susceptible to a toxic reaction owing to reduced liver function. Supplemental doses of vitamin A, below those that cause toxic reactions, will probably cause no harm. To increase carotene consumption, recommendations for two servings daily of vitamin-A rich plant foods have been suggested.

There is little conclusive evidence that vitamin C protects against human cancer (43). However, Vitamin C does inhibit the conversion of nitrates and related compounds to carcinogens in the stomach. This process may be especially important with respect to gastric cancer. In vitro and animal studies have shown that large amounts of vitamin C enhance tumor growth and help certain cancer cells survive radiation (3). One study on humans showed that 2 g of vitamin C daily reduced the body's ability to fight infection (44). Supplemental vitamin C, below 1000 mg/day, is not harmful since some epidemiological evidence suggests that low intakes are associated with higher risks of certain cancers. Larger supplemental doses should be discouraged, especially in older patients who may have impaired renal clearance.

Like vitamin C, vitamin E has been suggested as a potential cancer inhibitor. Vitamin E is an important intracellular antioxidant and thus deserves further study as an anticancer agent. Current epidemiological data provide no conclusive evidence that vitamin E, as it is currently used, has efficacy in preventing cancer (3). However, daily vitamin E supplements of 800 IU or less have resulted in no adverse effects, though this nutrient may offer little more than a placebo effect.

Epidemiologic data do support the idea that selenium deficiency increases the risk of certain cancers in middle-aged persons (45). Blood selenium levels are usually depressed in cancer patients. Animal and tissue culture studies further support the idea that selenium is protective against cancer (46). Supplementation recommendations, however, are difficult to define. Toxic levels of trace minerals, like selenium, may be only a few times the suggested intake (0.05–0.2 mg/day). Eating food sources—meat, seafood, and cereals—is a safer way to ensure an ample intake.

Patients should be encouraged to discuss nutrient supplementation since many chemotherapeutic agents function as vitamin antagonists or chelating agents. This interference with biologic reactions in normal and neoplastic cells can be essential to the drug's antitumor action (47). Self-prescribed nutrient supplementation may be detrimental in some instances.

Modification of diet is another approach to cancer prevention. Low-fat, high-fiber, low-protein, low-calorie, and vegetarian diets have all been suggested as helpful in reducing risks (46). For treatment of cancer, many unusual dietary plans have been prescribed, from total fast, to raw vegetables, to a macrobiotic diet (48). Clinical trials have not shown these unusual diets to be effective (49). Patients can choose any diet plan they wish as long as it maintains a positive nutritional state. Raw foods and vegetarian plans may be difficult to eat owing to side effects of treatment and, when early satiety and fatigue are factors, may not supply adequate calories to meet needs.

Patient aids:

A Guide to Good Nutrition During and After Chemotherapy and Radiation, (2nd ed., 1979) by Sandra Aker and Polly Larson

available from:

> Research Dietary Services
> Division of Medical Oncology
> Fred Hutchinson Cancer Research Center
> 1124 Columbia Street
> Seattle, Washington 98104

Something's Got to Taste Good, The Cancer Patient's Cookbook, (1981), by Joan Fishman and Barbara Anrod

available from:

> Andrews and McMeel, Inc.
> Universal Press Syndicate Company
> Time and Life Building
> Suite 3717
> 1271 Avenue of Americas
> New York, New York 10020

REFERENCES

1. Cairns, J., Aging and the natural history of cancer, in: *Perspectives on Prevention and Treatment of Cancer in the Elderly*, R. Yancik, ed., N.Y.: Raven Press, 1983.

2. Wolf, G., Is dietary B-carotene an anti-cancer agent? *Nutr. Rev.*, 40(9):257, Sept. 1982.

3. Willett, W.C., MacMahon, B., Diet and cancer—An overview, Part I. *N. Engl. J. Med.* 310(10):633, March 8, 1984.

4. Willett, W.C., MacMahon, B., Diet and cancer—An overview, Part II. *N. Engl. J. Med.* 310(11):697, March 15, 1984.

5. Cameron, E., Pauling, L., Leibovitz, B., Ascorbic acid and cancer: A review, *Cancer Res.* 39:663, March 1979.

6. Greenwald, P., Manipulation of nutrients to prevent cancer, *Hosp. Pract.*, p. 119, May 1984.

7. Rivlin, R.S., Shils, M.E., Sherlock, P., Nutrition and cancer, *Am. J. Med.*, 75:843, Nov. 1983.

8. Pariza, M.W., A perspective on diet, nutrition and cancer, *JAMA*, 251(11):1455, March 16, 1984.

9. Kennedy, B.J., Clinical oncology: focus on the elderly in: *Perspectives on Prevention and Treatment of Cancer in the Elderly*, R. Yancik, ed. N.Y.: Raven Press, 1983.

10. Steel, K., Caring for the elderly person: Focus on cancer, in *Perspectives on Prevention and Treatment of Cancer in the Elderly*, R. Yancik, ed. N.Y.: Raven Press, 1983.

11. Herbsman, H., et al., Survival following breast cancer in the elderly, *Cancer*, 47:2358, 1981.

12. Francis, G.M., Cancer: The emotional component, *Am. J. Nurs.*, 69(8):1677, 1969.

13. Cimino, J.E., Feeding the patients with advanced cancer, *Diet. Currents* 10(5):1, Sept.-Oct. 1983.

14. Mount, B.M., Palliative Care of the Terminally Ill, lecture presented at the Annual Meeting of the Royal College of Physicians and Surgeons of Canada, Vancouver, British Columbia, January 27, 1978.

15. Lauer, P., et al., Learning needs of cancer patients: A comparison of nurse and patient perceptions, *Nurs. Res.*, 31(1):11, Jan.-Feb. 1982.

16. Shils, M.E., How to nourish the cancer patient, *Nutr. Today* 4:16, 1981.

17. Gildea, J.L., et al., A systematic approach to providing nutritional care to cancer patients, *Nutr. Support Serv.* 2(9):24, Sept. 1982.

18. Kark, A.E., Gueret-Wardle, D.F., Management of malignant disease in old age, in *the Treatment of Medical Problems in the Elderly*, M.J. Denham, ed. Baltimore: University Park Press, 1980.

19. Frame, R.T., The dentist, the nutritionist and the cancer patient, *Nutr. Support Serv.*, 4(9):10, Sept. 1984.

20. Palmer, C.A., Nutrition and patients with head and neck cancer, *R.D.* 2(2):4, 1982.

21. Kahn, H.A., Colorectal carcinoma: Risk factors, screening, early detection, *Geriatrics*, 39(1):42, Jan. 1984.

22. Dietary Management of the ostomy patient, *Nutrition & the M.D.* 4(7):2, 1978.

23. Harden, W.B., Should we support the cancer patient until the end? *Nutr. Support Serv.*, 2:7, April 1982.

24. Ching, E. et al., Nutritional deficiences and nutritional support therapy in geriatric cancer patients, *J. Am. Geriatr. Soc.* 27:491, Nov. 1979.

25. Heslin, J., Nutritional care of the older cancer patient, *J. Nutr. Elderly* 2(3):27, Spring 1983.

26. Kaminski, M.V., et al., Nutritional status, immunity and survival in neoplastic disease, *Nutr. Support Serv.* 2:7, April 1982.

27. Dominioni, L., et al., Evaluation of possible delayed hypersensitivity impairment in cancer patients, *J. Parenteral Enteral Nutr.* 5:300, July-Aug. 1981.

28. Oberfell, M.S., Ometer, J.L., Quality assurance, II. Application of oncology standards against levels of care model, *J. Am.. Diet. Assoc.* 81:132, Aug. 1982.

29. Trant, A.S., et al., Is taste related to anorexia in cancer patients? *Am. J. Clin. Nutr.* 36:45, July 1982.

30. Daly, J.M., Nutritional support and the cancer patient, *Clin. Consult.* 3(2):1, April 1983.

31. Seltzer, M.H., Specialized nutrition support: The standard of care, *J. Parenteral Enteral Nutr.*, 6:185, 1982.

32. Rosenbaum, E.H., *Nutrition for Cancer Patient*, Palo Alto, CA.: Bull Publishing Co., 1980.

33. Daeffler, R., Oral hygiene measures for patients with cancer, Part I, *Cancer Nurs.*, 3:347, Oct. 1980.

34. Morrow, G.R., Morrell, C., Behavioral treatment for the anticipatory nausea and vomiting induced by cancer chemotherapy, *N. Engl. J. Med.* 307(24):1476, Dec. 9, 1982.

35. Carson, J.A.S., Gormican, A., Taste acuity & food attitudes of selected patients with cancer, *J. Am. Diet. Assoc.* 70:361, 1977.

36. Whitworth, F.M., Consultation: Feeding the cancer patient, *Nursing '78*, p. 87, Oct. 1978.

37. Vickers, Z.M., et al., Food preference of patients with cancer, *J. Am. Diet. Assoc.* 79(4):441, Oct. 1981.

38. Fishman, J., Anrod, B., *Something's Got to Taste Good: The Cancer Patient's Cookbook*, New York: Andrews and McMeel, Inc., 1981.

39. Handron, K.T., Taste—The unnecessary sense? (letters), *N. Engl. J. Med.*, 308(9):529, March 3, 1983.

40. Meyer, C.D., Consultation: Treating Laetrile toxicity, *Nursing '80*, p. 90, Sept. 1980.

41. Moertel, C.G., et al., A clinical trial of amygdalin (Laetrile) in the treatment of human cancer, *N. Engl. J. Med.* 306(4):201, Jan. 28, 1982.

42. Eisele, J.W., Deaths related to coffee enemas, *JAMA*, 244(14):1608, Oct. 3, 1980.

43. Willet, W.C., et al., Relation of serum vitamins A and E and carotenoids to the risk of cancer, *N. Engl. J. Med.*, 310(7):430, Feb. 16, 1984.

44. Shilotri, P.G., Bhat, K.S., Effect of mega doses of vitamin A bactericidal activity of leucocytes, *Am. J. Clin. Nutr.* 30:1077, 1977.

45. Salonen, J.T., et al., Association between serum selenium and the risk of cancer, *Am. J. Epidemiol.* 120(3):342, September 1984.

46. Willett, W.C., MacMahon, M.D., Diet and cancer—An overview, Part 2, *N. Engl. J. Med.* 310(11):697, March 15, 1984.

47. Ohnuma, T., Holland, J.F., Nutritional consequences of cancer chemotherapy and immunotherapy, *Cancer Res.* 37(7):2395, July 1977.

48. Burkhalter, P.K., Cancer quackery, *Am. J. Nurs.* 77(3):451, March 1977.

49. Bowman, B.B., et al., Macrobiotics for cancer treatment and prevention, *J. Clin. Oncol.*, 2(6):702, June 1984.

Chapter 10

CARDIOVASCULAR DISEASE

Cardiovascular diseases are those involving the heart and blood vessels, including myocardial infarction (heart attack), hypertension, stroke, congestive heart failure, claudication, and angina pectoris. Most people in this country who suffer from these diseases have atherosclerosis—the development of widespread fatty plaques on the inside of the arteries. There is strong evidence linking dietary practices to the development of atherosclerosis, and dietary manipulation therefore is assuming increasing importance even though very little in the way of a clear-cut cause-and-effect relationship between the two has been proven.

Ischemic heart disease remains the leading cause of death in the United States (1). Most deaths from heart disease (76%) occur in those over 65; however, 23% of all heart disease deaths occur in persons 35–65 years of age (2). The first decline in age-specific coronary mortality in the United States was observed in 1964, the year the Surgeon General first warned about the hazards of cigarette smoking. That same year, the American Heart Association recommended a general change in diet, aimed at lowering dietary cholesterol and saturated fat, in the hope of reducing the risk of heart attack. The continued decline in heart disease over the last 20 years has been accompanied by a reduced per capita consumption of tobacco, milk, cream, butter, eggs, and animal fats.

Although atherosclerosis is a multifactorial disease, continued decline in coronary and cerebrovascular mortality depends on even more

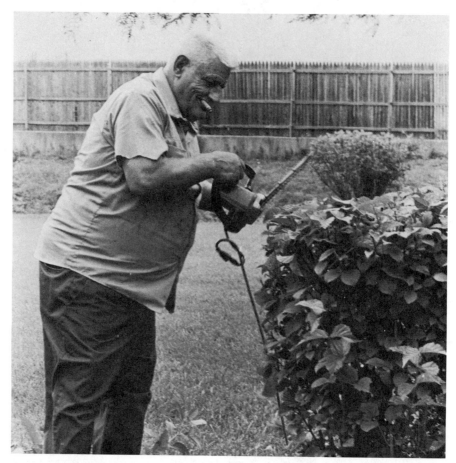

Some older adults exhibit multiple risk factors for cardiovascular disease. Photograph by L. Miller.

effective treatment of hypertension, continued reduction of cigarette smoking, and aggressive manipulation of dietary risk factors (1). In order to achieve control of ischemic heart disease, high-risk persons must be identified and treated with individual medical and dietary intervention. Concurrently, total-population-oriented preventive measures must be established (3). The mature adult will benefit from this approach, first through screening to identify risks, then from prevention protocols to reduce or control risk factors, and finally from the proper management of chronic problems, such as hypertension, to reduce mortality. Some have felt that older individuals will not benefit from life style changes, arguing that the coronary artery damage has already taken place and cannot be reversed. Recent evidence disputes this, demonstrating that if people 70 and older are willing to make significant changes in their life style, they can improve their functional capacity and health status (4).

HYPERLIPIDEMIA

Hyperlipidemia is an elevation of one or more of the lipids in the blood. It generally refers to increased levels of cholesterol or triglycerides. Hyperlipidemia is considered a major risk for coronary heart disease. In this respect, hypercholesterolemia is a more significant risk factor than hypertriglyceridemia.

There are differing opinions about what constitutes hypercholesterolemia. "Overt hypercholesterolemia" has been defined as concentrations over 260 mg/dl, which is the upper limit of normal for American adults (see Table 10-1). However, there is considerable evidence that plasma cholesterol contributes to atherogenesis at levels far below 260 mg/dl (5). The relationship between coronary heart disease (CHD) incidence and cholesterol is most significant above a level of 230 mg/dl (6). Furthermore, the Framingham data, derived from an older population, showed no myocardial infarction in those with plasma cholesterol levels under 180 mg/dl (7).

Although numerous epidemiologic studies have shown a positive correlation between plasma cholesterol levels and CHD, no one has yet defined precisely what this relationship is. The relationship may be linear over a broad range of values, with low levels constituting little risk and high levels accelerating atherogenesis rapidly (5). Current epidemiological evidence suggests that adult men should be considered as having mild hypercholesterolemia at levels in the range of 200–260 mg/dl (8). The impact of plasma cholesterol values must be considered concurrently with the presence or absence of other risk factors (e.g., hypertension, obesity, smoking, diabetes mellitus, and family history). Currently, it is widely believed that the increase in total cholesterol observed in Americans from adolescence through middle age is not a reflection of a biological phenomenom and therefore can be altered (3).

There are a number of tests that can help to determine how to handle a client with hypercholesterolemia. A plasma cholesterol level of less than 200 mg/dl requires no further immediate evaluation (5). Reevaluation on a yearly basis and reinforcement of good eating habits are all that is necessary.

Evaluation of plasma triglycerides is also important to establish a benchmark for continued care. In the presence of normal cholesterol levels, mild elevations of plasma triglycerides (less than 250 mg/dl) do not necessarily increase the risk for cardiovascular disease. The same is

Table 10-1   Serum Lipoprotein Values for Individuals 35 and Older

Age (yr)	Males (Percentiles)			Females (Percentiles)		
	5	50	95	5	50	95
Cholesterol Levels in Adults (mg/dL)*						
35–39	146	197	270	140	182	242
40–44	151	203	268	147	191	252
45–49	158	210	276	152	199	265
50–54	158	210	277	162	215	285
55–59	156	212	276	173	228	300
60–64	159	210	276	172	228	297
65–69	158	210	274	171	229	303
70 +	151	205	270	169	226	289

Age (yr)	Males (Percentiles)			Females (Percentiles)		
	5	50	95	5	50	95
Triglyceride Levels in Adults (mg/dL)						
35–39	54	113	321	40	73	176
40–44	55	122	320	45	82	191
45–49	58	124	327	46	87	214
50–54	58	124	320	52	97	233
55–59	58	119	286	55	106	262
60–64	58	119	291	56	105	239
65–69	57	113	267	60	112	243
70 +	58	111	258	60	111	237

*Values obtained from 10 communities in the USA and Canada.

true for normocholesterolemic adults with borderline hypertriglyceridemia (250–500 mg/dl) who have no risk factors for or family history of cardiovascular disease. Ranges of 250 to 500 mg/dl can be a marker for a subset of patients with a hereditary form of hyperlipoproteinemia. Dietary intervention as a primary approach is the usual course for this subgroup. Drug treatment may be needed for persons in this subgroup who do not respond to dietary treatment. Frank hypertriglyceridemia (triglyceride levels greater than 500 mg/dl) requires intervention by diet, adding drugs when necessary (9).

Unusually high triglyceride levels may be initiated by excessive caffeine intake, supplementation with vitamin A, or alcohol abuse.

Dietary intervention encourages the overweight patient to lose weight, increase physical activity, restrict alcohol intake, reduce the use of concentrated sweets, and adhere to a fat-restricted diet. In patients with severe hypertriglyceridemia, several months to a year must elapse before dietary and life style manipulations will effect a change in plasma values (10).

Table 10-1   *(Cont.)*

Age (yr)	Males (Percentiles)			Females (Percentiles)		
	5	50	95	5	50	95
*HDL Cholesterol in Adults (mg/dL)**						
35–39	29	43	62	34	52	82
40–44	27	43	67	33	55	87
45–49	30	45	64	33	56	86
50–54	28	44	63	37	59	89
55–59	28	46	71	36	58	86
60–64	30	49	74	36	60	91
65–69	30	49	78	34	60	89
70 +	31	48	75	33	60	91

Age (yr)	Males (Percentiles)			Females (Percentiles)		
	5	50	95	5	50	95
*LDL Cholesterol Levels in Adults (mg/dL)**						
35–39	81	131	189	76	116	172
40–44	87	135	186	77	120	174
45–49	98	141	202	80	127	187
50–54	89	143	197	90	141	215
55–59	88	145	203	95	148	213
60–64	83	143	210	100	151	234
65–69	98	146	210	97	156	223
70 +	88	142	186	96	146	207

*Values obtained from 10 communities in the USA and Canada.

Source: The Lipid Research Clinics Population Studies Data Book, US Dept. of Health and Human Services, publication No. (NIH) 80–1527, 1980.

As estimation of high-density lipoprotein (HDL) cholesterol is useful in patients with any degree of hypercholesterolemia. Because cholesterol is insoluble in aqueous solutions, unique proteins, called lipoproteins, solubilize lipids and complex with them to achieve transport in the plasma. The major cholesterol-carrying substance is low-density lipoprotein (LDL). LDL's carry two-thirds of the plasma cholesterol; the remainder is transported by HDL. Plasma LDL is derived from very low density lipoprotein (VLDL) after lipolysis of triglyceride. The most atherogenic lipoprotein is LDL, which can filter into the subintimal space of the arterial wall and deposit cholesterol (5).

Data from the Framingham study suggest that HDL cholesterol is the most predictive of all lipoprotein measurements for development of coronary heart disease (7). Numerous reports have suggested that high levels of HDL may protect against coronary heart disease. Although the function of HDL's has not been clearly defined, it is believed that it facilitates removal of cholesterol from peripheral tissues to the liver where it is catabolized and excreted (11). In adult men, an HDL level less than 35–40 mg/dl is considered abnormally low (5). Strenuous exercise, decrease in body weight, reduction of smoking, and a moderate alcohol intake all increase HDL levels. Higher HDL levels are found in females at all ages.

Patient management depends on many factors. For elderly patients, theoretically, lowering of lipid levels should prevent further development of atherosclerosis. Care of the individual patient will depend on age, past cardiac history, family history, and other medical problems. For the mature adult, aged 40–60, diet therapy should be more rigorous. Even though investigators are still not completely sure that lowering lipid levels will retard atherosclerosis and subsequently reduce the risk of coronary heart disease, the prevalence of heart disease is so high in patients with hyperlipidemia that treatment is wise (5, 11, 12).

Patient Management for Hyperlipidemia

As stated earlier, coronary heart disease is multifactorial so that maximum risk reduction should be achieved by multiple-risk-factor intervention. A patient's plasma lipid levels can be lowered in many ways—weight reduction, increased exercise, and dietary manipulations.

A number of studies have shown a large patient-to-patient variation in response to changes in dietary cholesterol intake (13, 14). Most patients, however, demonstrate a lowering of plasma cholesterol when dietary fat intake is lowered and changed from a low to a high P/S ratio (polyunsaturated/saturated) (15).

The American Heart Association (AHA) has developed a stepwise approach to lowering serum lipid levels (see Table 10–2). Phase 1 is designed primarily as a preventive approach for a person whose cholesterol level is higher than average and/or who has a family history of hyperlipidemia and/or other coronary heart disease risk factors. Phase 2 is advised as initial dietary treatment for those with cholesterol levels of 250 mg/dl or more, or for those who do not respond to Phase 1. Phase 3 is designed to achieve serum cholesterol reduction (15–20%) in patients with cholesterol levels over 275 mg/dl and/or high LDL levels (170 mg/dl or greater). If weight loss is necessary, any phase can be adjusted to a low-calorie pattern (16). Evaluations of the AHA recommendations are beginning to be reported in the literature, and not all are favorable (17). The diet pattern, however, is a balanced low-fat, low-cholesterol plan that can serve as the basis for diet counseling. Its effectiveness in reducing the risk of coronary heart disease may be proven over time.

Table 10-2 American Heart Association Stepwise Approach
for Lowering Blood Lipids

	Dietary goals for phases 1, 2, and 3		
	1	2	3
Fat	30–35%	30%	20–25%
Carbohydrate	45–50%	50%	55–60%
Protein	20%	20%	20%
Cholesterol (mg)	300	200–250	100
P/S ratio	1	1	1–2*

*At this level total fat intake, P/S ratio decreases because the limited
dietary fat sources contain primarily saturated fat, such as meat and
dairy products.

A major problem in treating clients with hyperlipidemia is dietary
compliance (6). Education, continued follow-up, and reevaluation are
essential (18). The client needs time and careful instruction to compre-
hend what a low-fat diet means. Consumers are often confused about
cholesterol and its major sources and do not recognize differences between various sources of fat. In addition, the effect of a low-fat diet
may not be seen for 2–3 months. Tables 10–3 and 10–4 will be useful for
client education.

Table 10-3 Eating Tips for a Low-Fat Diet

- Use liquid vegetable oils. Corn, soybean, sunflower, safflower, cottonseed
  (labeled Vegetable Oil), peanut, and olive oils.
- Choose margarines with "liquid vegetable oil" as their first ingredient.
  When margarines are high in polyunsaturated fat, they give this information
  on their label.
- Limit beef, lamb, pork, or ham. These foods should be eaten (in small
  amounts, 3–4 oz) only three times weekly. Use more fish, chicken, turkey,
  and veal. Shellfish can be substituted for meat. Do not use liver or other
  organ meats. Use dried peas and beans and lentils in place of meat two or
  more times weekly.
- Use lean cuts of meat. Trim off all visible fat. Cook without added fat.
  Bake, broil, or roast to further reduce fat.
- Use skim milk and skim milk cheese and yogurt. No butter, cream, sour
  cream, or whole milk should be used.
- Avoid nondairy creamers and whipped toppings. Coffee whiteners and
  nondairy whipped toppings are high in saturated fat.
- Use fruits and vegetables. Use all types raw or cooked, without added butter,
  cream, or sauce. Avoid avocado, olives, and coconut.
- Limit eggs. Eggs should be limited to three a week, cooked without butter.
  Egg whites can be used as desired: 2 egg whites = 1 egg.
- Use cereals, rice, macaroni. Whole-grain varieties offer fiber and nutrients.
  Avoid granola cereals and sauces made with fat.
- Use sparingly nuts, seeds, chocolate, peanuts, and peanut butter, all of
  which are high in fat.

Table 10–4 Improving the Nutritional Quality of Recipes

If the ingredient is . . .	Try this . . .	Nutritional benefits
Shortening	Oil (¾ cup oil = 1 cup shortening) Margarine made with liquid vegetable oil Reduce amount by one-fourth	Reduce saturated fat Reduce fat
Butter	Same as for shortening	Reduce saturated fat Reduce cholesterol Reduce fat
Eggs	Substitute egg whites (2 egg whites = 1 egg)	Reduce saturated fat Reduce cholesterol Reduce fat
Milk	Skim milk	Reduce saturated fat Reduce cholesterol Reduce fat
Sour cream	Low-fat plain yogurt, buttermilk, imitation sour cream	Reduce saturated fat Reduce fat
Red meat	Reduce amount Trim all visible fat	Reduce saturated fat Reduce fat
Poultry	Remove skin	Reduce fat
Salt	Reduce or eliminate Substitute herbs or spices	Reduce sodium
Sugar	Reduce amount by one-half	Reduce calories
Honey, molasses, maple syrup	Substitute frozen, concentrated, unsweetened fruit juice	Reduce calories Increase nutrients
Flour	Substitute with one-half whole-grain flour	Increase fiber Increase nutrients

A low-fat diet with a high ratio of polyunsaturated to saturated fatty acids is effective in lowering total serum cholesterol in middle-aged adults (19). Clients need to be counseled about fat distribution in common foods and to establish eating behaviors that rely on food choices with a ratio of polyunsaturated to saturated fat of 1 or greater (see Table 10–5). The ratio of saturated to unsaturated fat in the total diet is also important. It is generally agreed that dietary fat should be divided one-third from saturated fat, one-third from monounsaturates, and one-third from polyunsaturates. Saturated fats, mainly from animal sources, raise serum cholesterol levels. Polyunsaturates mainly from plant sources lower serum cholesterol and reduce clotting tendencies (platelet aggregation). Coconut and palm oils are the major exceptions in this group, being highly saturated. Monounsaturates were long considered as not affecting serum cholesterol, but recent evidence suggests that they too may have a beneficial effect (20). Olive and peanut oils and poultry fat are major sources of monounsaturated fatty acids.

Additional Dietary Considerations

Dietary modifications to manipulate lipogenic processes and affect blood lipid parameters are the subject of much ongoing research. These modifications in some cases may be impractical or may have adverse health consequences that must be considered in light of suspected benefits. Today, noteworthy scientific findings are often reported in the media. Clients may question the efficacy of these new treatments and/or attempt self-treatment when results may be preliminary. This underscores the need for the health professional to be conversant with, and capable of evaluating, recent research. Following is a brief description of several recent research findings worthy of note.

Investigators have been comparing the lipid-lowering effect of the omega-3 family of essential fatty acids (found mostly in fish oils) with the omega-6 essential fatty acids (found mainly in vegetable oils). Oilier, fattier fish are rich in omega-3 fatty acids—eicosapentaenoic acid (EPA) and docosahexaenoic acid (DHA). Greenland Eskimos who eat diets rich in fish oils have a low incidence of cardiovascular disease as well as increased bleeding times (21). Clinical trials have supported the theory that EPA can lower serum cholesterol more effectively than vegetable oils (22, 23). Use of EPA, sold in capsule form as Maxepa, cannot be recommended at this time because of the interferences with blood clotting. Increasing the consumption of fish high in EPA (salmon, mackerel, sea herring, anchovies, mullet, trout, catfish, smelt, canned sardines) may be beneficial and should pose no harm (24).

Variations in levels of dietary fiber consumption have been epidemiologically linked to variations in susceptibility to atherosclerosis. Studies have shown that food fiber is not a single substance and not all types have the same effect on lipid levels. Water-soluble fiber, oat bran, pectin, and guar gum have been shown to be most effective in lowering serum cholesterol levels in hyperlipidemic subjects (25, 26, 27). Increasing fiber in the diet may have many healthful benefits for the older adult, and it is a diet modification that should be encouraged. For guidelines on how to accomplish this change see Chapter 6.

Table 10–5 Distribution of Fats in Common Foods

Food	Amount	Total fat (g)	Total poly. fat (g)	Sat. fat	Mono. fat	P/S ratio	Chol
Cheese							
American cheese	1 slice	9	.2	5.6	2.1	1:28	27
Cheddar cheese	1 oz	9.2	0.28	5.4	3.52	1:19	45.5
Cream cheese	2 tbsp	10	.2	6.2	2.4	1:31	27
Creamed cottage cheese	4 oz	4.8	0.0	2.4	2.4	—	12
Egg							
Whole egg, large	1 large	6.2	0.5	2.2	3.5	1:4	253
Fats							
Butter	1 tsp	4	0.1	2.3	1.6	1:23	14
Coconut oil	1 tbsp	14	0.3	12.2	1.5	1:41	—
Corn oil	1 tbsp	14	7.1	1.7	5.2	4:1	—
Cottonseed oil	1 tbsp	14	7.0	3.5	3.5	2:1	—

	Serving					Ratio	
French dressing	1 tbsp	5.8	3.0	1.0	1.8	3:1	—
Italian dressing	1 tbsp	9	4.6	1.5	2.9	3:1	—
Lecithin	1 tsp	3.5	1.9	0.5	1.1	3.8:1	—
Margarine, stick	1 tsp	4	0.4	1.1	2.5	1:2.8	—
Mayonnaise	1 tbsp	12	6.0	2.1	3.9	2.8:1	8
Olive oil	1 tbsp	14	1.0	1.5	11.5	1:1.5	—
Peanut oil	1 tbsp	14	4.1	2.5	7.4	1.6:1	—
"Promise", stick	1 tbsp	11	4.62	1.76	4.62	2.6:1	—
"Promise," tub	1 tbsp	11	6.0	1.7	3.3	3.7:1	—
Russian dressing	1 tbsp	8.1	4.2	1.4	2.3	3:1	—
Safflower oil	1 tbsp	14	10.1	1.1	2.8	10:1	—
Soybean oil	1 tbsp	14	7.3	2.1	4.6	3.5:1	—
Sunflower oil	1 tbsp	14	10.0	2.0	2.0	5:1	—
Fish							
Lean fish	3.5 oz	3.1	0.6	0.5	2.0	1:1	70
Lobster	3.5 oz	1.5	0.2	0.5	0.8	1:2.5	85
Shrimp	3.5 oz	1.1	0.2	0.4	0.5	1:2	100
Tuna salad	3.5 oz	10.5	3.0	3.0	4.5	1:1	100
Tuna in water	3.5 oz	4.0	0.8	0.7	2.5	1:1	75

Table 10–5 (*Cont.*) Distribution of Fats in Common Foods

Food	Amount	Total fat (g)	Total poly. fat (g)	Sat. fat	Mono. fat	P/S ratio	Chol
Meats							
Bologna	1.5 oz	13.8	1.0	5.0	7.8	1:5	50
Beef liver	3.5 oz	5.1	0.0	1.3	3.8	—	250
Club steak, tr	3.5 oz	13.4	0.0	6.0	7.4	—	90
Club steak, untr	3.5 oz	39.4	1.0	18.0	20.4	1:18	100
Frank	2.0 oz	15.0	1.2	5.6	6.5	1:5	50
Ham, tr	3.5 oz	8.8	1.0	3.0	4.8	1:3	90
Ham, untr	3.5 oz	22.1	2.0	9.0	11.1	1:4.5	100
Leg of lamb, tr	3.5 oz	7.5	0.0	4.0	3.5	—	90
Leg of lamb, untr	3.5 oz	18.9	1.0	12.0	5.9	1:12	100
Pork loin, tr	3.5 oz	14.2	1.3	5.1	7.8	1:4	90
Pork loin, untr	3.5 oz	30.5	2.7	11.0	16.8	1:4	100
Round steak, tr	3.5 oz	7.0	0.0	4.0	3.0	—	90
Round steak, untr	3.5 oz	15.7	0.3	7.5	7.9	1:25	100
Rump roast, tr	3.5 oz	10.5	0.0	5.0	5.5	—	90
Rump roast, untr	3.5 oz	28.1	1.0	14.0	13.1	1:14	100
Sirloin, tr	3.5 oz	10.5	0.0	5.0	5.5	—	90
Sirloin, untr	3.5 oz	36.7	1.0	17.0	18.6	1:17	100
Spare ribs	3.5 oz	38.9	3.5	14.0	21.4	1:4	100
Veal breast, tr	3.5 oz	9.9	0.4	4.9	4.6	—	90
Veal breast, untr	3.5 oz	20.3	0.0	9.0	11.3	—	100

	Serving						
Veal, chuck, untr	3.5 oz	13.4	0.0	6.0	7.4	—	100
Veal, lean, tr	3.5 oz	6.0	0.0	2.8	3.2	—	90
Veal riblets, untr	3.5 oz	32.0	1.0	15.0	16.3	1:15	100
Milk and ice cream							
Ice cream	3.5 oz	12.5	0.0	7.0	5.5	—	60
Ice milk	3.5 oz	5.1	0.0	3.0	2.1	—	5
Sherbet	3.5 oz	1.2	0.0	0.7	0.5	—	—
Skim milk	1 cup	1	Trace	0.4	0.1	—	5
Sour cream	1 tbsp	3	0.1	1.6	0.6	1:16	5
Whole milk	1 cup	8	0.2	5.1	2.1	1:25	34
Nuts							
Almonds	1 oz	16.2	3.4	1.4	11.4	2.4:1	—
Cashews	1 oz	12.8	0.8	2.2	9.8	1:2.8	—
Peanut butter	1 tbsp	7.9	2.2	1.4	4.3	1.6:1	—
Peanuts	1 oz	13.9	2.5	2.0	9.4	1.3:1	—
Walnuts	1 oz	17.9	11.2	1.1	5.6	10:1	—
Poultry							
Chicken fryer, no skin	3.5 oz	3.6	1.1	1.1	1.4	1:1	75
Chicken with skin	3.5 oz	6.8	1.3	2.7	2.8	1:1	75
Turkey, no skin	3.5 oz	6.1	1.0	2.0	3.1	1:2	75
Turkey, with skin	3.5 oz	9.6	2.0	2.8	4.8	1:1.4	75

Poly = polyunsaturated; sat = saturated; mono = monounsaturated; chol = cholesterol; tr = trimmed; untr = untrimmed.

A study based on 20 healthy individuals and 68 patients with coronary heart disease measured the effects of essential oil of garlic on blood lipids over a 20-month period of time. The results indicated that both groups had significant reductions in serum cholesterol, triglycerides, and low-density lipoproteins (LDL), as well as increases in high-density lipoproteins (HDL). The precise mechanism of this effect of garlic is not known. The drawbacks to this finding are that the subjects had to eat the garlic 8 months or longer before results were evident, and they had to eat 30 g of raw garlic daily (the equivalent of 20 peeled, medium garlic cloves) (28).

Sucrose polyester, a synthetic lipid, is currently under investigation. It has the physical and culinary properties of dietary fat but is totally nonabsorbable. In a carefully controlled study with chronically obese subjects, both weight loss and positive change in serum lipids were demonstrated (29). In familial hypercholesterolemic subjects the cholesterol-lowering effect was small but statistically significant (30). There are some mild gastrointestinal side effects with subjects consuming 40 g/day or more of sucrose polyester. With FDA approval, which is anticipated shortly, sucrose polyester may be a new and effective treatment for obesity and hyperlipidemia.

Suggestions that chelation therapy or large doses of nutrients will retard or cure coronary disease or arterial atherosclerosis have not been proven (31, 32, 33). In some instances the treatment may be dangerous, particularly for an older adult and/or may have a negative impact on serum lipids (34, 35).

HYPERTENSION

Hypertension (high blood pressure) or elevated systolic or diastolic arterial pressure is found in persons of all ages. It has been estimated to affect 20% of the total population in the United States. It is, however, more prevalent in older than younger persons (36). Eleven percent of the population between the ages of 35 and 45 have hypertension. The prevalence rises to 30% between ages 60 and 65, and in men over 70 the incidence of hypertension ranges between 40 and 65%. Hypertension causes increased cardiovascular morbidity and mortality. The risk is greater in the old than in the young, as great for older women as for older men, and most prevalent in blacks in later years (37).

The cause of the elevation in blood pressure is, in about two-thirds of all cases, unknown. These cases of hypertension are termed ''essential'' or idiopathic. In other situations, the cause of hypertension is secondary to renal and endocrine disorders. In these cases the causative disorder must be treated as well as the blood pressure. In cases of unknown etiology, only the high blood pressure symptom is treated.

Healthy young adults have arterial pressure readings of about 120 mm Hg for the systolic (given as the upper figure in the reading) and 80 mm Hg for the diastolic. For most people in Western societies there is an increase in these readings with age, but the increase is variable. There is a possible physiological need for higher pressure to compensate for decreased cardiac output that might otherwise result in inadequate perfusion of the brain, kidneys, and heart. In addition, the patient's weight and other conditions at the time of examination affect the blood pressure readings. For these reasons, it is hard to define precisely what blood pressure levels in an elderly individual constitute hypertension that requires treatment.

A National Health Examination Survey has shown that systolic blood pressure tends to rise slowly during early adulthood with a steep rise after age 40. Diastolic pressure rises steadily until age 60 after which there tends to be a slight decline (38). Today most practitioners feel that the goal of hypertensive therapy for the older adult is to maintain systolic pressure between 140 and 160 mm Hg and diastolic between 90 and 104 mm Hg (39, 40). Elevation in blood pressure, coupled with increasing age, shortens survival. There is clear evidence that older hypertensive patients are at greater risk for coronary heart disease, congestive heart failure, and stroke. For this group as well as for middle-aged men systolic pressure appears to be a better predicter of cardiovascular morbid events than diastolic pressure (37, 39). Frequently health practitoners debate the validity of treating asymptomatic older hypertensive patients. Recent evidence suggests that further debate is fruitless since therapy delays morbid events and fatal complications making it beneficial to lower blood pressure at any age (36, 37).

Nutrition and Hypertension

In recent years, considerable evidence has developed about the effectiveness of nonpharmacological treatment for hypertension. In the Hypertension Detection and Follow-Up Program, subjects 60–69 years of age had a 16.4% reduction in mortality owing to a stepped-care approach to treatment (41). A similar program in Chicago aimed at middle-aged men (aged 40–59 years at entry) demonstrated that long-term improvements in eating and exercise yielded a moderate sustained weight loss preventing high blood pressure in hypertension-prone persons and controlling high blood pressure in persons with established mild hypertension (42). This hygienic treatment—weight loss, simple changes in diet and life style—is beneficial to older persons who often suffer side effects from drug therapy for high blood pressure. For younger, mature adults, hygienic treatment can delay the need for pharmacological intervention. These community-based, long-term population studies showed that all groups benefited from treatment—whites, blacks, men, and women (37).

Although it is well known that weight loss reduces blood pressure, it is not widely appreciated that this mechanism operates independent of sodium intake (43, 44). The correlation between increases in body weight and increases in blood pressure is particularly strong in middle-aged adults. In addition, it is becoming increasingly evident that the distribution of calories in the diet may have an impact on blood pressure. Percent of total fat, reduction of saturated fat, and adjusting polyunsaturated-saturated fat ratio to exceed 1 all have been associated with lower blood pressure (36, 45). Heavy alcohol intake, in excess of 2 oz ethanol/day, may initiate hypertension (46, 47). (One ounce of ethanol is equal to 2 oz of 100-proof whiskey, 8 oz of wine or 24 oz of beer.) Moderate alcohol intake does not appear to affect hypertension so that it is not necessary for the older adult to be abstinent unless alcohol is contraindicated by antihypertensive medications.

The efficacy of using a sodium-restricted diet to manage hypertension has come under question recently. Many issues still need to be resolved.

The first known effective treatment for hypertension with salt restriction was reported in 1904 (48). This and other early experiences used drastic salt restriction in patients with established hypertension. One of the most famous, originating in the early 1940s, was the Kempner rice-fruit diet (44). As antihypertensive agents were discovered and used effectively in the 1950s, salt restriction became a less popular approach to treatment (48).

Currently no ideal drug regimen has been found so there is renewed interest in determining whether and how much dietary sodium will influence blood pressure control. Furthermore, it is clear from epidemiological studies that the majority of hypertensive individuals are in the mild range. There is concern and controversy about the wisdom of subjecting these asymptomatic patients to a lifetime of medication when they have only mild disease (48). The bulk of research on salt restriction has shown blood pressure reduction with severe salt restriction. This has led to the misconception that salt abstinence is needed for a significant antihypertensive effect. Experience with moderate salt restriction as the primary therapy of hypertension is not extensive but does show a small but significant lowering of pressure (44). To confuse the issue even further, researchers now realize that some hypertensive patients are salt sensitive whereas others are salt resistant. There is no way of predetermining whether an individual is salt sensitive or salt resistant. Nonetheless, a fraction of hypertensive patients do react favorably to salt restriction with a normalization of pressure (47).

Low-Sodium Diets for Older Adults

Even though all the questions regarding sodium restriction and hypertension have not been answered, it still seems prudent to advise older clients to restrict sodium intake. A recent study indicated that reductions from 13 g of salt intake to 10 g a day can cause a 5-to-10-mm reduction in blood pressure. This may not appear to be a significant reduction. However, for the older mild hypertensive patient, it could reduce borderline hypertension to the normal range and/or decrease the amount of medication needed to lower blood pressure (43). A study of a nursing home population showed the same degree of blood pressure control on a 2- or 4-g sodium diet. The 4-g-sodium diet is easier to prepare and more palatable for the residents (49). Most individuals over 50 require some type of medication to help control blood pressure. If diurectics are given, reducing sodium intake will enhance their effect (48). For elderly patients with isolated systolic hypertension, sodium restriction and weight control is a preferred therapy (36).

Moderate sodium restriction—intake of 2–4 g of sodium/day (5–9 g of salt) will usually produce a modest but definite fall in blood pressure. This diet is sometimes referred to as the "no-salt-shaker diet" because, although small amounts of salt may be used in cooking, no salt is added at the table. In addition, all prepared and processed foods to which salt has been added as a preservative or flavoring are excluded. These include all salted and smoked meats and fish such as bacon, ham, bologna, and other luncheon meats, anchovies, salt cod, and condiments such as seasoned salt, bouillon cubes, catsup, pickles, olives, soy cause, and Worcestershire sauce. Salted snacks such as chips, nuts, popcorn and pretzels may not be eaten. Some ordinarily salty foods such as cheese and peanut butter and now readily available (and tasty) in low-sodium versions, and these should be used in place of the usual salty types.

A major problem with a low-sodium diet is adherence on the part of the client. The use of client education materials along with follow-up by health care professionals may increase long-term adherence (50). Tables 10–6, 10–7, and 10–8 should be helpful in client counseling. For a listing of the sodium content of common antacids see Table 6–2, page 94.

Table 10–6 Sodium Content of Common Foods

Food	Sodium (mg)	Portion
Corn, fresh	1	1 ear
Peanuts	1	4 tbsp
Oatmeal, regular, cooked, no salt added	1	¾ cup
Pineapple, canned	1	1 slice
Butter, sweet	2	1 tbsp
Coffee	2	6 oz
Herb-Ox Low-sodium Beef Broth	9	1 packet
Celery, raw	25	1 stalk
Campbell's Low-Sodium Corn Soup	30	10¾ oz
Carrots, raw	34	1 medium
Saltine	35	1 cracker
Butter, salted	50	1 tsp
Chicken	57	3 oz
Fudge	60	1 oz
Egg	70	1 medium
Graham cracker	95	1 large
Peas, frozen	106	½ cup
Pepperidge Farm White Bread	117	2 slices
Whole milk	130	1 cup
Planters Cocktail Peanuts	132	1 oz
White bread	140	1 slice
Heinz Tomato Ketchup	154	1 tbsp
Skippy Creamy Peanut Butter	167	2 tbsp
Lay's Potato Chips	191	1 oz
Worcestershire sauce	206	1 tbsp
Kraft American Cheese	238	1 slice (1 oz)
Kellogg's Corn Flakes	260	1 oz
Peanuts, salted	275	¼ cup
Taco Bell Bean Burrito	288	Entire serving
Campbell's Tomato Juice	292	4 oz
Oscar Mayer Bacon	302	3 slices
Wish-Bone Italian Salad Dressing	315	1 tbsp
Tomato juice	320	½ cup
Del Monte Sweet Peas, canned	349	½ cup
Beef	381	3 oz
Jell-O Chocolate Instant Pudding	404	½ cup
Devil's Food Pudding Cake Mix	435	1/12 of a cake
Frankfurter	495	1
English muffin, buttered	466	Entire muffin
Oscar Mayer Bologna	672	3 slices
Burger King Whaler	735	Entire serving
Herb-Ox Instant Broth, beef	818	1 packet

Table 10–6   (*Cont.*)

Food	Sodium (mg)	Portion
Burger King Whopper	909	Entire serving
Campbell's Beans & Franks	958	8 oz
Heinz Dill Pickles	1137	1 large pickle
Swanson Fried Chicken Dinner	1152	Complete dinner
Chef Boy-Ar-Dee Beefaroni	1186	8 oz
Soy sauce	1320	1 tbsp
McDonald's Big Mac	1510	Entire serving
Kentucky Fried Chicken Dinner, extra crispy	1915	Dinner for 1 person
Kentucky Fried Chicken Dinner, original recipe dinner	2285	Dinner for 1 person

Foods naturally high in sodium

Artichokes	Greens	Milk
Celery	Spinach	Beets
Carrots	Egg white	White turnip

Foods naturally low in sodium

Fruits	Shredded wheat	Rice
Coffee and tea	Puffed rice	Pasta
Jelly	Fresh fish	Oatmeal

A method of urine testing has recently been described that improves adherence to dietary sodium restriction by offering immediate feedback to the patient on the amount of sodium being excreted in the urine. When patients were instructed on this technique, which involves overnight urine collections, two-thirds of the group studied were able to decrease their dietary sodium intake by one-third or more (51).

If the individual is taking a diuretic, potassium balance must be considered. For the older patient, both hypokalemia and hyperkalemia can be life-threatening. Most often balance can be maintained by dietary means. See Table 10–9 for a list of the potassium content of common foods. A maintenance dose potassium supplement is 900 mg. The client should be advised to have the equivalent in dietary sources.

A study of the usefulness of potassium-containing salt substitutes to replace the potassium lost in diuretic therapy found them to be uniform from sample to sample of each brand as well as among different brands. They are less expensive than prescription potassium supplements, which may also be unpleasant to take. Thus, potassium-containing salt substitutes might serve a dual function: seasoning food

Table 10–7   Sodium-Containing Additives

Additive	Use
Sodium saccharin	Artificial sweetener
Monosodium glutamate (MSG)	Seasoning, flavor enhancer, sold under brand names—Accent, Lawry's, McCormick
Sodium pyrophosphate	Buffer and texturizer used in tuna and instant pudding mix
Sodium silicate	Anticaking agent in salt
Sodium nitrite	Preservative in cured meats
Sodium ascorbate	Vitamin C
Sodium benzoate	Preservative in soda, relishes, sauces, salad dressings
Sodium carboxymethyl cellulose	Stabilizer in frozen deserts, salad dressings, chocolate milk
Sodium sulfite	Used to bleach maraschino cherries or to preserve some dried fruits
Sodium hydroxide	Used in processing ripe olives, fruits, and vegetables to soften skins
Sodium propionate	Mold inhibitor used in bread, cake, pasteurized cheese
Sodium erythorbate	Preservative in processed meat such as hot dogs

Table 10–8   How to Break the Salt Habit

Empty your salt shaker and don't refill it.

Reduce or eliminate salt used in cooking. Don't add salt when cooking rice, pasta, or vegetables; it is not needed.

Limit the use of processed foods, especially "convenience" foods like TV dinners, pot pies, canned soups, gravies, sauces, and seasoned rice mixes.

Substitute low-salt snacks like fresh fruit; vegetable sticks; unsalted nuts, pretzels, or popcorn for the usual salty nibbles.

Stay away from salt-preserved foods like bacon, bologna, anchovies, sardines, pickles, sauerkraut, and olives.

Watch out for salty condiments like soy sauce, ketchup, Worcestershire sauce. Use lemon, vinegar, herbs, spices (not garlic, onion, and celery salt) instead.

In restaurants, ask them not to salt or use MSG when food is prepared.

Use low-salt varieties of cheeses, canned tuna, peanut butter, and unsalted margarine and sweet butter.

Table 10-9 *500 Milligrams Potassium from Common Food Sources*

1 medium banana	1 ¼ cups orange juice
1 ¼ cups grapefruit juice	1 cup prune juice
½ cantaloupe	1 large white or sweet potato
⅓ cup lentils	¾ cup kidney beans
1 ¼ cups milk	2 small tomatoes

and combating the hypokalemia that may result from diuretic therapy (52). The salt substitutes should be used with caution and under a physician's supervision. Potassium salt substitutes are not appropriate for individuals with impaired renal function.

Some recent evidence has shown an important interface between calcium and sodium metabolism in blood pressure regulation. Although it is too early to make specific therapeutic recommendations, it appears that low calcium intakes are negatively correlated with blood pressure in man. In experimental models dietary modification of calcium altered blood pressure in both normotensive and hypertensive humans (53). Because of this, it would be wise to determine whether a hypertensive client has a low dietary calcium intake and encourage an intake in line with recommendations set forth in Chapter 11. This increased calcium may have an impact on blood pressure regulation while also offering other health benefits.

On occasion a strict sodium restriction may be ordered by the physician such as in the case of congestive heart failure (54). Diet usually consists of 1000 mg sodium/day. In addition to following the guidelines for a moderate sodium restriction, no salt is used in cooking. There is also limited intake of vegetables that are high in sodium, such as beets, carrots, celery, kale, white turnips, dandelion, mustard and beet greens, spinach, and Swiss chard. Regular canned vegetables, vegetable juices, soups, meat, and fish may not be used. There are several varieties of canned soups, vegetables, and tuna processed without added salt and these are allowed. All commercially prepared baked products, other than those labeled low sodium, should not be eaten. Because meat, milk, and milk products like yogurt are high in natural sodium, their use is limited as well.

NUTRITIONAL MANAGEMENT OF MYOCARDIAL INFARCTION

Nutritional management of the postmyocardial infarction patient begins in the intensive care unit and continues for the patient's lifetime (55).

Once a person has had a myocardial infarction, dietary measures must be taken to help ensure recovery and to help decrease the risk of infarction in the future. During the first few hours after a myocardial infarction, the patient may have nausea from increased vagal tone, from ongoing pain, or from medications given. Thus solid food should be withheld until any nausea has subsided. For at least a few days, after infarction, extremes of hot and cold should be avoided in the food served, as these may set up vagal reflexes that might slow the heartbeat or decrease blood pressure. There is little or no good evidence supporting the idea that coronary care unit patients should avoid drinking tea or coffee, but these beverages are commonly withheld (56). If restriction of caffeine-containing beverages is causing the patient undue anxiety, they may be included in moderation (<2 cups/day) unless the patient is experiencing arrhythmias (55).

A diet restricted to 2–4 g of sodium/day is advisable as congestive heart failure may be caused by excess sodium, especially in the setting of a recent myocardial infarction. A somewhat high dietary fiber content is advisable for those patients who can tolerate it, since constipation is a frequent problem for bedridden individuals, and it is especially important that coronary patients not increase vagal tone unnecessarily as would happen with straining to have a bowel movement. The coronary care unit is a stressful place to be, with little to offer clear distinction between day and night, and little or no available contact with family or friends. Therefore, every effort should be made, within reason, to allow the patient the opportunity to choose meals that are similar to his usual, so as to allow some elements of familiarity in a very unfamiliar environment.

After leaving the coronary care unit, a moderate sodium-restricted diet is almost always continued and is advisable. See Table 10–8 for patient teaching strategies. Little or no alcoholic beverages should be consumed as ethanol is a depressant to the myocardium and may precipitate an episode of congestive heart failure. If angina continues to be a problem, especially if occurring soon after eating, small frequent meals, eaten slowly, and the avoidance of very cold food will usually alleviate the problem. Further dietary recommendations depend on the patient's serum lipid levels and the presence of any other disease processes (56). Potassium levels must also be monitored (see Table 10–9). The majority of cardiac rehabilitation patients will require nutrition counseling for the modification of cholesterol and saturated fat intake. Follow-up and support in a nutrition education program tailored to their needs can affect a sustained positive change in eating behavior (55, 57).

Patient aids:

Grocery Guide: Tips on Wise Food Selection

available from:

American Heart Association
National Center
7320 Greenville Ave.
Dallas, TX 75231

Sodium: Facts for Older Citizens

available from:

U.S. Department of Health and Human Services
Public Health Services
Food and Drug Administration
5600 Fishers Lane
Rockville, Maryland 20857
HHS No. 83–2169

A Word About Low-Sodium Diets

available from:

U.S. Department of Health & Human Services
Public Health Services
Food and Drug Administration
5600 Fishers Lane
Rockville, Maryland 20857
HHS No. 84-2179

REFERENCES

1. Walker, W.J., Changing U.S. life style and declining vascular mortality—A retrospective, *N. Engl. J. Med.* 308:649, March 17, 1983.

2. Harper, A.E., Coronary heart disease—an epidemic related to diet? *Am. J. Clin. Nutr.* 37:669, April 1983.

3. Tyroler, H.A., Cholesterol and cardiovascular disease, *Am. J. Cardiol.* 54:14C, August. 27, 1984.

4. Weber, P., Barnard, J.R., Roy, D., Effects of a high-complex-carbohydrate, low-fat diet and daily exercise on individuals 70 years old and older, *J. Gerontol.* 38:155, 1983.

5. Grundy, S.N., Questions and answers on hyperlipidemia, *Geriatrics* 36: 101, Sept. 1981.

6. McNamara, D.J., Dietary and serum cholesterol and coronary heart disease, *Nutr. & M.D.* XI:1, Jan. 1985.

7. Kannel, W.B., Castelli, W.P., Gorden, T., Cholesterol in the prediction of atherosclerotic disease: New perspectives on the Framingham study, *Ann. Intern. Med.* 90:85, 1979.

8. The Pooling Project Research Group, Relationship of blood pressure, serum cholesterol, smoking habit, relative weight and ECG abnormalities to incidence of major coronary events: Final report of the pooling project research group, *J. Chronic Dis.* 31:201, 1978.

9. Treatment of hypertriglyceridemia, Consensus Conference, *JAMA* 251: 1196, March 2, 1984.

10. Hypertriglyceridemia, *Nutri. & M.D.* XI:4, Jan. 1985.

11. Hyperlipidemia, what to do about the lipid to-do, *Patient Care* 14:14, Oct. 30, 1980.

12. Nash, D.T., Cholesterol and atherosclerosis—Fact or fiction? *Geriatrics* 36:128, January 1981.

13. Roberts, S.I., McMurry, M.P., Connor, W.E., Does egg feeding (i.e. dietary cholesterol) affect plasma cholesterol levels in humans? The results of a double-blind study, *Am. J. Clin. Nutr.* 34:2092, Oct. 1981.

14. Ahrens, E.H., The Evidence relating six dietary factors to the nation's health, *Am. J.Clin. Nutr.* 32:2621, 1979.

15. Samuel, P., McNamara, D.J., Shapiro, J., The role of diet in the etiology and treatment of atherosclerosis, *Ann. Rev. Med.* 34:179, 1983.

16. *AHA Recommendations for the Treatment of Hyperlipidemia*, Dallas, Texas: American Heart Association, 1984.

17. Reiser, R., A commentary on the rationale of the diet-heart statement of the American Heart Association, *Am. J. Clin. Nutr.* 40:654, 1984.

18. Majonnier, M.L., et al., Experience in changing food habits of hyperlipidemic men and women, *J. Am. Diet. Assoc.* 77:140, Aug. 1980.

19. Ehnholm, C., et al., Effect of diet on serum lipoproteins in a population with a high risk of coronary heart disease, *N. Engl. J. Med.* 307:850, Sept. 30, 1982.

20. Mattison, F.H., Grundy, S.M., Comparison of effects of dietary saturated, monounsaturated and polyunsaturated fatty acids on plasma lipid and lipoproteins in man, *J. Lipid Res.* 26:194, 1985.

21. Gunby, P., It's not fishy: Fruit of the sea may foil cardiovascular disease, *JAMA* 247:729, 1982.

22. Gutafson, T.M., Effects of 11-week increases of dietary eicosapentantoic acid and bleeding time, lipids and platelet aggregation, *Lancet* 2:1190, 1981.

23. Illingworth, D.R., Harris, W.S., Connor, W.E., Inhibition of low density lipoprotein synthesis by dietary omega-3 fatty acids in humans, *Arteriosclerosis* 4:270, May/June 1984.

24. Fish oils, serum lipids and platelet aggregation, *Nutr. & M.D.* XI:5, Jan. 1985.

25. Kirby, R., et al., Oat-bran intake selectively lowers serum low-density lipoprotein cholesterol concentrations of hypercholesterolemic men, *Am. J. Clin. Nutr.* 34:824, May 1981.

26. Story, J.A., The role of dietary fiber in lipid metabolism, *Adv. Lipid Res.* 18:229, 1981.

27. Jenkins, D.J., et al., Dietary fiber blood lipid: Treatment of hypercholesterolemia with guar crisp bread, *Am. J. Clin. Nutr.* 33:575, 1980.

28. Bordia, A., Effect of garlic on blood lipids in patients with coronary heart disease, *Am. J. Clin. Nutr.* 34(10):2100, 1981.

29. Glueck, C.J., Sucrose polyester and covert delution, *Am. J. Clin. Nutr.* 35:1352, June 1982.

30. Glueck, C.J., et al., Sucrose polyester: Substitution for dietary fat in hypocaloric diet in the treatment of hypercholesterolemia, *Am. J. Clin. Nutr.* 36:347, 1983.

31. Hooper, P.I., et al., Vitamins, lipids and lipoproteins in healthy elderly population, *Int. J. Vitamin Res.* 53:412, 1983.

32. Johnson, G.E., Obenshain, S.S., Nonresponsiveness of serum high-density lipoprotein-cholesterol to high dose ascorbic acid administration in normal men, *Am. J. Clin. Nutr.* 34:2088, 1981.

33. Crouse, S.F., et al., Zinc ingestion and lipoprotein values in sedentary and endurance-trained men, *JAMA* 252:785, Aug. 10, 1984.

34. Hooper, P. L., et al., Zinc lowers high-density lipoprotein cholesterol levels, *JAMA* 244:1960, Oct. 1980.

35. Chelation therapy, *JAMA* 250:672, Aug. 5, 1983.

36. *The 1984 Report of the Joint National Committee on Detection, Evaluation and Treatment of High Blood Pressure*, U.S. Dept. of Health and Human Services, NIH, No. 84–1088, June 1984.

37. Kirkendall, M.N., Hammond, J.J., Hypertension in the elderly, *Arch Intern. Med.* 140:1155, Sept. 1980.

38. Garvas, I., Garvas, H., Special considerations in treating hypertension in the elderly, *Geriatrics* 35:34, July 1980.

39. Tucker, R.M., Is hypertension different in the elderly? *Geriatrics* 35:28, May 1980.

40. Lucas, C.P., Omar, M., Pretreatment assessment of the hypertensive patient, *Geriatrics* 35:51, Jan. 1980.

41. Gifford, R.W., Dustan, H.P., Management of hypertension in the elderly (letter), *N. Engl. J. Med.* 303:1233, Nov. 20, 1980.

42. Stamler, J., et al., Prevention and control of hypertension by nutritional-hygienic means, *JAMA* 243:1819, May 9, 1980.

43. Hypertension in the elderly: A pathophysiologic approach to therapy, *J. Am. Geriatr. Soc.* 30:352, May 1982.

44. Laragh, J.H., Pecker, M.S., Dietary sodium and essential hypertension: Some myths, hopes and truths, *Ann. Intern. Med.* 98(Part 2):735, May 1983.

45. Puska, P., et al., Controlled, randomized trail of the effect of dietary fat on blood pressure, *Lancet* 1:1, 1983.

46. Friedman, G.D., Klatsky, A.L., Siegelaub, A.B., Alcohol intake and hypertension, *Ann. Intern. Med.* 98(Part 2):846, 1983.

47. Dustan, H.P., Nutrition and hypertension, *Ann. Intern. Med.* 98(Part I):660, May 1983.

48. Wilbur, J.H., The role of diet in the treatment of high blood pressure, *J. Am. Diet. Assoc.* 80:25, Jan. 1982.

49. Hadler, M.H., The lack of benefit of modest sodium restriction in the institutionalized elderly, *J. Am. Geriatr. Soc.* 32:235, March 1984.

50. Morisky, D.M., et al., Five-year blood pressure control and mortality following health education for hypertensive patients, *Am. J. Pub. Health* 73:153, Feb. 1983.

51. Kaplan, N.M., et al., Two techniques to improve adherence to dietary sodium restriction in the treatment of hypertension *Arch. Intern. Med.* 142:1638, 1980.

52. Sopko, J.A., Freeman, R.M., Salt substitutes as a source of potassium, *JAMA* 238:608, 1977.

53. Mc Carron, D.A., Calcium, magnesium and phosphorus balance in human and experimental hypertension, *Hypertension* 4(Suppl. III): 27, Sept.-Oct. 1982.

54. Feldman, E.B., Does nutrition play a role in cardiovascular disease? *Geriatrics* 37:65, July 1980.

55. Palmer, S., Sonnenberg, L., Cardiac rehabilitation: role of the dietetian in a multidisciplinary team, *Am. J. Intravenous Ther. Clin. Nutr.*, 11(3):9, March 1984.

56. Wenger, N.K., Guidelines for dietary management after myocardial infarction, *Geriatrics* 34:75, Aug. 1979.

57. Kris-Etherton, P.M., et al., Modifications of food intake by myocardial infarct patients, *J. Am. Diet. Assoc.* 83:39, July 1983.

Chapter 11

OSTEOPOROSIS, GOUT, AND ARTHRITIS

Osteoporosis, osteomalacia, gout, and arthritis are a group of disparate conditions often grouped together because they all involve some aspect of the skeletal system. Osteoporosis, osteomalacia, and gout are often the result of metabolic derangements, certain medications, or dietary practices. Nutritional factors may be important aspects of their cause, or at least part of their exacerbation. Thus, it follow that nutritional considerations are an important part of the prevention or treatment of these conditions.

Arthritis, itself encompassing a wide range of disparate conditions, is less clearly due to specific metabolic derangements or other factors that would lead nutritional intervention to logically be a part of its treatment. Nonetheless, probably because currently accepted treatment of many of the conditions lumped into the category of "arthritis" is often inadequate, many arthritis sufferers turn to nutritional "treatments" in hope of obtaining relief from discomfort or deformity.

OSTEOPOROSIS

Osteoporosis, the most common bone disease affecting older adults, refers to decreased bone mass that leads to an increased number of fractures. Bones may become so brittle and weak that stepping off a curb or even repositioning the body may cause a fracture. Some authorities use the term *osteoporosis* only after fractures have developed, while *osteopenia* is used to describe gradual adult bone loss (1). It is estimated that 1.3 million fractures yearly in persons over 45 are due to osteoporosis (2). Severe bone loss can be present for many years before clinical or laboratory signs appear. Symptoms include persistent, nonradiating low-back pain, loss of height, and increased kyphosis of the dorsal spine. Often the individual will have no symptoms at all until the first fracture occurs. Three or four out of every 10 women over age 65 have fractures, often of the hip, and 12 to 20% of those with hip fractures die within 6 months (3).

Vertebral bone loss begins in young adulthood and continues throughout life (4). There is an accelerated loss of bone in many women during and after menopause and a similar, but less extensive, loss of bone in the aging male. By the end of a woman's life, she has lost 42% of the bone mass from her spine while men lose 10%. Only 10 to 15% of men develop osteoporosis, and then usually after age 60 or 70. Women are afflicted more frequently, and at an earlier age, often in their 50s.

As much as 30–35% of the bone may be lost before it can be detected on routine skeletal X rays (5). Bone loss also affects the teeth-bearing bone of the upper and lower jaw. This loss of peridontal bone is estimated to affect 80% of adults in the United States and is a major cause of tooth loss (6).

The earlier the age of menopause, the greater is the subsequent risk for osteoporosis and hip fracture. Calcium is not well absorbed and is readily excreted when estrogen is lacking, resulting in negative calcium balance (7). Recent studies suggest that it is the estrogen deficiency, not aging, that may be the main cause of bone loss during the first two decades after menopause (8). Premenopausal women who have amenorrhea associated with vigorous exercise frequently have decreased circulating estrogen levels and decreased bone mass (9). Estrogen treatment after oophorectomy or menopause reduces bone loss.

The amount of bone mass at maturity, age 30–35, is another factor in the etiology of osteoporosis. It may be that individuals who have had high calcium intakes since childhood reach adulthood with more bone quantity. Blacks, in general, have greater skeletal mass than whites, who therefore are at greater risk for osteoporosis. Short women and both men and women who are slender are also at greater risk (10, 11). Obesity, along with the thicker skeleton needed to support the weight, and perhaps increased circulating estrogens, may protect against excess calcium loss and bone resorption. Physical activity is a likely factor in the progression of osteoporosis as there is a positive correlation between muscle weight and bone mass (12). Mechanical stress is needed to maintain bone mass, and physical exercise can inhibit or reverse bone loss in areas where skeletal forces are exerted (13). Prolonged bedrest and immobilization increases bone loss.

Smoking has been associated with an increased risk of hip fractures, possibly because women who smoke have earlier menopause, which puts them at greater risk (14). Alcohol use, especially when coupled with smoking puts the individual at increased risk of developing osteoporosis (10).

Hyperthyroidism and hyperparathyroidism lead to general loss of bone, as does long-term use of corticosteroids (15, 16). Overuse of magnesium-containing antacids (Maalox or Mylanta) impairs calcium absorption, while high levels of aluminum-containing antacids (Gelusil) taken for a long period of time can block the absorption of phosphates by bone.

Dietary Factors

Deficiences of calcium and vitamin D, as well as increased acid and phosphate loads resulting from high intake of meat, soda, and processed foods, all have been found to be involved in the development of osteoporosis. Persons who eat large amounts of meat have decreased bone density when compared to vegetarians. The increased acid loads that are formed from meat and soda are buffered partially at the expense of bone minerals. High-protein diets cause increased urinary excretion of calcium, which may add to this effect (17).

CALCIUM

High calcium intake throughout life may be protective against osteoporosis. It has been shown that higher bone mineral content and resistance to hip fractures are associated with a calcium intake of from 800 to 1100 mg, rather than intakes of 350 to 500 mg. (18). This latter intake is typical of women in the United States. With aging, there is a decline in intestinal absorption of calcium and a more negative calcium balance (19). Young adults can accommodate a lower calcium intake by absorbing more. Those with osteoporosis and nonosteoporotic persons over age 65, are not able to adapt to low dietary calcium intakes by increasing absorption.

After menopause, the amount of calcium needed to maintain calcium balance increases from about 1000 mg a day to nearly 1500 mg. This is about three times the amount that is commonly ingested. Some experts believe that this increase in calcium could reduce the incidence or severity of osteoporosis in most people (20). Treatment with 1.2 g daily of calcium was found to decrease bone loss and the incidence of vertebral fractures in postmenopausal women. Calcium balance was improved as well. Another prospective study showed that giving 1.5 g/day of elemental calcium for 2 years reduced the rate of bone loss and improved calcium balance (21). Another study of a group of subjects with an average age of 70, showed that even the elderly can benefit from supplementary calcium and calcium-rich foods (22). Although some studies do not show a beneficial effect from calcium supplementation, the majority suggest improvement in calcium balance, reduced skeletal demineralization, and compensation for the increased calcium requirements imposed by menopause.

Few foods are rich sources of calcium (see Table 11–1). Many of the richest sources—milk, cheese, and ice cream—are avoided by many adults because they believe them to be ''fattening'' or ''bad'' for them because of their saturated fat and cholesterol content. Milk, cheese, and many other dairy products are available in low-fat forms that contain all the calcium and other minerals in milk but much less fat. Fortified skim milk has even more calcium than regular milk, as it has dry milk solids added to improve the flavor.

The vegetable sources of calcium are not as valuable as they might appear based on the amounts listed in Table 11–1. Spinach, rhubarb, collards, mustard greens, Swiss chard, okra, beets, and beet greens contain oxalic acid, which can chelate calcium and make it unavailable for absorption. Phytic acid, which is found in the bran of cereals, can also complex with calcium so that it is not absorbed. Sardines and canned salmon are excellent sources of calcium only when eaten with their softened bones.

Calcium is absorbed best in adults when the ratio of calcium to phosphorus in the diet is 1:1. In most foods, there is much more phosphorus than calcium. Meat, poultry, and fish average 15 to 20 times as much phosphorus as calcium, while eggs supply 4 times as much. Only milk, most natural cheese, and green leafy vegetables contain more calcium than phosphorus. In view of these facts and keeping in mind the high intake of phosphate-containing soda and additives like disodium phosphate, calcium phosphate, and sodium pyrophosphate, many Americans take in four times as much phosphorus as calcium.

Besides interfering with calcium absorption, high-phosphorus, low-calcium diets have been shown to cause soft-tissue calcification and bone loss in some lower animal species. This may not be true in man as it is not seen in nonhuman primates. In fact, 1 g phosphorus supplements has resulted in increased calcium retention in osteoporotic postmenopausal women (23). The role of phosphorus in osteoporosis is con-

Table 11–1 Food Sources of Calcium

Food	Portion	Calcium (mg)
Almonds	12 nuts	38
Beef	3 oz	10
Beet greens	1 cup	144
Bread, white enriched	1 slice	24
Bread, whole wheat	1 slice	24
Broccoli	½ cup	68
Butter	1 tbsp	3
Cheese, American	1 oz (1 slice)	195
Cheese, cheddar	1 oz	204
Cheese, cottage, creamed	¼ cup	34
Cheese, cream	1 oz	23
Cheese, mozzarella (whole milk)	1 oz	163
Cheese, Swiss	1 oz	259
Collards	1 cup	357
Crackers, graham	2 crackers	10
Custard	½ cup	161
Egg	1 medium	28
Figs	2 figs	40
Ice cream	½ cup	99
Kale	1 cup	157
Margarine	1 pat	2
Milk, buttermilk	1 cup	296
Milk, nonfat dry (reconstituted)	1 cup	298
Milk, skim (1% fat)	1 cup	300
Milk, skim plus milk solids (protein fortified)	1 cup	349
Milk, whole	1 cup	291
Mustard greens	1 cup	193
Nuts, Brazil	4 nuts	28
Oatmeal, cooked	½ cup	11
Okra	10 pods	98
Orange juice	1 cup	25
Peanuts, roasted without skin	1 tbsp	5
Peas, cooked	½ cup	22
Perrier water	1 cup	32
Rhubarb	1 cup	211
Salmon	3 oz	167
Sardines	3 oz	372
Shrimp	3 oz	98
Spinach	1 cup	51
Swiss chard	1 cup	130
Tofu	3 oz	128
Tuna	3 oz	7
Tums (antacid)	1 tablet	200
Turkey	3 oz	7
Walnuts	¼ cup	41
Yogurt	1 cup	293

troversial and complex. Meat, which is high in both phosphorus and protein, has its effect on calcium metabolism moderated.

Because of the difficulty of achieving calcium intakes of 1000–1500 mg from foods, calcium supplements should be used in addition to rich food sources to reach the desired level. As the calcium content of supplements is low, it is necessary to take several tablets daily. Calcium carbonate is the most concentrated form, 40% calcium. Other forms include calcium gluconate, which is about 9%, and calcium lactate, 15% (24).

Calcium carbonate is available as tablets or liquid. The often-used antacid Tums contains 200 mg of calcium in one tablet. Problems with calcium carbonate are that it is very insoluble, and its absorption is reduced when there is achlorhydria. Prolonged used may cause constipation. Calcium lactate and calcium gluconate are more soluble, but because they contain less calcium per weight they must be taken in larger quantities. As these tablets are large, crushing or breaking them will make swallowing easier. The crushed tablet can be mixed into food. Taking the tablet with a little milk may increase absorption because of the lactose in the milk. Liquid forms of calcium carbonate and calcium glubionate are available, but are relatively expensive.

Bone meal and dolomite (calcium magnesium carbonate) are often promoted as "natural" calcium supplements. They can be dangerous because of the possibility of contamination with toxic minerals such as lead, arsenic, mercury, and aluminum. It is not true that the magnesium content of dolomite allows better absorption of the calcium. The only beneficial effect of magnesium is that it counteracts the constipating effect of calcium carbonate.

Daily intakes of up to 2500 mg of elemental calcium are safe for normal persons, including the elderly. Such intakes do not result in hypercalcemia, kidney stones, or calcification of soft tissue (20). If a patient has a history of forming calcium stones, a thiazide diuretic is often given to decrease the urinary concentration of calcium (25).

FLUORIDE

Sodium fluoride is the only substance that can actually increase bone formation. It increases bone matrix production, which then becomes mineralized if sufficient calcium is given. Fluoride has not been approved by the Food and Drug Administration for use in the treatment of osteoporosis. Its use is restricted to investigative studies at the present. Epidemiological studies show that persons living in areas where the water is fluoridated have greater bone densities than those living where the water contains low fluoride levels (26). Fluoride given alone results in defective bone formation, but adding fluoride to a calcium-and-estrogen-treated group of osteoporotic postmenopausal women virtually abolished fractures after 1 year of treatment (27). Fluoride at levels used for treating osteoporosis can cause side effects of nausea, vomiting, gastric ulcers, and joint pain or swelling (28).

VITAMIN D

Vitamin D is another nutrient studied in the treatment of osteoporosis. This vitamin can be obtained in some foods—fortified milk and margarine, yeast, fish liver oils. Ultraviolet radiation on the skin converts 7-dehydrocholesterol to vitamin D. The biologically active form of the vitamin, 1,25-dihydroxy vitamin D [1,25-$(OH)_2$D], is formed by the hydroxylation of "D" in the liver and kidney. This hormonelike vitamin is responsible for regulating the absorption of calcium and phosphorus and its subsequent deposition in the mineralization of bone.

Severe and prolonged deficiency of vitamin D leads to osteomalacia, where the bones are not mineralized normally. Some researchers believe that disturbances in the metabolism of vitamin D might be a factor in osteoporosis as well.

Studies have reported lower blood levels of 1,25-dihydroxy vitamin D in elderly subjects than in young adults. This corresponds to a fall in calcium absorption seen in aging (20). Other studies show lower blood levels of 1,25-dihydroxy vitamin D in persons who have osteoporosis (29). It is hypothesized that there may be some problems converting vitamin D to its active form, and this in turn prevents the older adults from adapting to low calcium intakes.

Administering 0.5 mcg a day of synthetic 1,25-dihydroxy vitamin D to older patients and postmenopausal osteoporotic women increases calcium absorption and improves calcium balance (30). Because of the dangers of toxicity with hypercalcemia and hypercalciuria, active vitamin D is not believed to be useful as a preventive measure. It may have potential as a treatment for severe osteoporosis, but when used for that purpose it requires careful monitoring of serum calcium.

Elderly persons may consume little vitamin D in food and also may have little exposure to sunlight coupled with a reduced ability to convert the vitamin to its active form. Therefore, many elderly persons should be given a supplement of vitamin D, particularly in the winter. Studies show that the elderly have significantly higher levels of vitamin D in their plasma in summer than in winter (31). Because toxic effects from vitamin D supplementation have occurred at levels as low as 2000–5000 IU (50 to 125 mcg) daily, no one should consume more than 600–

800 IU (15 to 20 mcg) daily unless specifically recommended by a physician (32).

Osteomalacia

In 1885, when osteopenia was first described, osteomalacia and osteopenia were not clinically separated from one another. Indeed, it is often difficult to tell them apart. *Osteopenia* is bone thinning with no change in the mineral composition of the bone whereas *osteomalacia* refers to impaired mineralization of the bone matrix (1). Bone volume can be normal, increased or decreased, but mineralization is reduced. Osteomalacia is due to metabolic abnormalities such as vitamin D deficiency, vitamin D resistance, or hypophosphatemia.

   Long-term use of high levels of aluminum-hydroxide-containing antacids can block bone absorption of phosphates and is the most common cause of osteomalacia, developing in as little as 3 weeks. Substitution of antacids that do not contain aluminum can reverse the condition.

   Insufficient dietary intake of vitamin D and lack of exposure to sunlight is another cause of osteomalacia in older adults (33). It can be cured by 20-minute exposure to ultraviolet light daily, which causes a rapid increase in plasma 25-hydroxy vitamin D (34).

GOUT

Gout is an error of metabolism in which an excess amount of uric acid appears in the blood. Uric acid in the body is synthesized from glycine and the degradation of purines. Those with gout do not eliminate uric acid normally, so that it can precipitate out of the blood into the tissues. Deposits of sodium urate crystals that occur in the small joints and surrounding soft tissue can be disfiguring, as well as disabling. In chronic gout, these deposits, called *tophi*, are often found in the helix of the ear. The disorder is found more often in males, who may first show symptoms around age 35. A smaller number of women are affected and usually do not show symptoms until after menopause (35). It is estimated that nearly two million persons in the United States have this disorder.

   Gout attacks most often manifest as sudden pain in the large toe radiating up the leg. Control of serum uric acid level is imperative. If levels are allowed to rise to 9.0 mg/dl or more (3 to 7 mg/dl is the normal range), there is an 83% chance that the patient will develop acute gouty arthritis, which leads to joint destruction and severe crippling. Gout can usually be controlled if treated appropriately.

Avoidance or correction of obesity is recommended, as is a diet low in fat and alcohol. The use of alcohol will not induce an attack; however, lactic acid, which appears during ethanol metabolism, disrupts the metabolism of uric acid and results in renal retention of urate. Overindulgence or moderate chronic use of alcohol is not advisable. When a person is found to have an elevated uric acid level for the first time, the individual should be questioned about alcohol use (36).

Fasting can precipitate a gouty attack. Many gout sufferers are overweight, and reducing will make their management easier. The weight loss plan should be formulated so that it is slow and gradual. A sudden weight loss may lead to the development of ketonemia and then precipitate a gout attack.

Diuretic therapy can also induce a gout attack. A gouty condition may surface for the first time as a result of a therapeutically increased fluid excretion when hypertensive treatment is initiated.

Although the effect of a low-purine diet in lowering blood uric acid is modest compared with the effect of drug therapy, excess intake of dietary purines should be avoided. Foods high in purines include organ meats, dried peas and beans, lentils, sardines, anchovies, bacon, beef, cod, halibut, perch, pork, turkey, and veal. The diet should be high carbohydrate, low fat, and moderate in protein. A high-carbohydrate diet has a tendency to increase uric acid excretion whereas a high-fat diet retards excretion. In a few persons with frequent attacks that are difficult to control and in whom drug therapy is poorly tolerated, a moderate restriction of protein to 50 g/day may be indicated (37). Caffeine, theophylline, and theobromine found in coffee, tea, and cocoa are metabolized to methylurates but are not deposited as gouty tophi. Thus these beverages need *not* be avoided (35). Liberal fluid intake of 10–12 cups/day is advised.

During an acute attack, a diet that is high in carbohydrate and low in fat and protein should be used. Fluids should be increased up to 3 liters/day to aid in the excretion of uric acid and to minimize the formation of renal stones.

ARTHRITIS

Arthritis is a major cause of disability commonly afflicting older adults; it occurs most often in the fifth and sixth decades of life. It is estimated that as many as 31 million people in the United States are affected by the more than 100 ailments grouped under the label arthritis. Osteoarthritis, rheumatoid arthritis, as well as scleroderma, lupus, and other arthritic conditions are often found in older adults.

The most common type of arthritis is osteoarthritis, degenerative joint disease. It affects mainly the large weight-bearing joints such as the hips and knees. Women with osteoarthritis have larger skinfolds, a higher proportion of body fat, and greater muscle girth compared to women with osteoporosis (9). Osteoarthritis occurs after the late fifties, and approximately 16 million people in the United States require some medical treatment for this disorder.

Another 6.5 million adults are afflicted with the more serious rheumatoid arthritis. It tends to recur with pain, swelling, and eventual deformities affecting many joints of the body but mainly in the hands. Three times as many women as men have rheumatoid arthritis. It usually starts in young and middle adulthood between the ages of 20 and 45.

A wide variety of nutritional interventions have been proposed as being useful for various forms of arthritis. With few exceptions, these treatments are based on little or no scientific information and have not been subjected to controlled clinical trials.

As early as the 1940s, vitamin preparations were studied for potential use in the treatment of arthritis (38). More recently, vitamin C and pyridoxine have been suggested as possibly helpful (39). Vitamin C depletion from tissues can occur with the use of high doses of aspirin such as those used for rheumatoid arthritis and should be replenished (40). In addition, vitamin A derivatives hold some promise as potential agents for future treatment of certain arthritides (41).

Several nonscientific publications have printed articles that purport to link arthritic conditions to food allergy. This has become particularly frequent since the advent of RAST (Radioallergosorbent Test) testing for food allergy, which almost invariably yields positive test results even in individuals who have no demonstrable food allergy. The medical literature has occasional reports linking rheumatoidlike arthritis to certain food allergies (42,43,44). However, most of these articles describe only individual cases. Nonetheless, several researchers have shown that certain food allergies can, in fact, in some cases, cause pain and swelling of the joints (45,46,47). thus although this idea cannot be fully discounted in all cases, it is safe to say that the vast majority of arthritis bears no relationship at all to food allergy. Therefore, elimination diets, including the popular diet that eliminates all nightshade vegetables, have no place in the treatment of arthritis.

It is common for arthritis sufferers to wear jewelry, especially bracelets, made from copper or zinc. Most people who wear such jewelry believe that the jewelry itself is useful in reducing their arthritic pain, especially in the nearby joints. There is some information about the antiinflammatory properties of copper that may explain how this actually happens (48, 49). In addition, some researchers have shown that oral copper or zinc supplements may be useful in decreasing the inflammation in rheumatoid arthritis (50, 51).

Despite the somewhat promising results mentioned in several of the above reports and studies, nutritional intervention other than maintaining a balanced diet, eliminating nutrient deficiencies, and preventing osteoporosis is not a major aspect of the treatment of arthritis. It is important to remind arthritis patients of this so that they are not led to disregard sound medical advice regarding nonnutritional treatment.

Patient aid:

Arthritis, Basic Facts That Can Help You

available from:

Arthritis Foundation
1314 Spring Street, N.W.
Atlanta, Georgia 30309

Patient aid:

Are You At Risk for Bone Disease?

available from:

National Dairy Council
6300 North River Road
Rosemont, Illinois 60018

REFERENCES

1. Thomson, D.L., Frame, B., Involutional osteopenia: Current concepts, *Ann. Intern. Med.* 85:789, 1976.
2. Peck, W.A., et al., *National Institutes of Health Consensus Development Conference statement: Osteoporosis*, April 2–4, 1984, Office of Medical Applications Research, NIH, Bethesda, MD.
3. Raisz, L.G., Osteoporosis, *J. Am. Geriatr. Soc.* 30(2):127, 1982.

4. Riggs, B.L., et al., Differential changes in bone mineral density of the appendicular and axial skeleton with aging: Relationships to spinal osteoporosis, *J. Clin. Invest.* 67:328, 1981.

5. Lachman, E., Osteoporosis: The potentialities and limitations of its roentgenologic diagnosis, *Am. J. Roentgenol. Radium Ther. Nucl. Med.* 74:712, 1955.

6. Albanese, A.A., et al., Problems of bone health—A ten year study, *N.Y. State J. Med.* 75:328, 1975.

7. Paganini-Hill, et al., Menopausal estrogen therapy and hip fractures, *Ann. Intern. Med.* 95:28,1981.

8. Richelson, L.S., et al., Relative contributions of aging and estrogen deficiency to postmenopausal bone loss, *N. Engl. J. Med.* 311:1273, 1984.

9. Cann, C.E., et al., Decreased spinal mineral content in amenorrheic women, *JAMA* 251(5):626, 1984.

10. Seeman, E., et al., Risk factors for spinal osteoporosis in men, *Am. J. Med.* 75:977, 1983.

11. Dequeker, J., et al., Osteoporosis and osteoarthritis (osteoarthrosis): Anthropometric distinctions, *JAMA* 249:1448, 1983.

12. Doyle, F., et al., Relationship between bone mass and muscle weight, *Lancet* 1:391, 1970.

13. Aloia, J.F., Exercise and skeletal health, *J. Am. Geriatr. Soc.* 29:104, 1981.

14. Williams, A.R., et al., Effect of weight, smoking and estrogen use on the risk of hip and forearm fractures in postmenopausal women, *Obstet. Gynecol.* 60(6):695, 1982.

15. Adinoff, A.D., Hollister, J.R., Steroid-induced fractures and bone loss in patients with asthma, *N. Engl. J. Med.* 309:265, 1983.

16. Hahn, T.J., Corticosteroid-induced osteopenia, *Arch. Intern. Med.* 138:882, 1978.

17. Lutz, J., Linkswiler, M., Calcium metabolism in postmenopausal and osteoporotic women consuming two levels of dietary protein, *Am. J. Clin. Nutr.* 34:2178, 1981.

18. Matkovic, V., et al., Influence of calcium intake, age and sex on bone, *Calcif. Tissue Res.* 22 (Suppl.) 393, 1977.

19. Bullamore, J.R., et al., Effects of age on calcium absorption, *Lancet* 2:535, 1970.

20. Heaney, R.P., et al., Calcium nutrition and bone health in the elderly, *Am. J. Clin. Nutr.* 36:986, 1982.

21. Recker, R., et al., Effect of estrogens and calcium carbonate on bone loss in postmenopausal women, *Ann. Intern. Med.* 87:649, 1977.

22. Lee, C.S., Effects of supplementation of the diets with calcium and calcium-rich foods on bone density of elderly females with osteoporosis, *Am. J. Clin. Nutr.* 34:819, 1981.

23. Goldsmith, R.S., et al., Effect of phosphorus supplementation on serum parathyroid hormone and bone morphology in osteoporosis, *J. Clin. Endocrinol. Metab.* 43:523, 1976.

24. Seeman, E., Riggs, B.L., Dietary prevention of bone loss in the elderly, *Geriatrics* 36(9):71, 1981.

25. Wasnick, R.D., et al., Thiazide effect on the mineral content of bone, *N. Engl. J. Med.* 309:344, 1983.

26. Bernstein, D.S., et al., Prevalance of osteoporosis in high and low fluoride areas in North Dakota, *JAMA* 198:499, 1966.

27. Riggs, B.L., et al., Effect of the fluoride-calcium regimes on vertebral fracture occurrence in postmenopausal osteoporosis, *N. Engl. J. Med.* 306:446, 1982.

28. Bikle, D.D., Fluoride treatment of osteoporosis: A new look at an old drug, *Ann. Intern. Med.* 98(6):1013, 1983.

29. Gallagher, J.C., et al., Impaired intestinal calcium absorption in postmenopausal osteoporosis: Possible role of vitamin D metabolites and PTH, *Clin. Res.* 24:360A, 1976.

30. De Luca, H., New developments in the vitamin D endocrine system, *J. Am. Diet. Assoc.* 80:231, 1982.

31. Dattani, J.T., et al., Vitamin D status of the elderly in relation to age and exposure to sunlight, *Hum. Nutr. Clin. Nutr.* 38C:131, 1984.

32. Osteoporosis—Consensus conference, *JAMA* 252(6):799,1984.

33. Corless, D., et al., Vitamin D status in long stay geriatric patients, *Lancet* 1:4044, 1975.

34. Jung, R.T., Ultraviolet light: An effective treatment of osteomalacia in malabsorption, *Br Med J.* 1:1668, 1978.

35. Bayles, T.B., Nutrition in diseases of the bones and joints, in: *Modern Nutrition in Health and Disease*, R.S. Goodhart and M. E. Shils, eds. Philadelphia: Lea & Febigier, 1973.

36. Drum, D.F., Elevation of serum uric acid as a clue to alcohol abuse, *Arch. Intern. Med.* 141:447, March 1981.

37. Kalman, E., Can diet help in the fight against arthritis? *Environment. Nutr. Newsletter* 4(4):1, 1981.

38. Freyberg, R.H., Treatment of Arthritis with vitamin and endocrine preparations, *JAMA* 119:1165, 1942.

39. Horrobin, D.F., et al., Treatment of the SICCA syndrome with EFA, pyridoxine and vitamin C, *Prog. Lipid Res.* 20:253, 1981.

40. Sahud, M.A., Cohen, R.J., Effect of aspirin ingestion on ascorbic acid levels in rheumatoid arthritis, *Lancet* 1:937, 1971.

41. Brinckerhoff, C.E., et al., Inhibition by retinoic acid of collagenase production in rheumatoid synovial cells, *N. Engl. J. Med.* 303:432, 1980.

42. Zussman, B.M., Food hypersensitivity simulating rheumatoid arthritis, *South. Med. J.* 59:935, 1966.

43. Parke, A.L., Hughes, G.R.V., Rheumatoid arthritis and food: A case study *Br. Med J.* 282:2027, 1981.

44. Catterall, W.E., Allergy and arthritis, *Ann. Rheum. Dis.* 36:594, 1977.

45. Millman, M., An allergic concept of the etiology of rheumatoid arthritis, *Ann. Allergy* 30:135, 1972.

46. Zeller, M., Rheumatoid arthritis—Food allergy as a factor, *Ann. Allergy*, 7:200, March-April, 1949.

47. Denman, A.M., et al., Joint complaints and food allergic disorders, *Ann. Allergy* 51:260, 1983.

48. Milano, R., et al., Concerning the role of endogenous copper in the acute inflammatory process, *Agents Actions* 9:581, 1979.

49. Whitehouse, M.W., Walker, W.R., Copper and inflammation, *Agents Actions* 8:85, 1978.

50. Conforti, A., et al., Copper and ceruloplasmin activity in rheumatoid arthritis, *Advances in Inflammation Research* Vol. 3, S. Gorini, et al., ed., N.Y., Raven Press, 1982, pp. 237–243.

51. Simkin, P., Oral zinc sulfate in rheumatoid arthritis, *Lancet* 2:539, 1976.

Chapter 12

NEUROLOGIC DISEASE

Neurologic diseases, following only cancer and heart disease in frequency, are a major cause of death and disability in the elderly (1). Patients with stroke, Parkinson's disease, and dementia not only have an impaired ability to feed themselves, but often also have specific nutritional requirements or restrictions as important aspects of their treatment. The following is a review of what is known about the effects of nutrients on brain function and the specific nutritional implications of the most common neurologic problems seen in the elderly.

For many years, people have believed that dietary intake has effects on the brain (2). Deficiencies of certain nutrients such as thiamin or vitamin B_{12} have long been known to affect the nervous system, but except for these isolated examples, researchers have not known until recently how the diet may affect the brain.

In elderly persons, low blood levels of riboflavin or folic acid have been correlated with poor abstract calculating ability, while low blood levels of vitamin C or B_{12} have been correlated with poor memory and poor abstract calculating ability (3). Furthermore, vitamin C supplements and multivitamin supplements have been shown to improve the mental status of long-term nursing home patients (4,5). Poor memory and poor reasoning ability often make the older person more prone to accidents or injury. These problems may be caused by poor nutrition and may be corrected by nutritional supplementation. Therefore, it is understandably very important to maintain good nutrition in the elderly, especially if there is a coexistent neurologic disease that may impair mental status.

Alterations in sleepiness, and in the craving for carbohydrates, and changes in brain serotonin levels have all been shown to be affected by the diet, specifically the carbohydrate and tryptophan intake (6,7). The true significance of these effects is not yet known, but it has been suggested that this information will lead to a better understanding of obesity and sleep disorders.

DEMENTIA

Most of us are not surprised when an elderly person is occasionally forgetful or is confused for a short period of time. In fact, adults of all ages are occasionally forgetful or confused, and this becomes more common with advancing age. With aging there is atrophy of the brain, and mild degrees of memory loss and confusion are considered a normal part of the aging process. (8,9)

Marked memory loss, along with confusion, poor judgment, and poor reasoning ability, is referred to as dementia and (although there is some dispute on this point) will probably occur in all persons if they live long enough (8,10). This decline in intellectual capacity is often associated with personality changes, such as decreased adaptability and suspiciousness toward change. These personality changes lead many older persons to have an increased need for a stable environment and also lead to a tendency toward conservative opinions. It is important to note that being conservative and disliking changes in the surroundings do not mean a person is demented. However, strictly speaking, most elderly persons have some degree of dementia, though it progresses at different rates in different people, and people differ in their ability to compensate for it.

There are many different causes of dementia, some of which are reversible, such as nutritional deficiencies (11). However, the most common cause of dementia, Alzheimer's disease, is irreversible, progressive, and of unknown origin. Alzheimer's disease is a major cause of death and disability among the elderly in the United States. At least 5% of persons over age 65 suffer severe dementia from Alzhemier's disease, and an additional 10% of persons over 65 suffer mild-to-moderate Alzheimer's disease (12). Alzheimer's disease is presently the fourth leading cause of death in the elderly, and it has been estimated that, with the proportion of elderly persons in our population growing, by the year 2050 Alzheimer's disease may be the leading cause of death in the

United States (13). Alzheimer's disease presently is also a major cause of disability in this country, with over 25% of all nursing home beds being occupied by these patients.

Maintaining adequate nutrition can be difficult in an individual who is very forgetful and has poor judgment. Persons with dementia do best in an uncluttered, well-organized environment and with consistent routines; therefore, it is a good idea to develop a daily routine for mealtimes and adhere to it strictly. The patient may forget that a meal was eaten and may try to eat again. Thus it may be necessary to keep food locked up between meals. Also, condiments may need to be locked up between meals to avoid the patient's consuming large amounts of ketchup or vinegar and becoming ill.

Having to choose from among a number of food selections may be quite confusing for the demented person, so it is best to minimize the number of food choices presented. It is also important not to serve food that is too hot since these patients often lack the judgment necessary to wait for food to cool off, and thus they may burn their mouth or throat.

As the disease progresses, the patient may develop poor coordination, balance, and mobility. This will increase the chance for accidents in the kitchen or dining area. It is important for the patient to wear washable clothes at mealtime, but bibs should *not* be used, as they cause embarrassment and frustration in the person with Alzheimer's disease.

It is best to serve food on plastic dishes. These may be purchased with suction cups on the underside and with vertical lips at the edge to aid the person with poor coordination. Finger foods should make up a major portion of the menu and are certainly preferable to pureed food or baby food for individuals who are still able to participate in their own feeding (14). Such foods include soft sandwiches, tomato wedges, French fries, hard-boiled eggs, canned sardines, fish fillet. Further discussion of feeding techniques for the patient with Alzheimer's disease can be found later in this chapter in the section on Feeding the Person with a Movement Disorder.

In advanced Alzheimer's disease, the patient is often unwilling or unable to feed himself or be fed. In this situation, placement of a gastrostomy tube may be the only alternative.

In caring for individuals with poor memory, poor judgment, and poor communication skills, it is important to be aware of the usual food intake. This is because a change in the amount of food eaten may be the only indication one has of a change in the patient's well-being. Illness, depression, or injury in a person with dementia may be manifest only as a decrease in food intake.

Although the exact cause of Alzheimer's disease is unknown, many experts believe it may be due to a low production of acetylcholine (a neurotransmitter) in certain parts of the brain (12,13). For this reason, persons with Alzheimer's disease have been given large amounts of lecithin (which is broken down to choline) in an attempt to increase the production of acetylcholine from choline in the brain. Others have proposed additional nutritional supplements as being potentially useful in Alzheimer's disease. At this time, however, it has not been conclusively shown that any treatment has a significant effect on Alzheimer's disease.*

STROKE

A stroke is damage to the brain from lack of blood supply. This may be caused by blockage of a blood vessel leading to the brain or by rupture of a blood vessel in the brain. Stroke is the third leading cause of death in the United States. The incidence of stroke increases with age. It has been estimated that at least two million people now alive in the United States have suffered a stroke, and one-third of them were rendered unemployable by their stroke (10). Unfortunately, most people have serious handicaps after a stroke, such as partial or complete paralysis, blindness or vision impairment, speech impairment, and coma. It is uncommon for these handicaps to completely resolve.

In an individual who has had a stroke, maintaining adequate nutrition may be quite difficult. However, it is crucial since adequate nutrition is needed to prevent muscle wasting and allow for recovery of as much strength as possible. Furthermore, meals should be planned so as to allow the psychologically important activity of eating to continue as normally as possible for a person who has suffered a major loss of body function and perhaps independence as well.

Specific recommendations about eating for the patient with a movement disorder will be discussed later in this chapter. Here, however, it should be noted that the stroke patient may have a wide range of neurologic problems that may interfere with normal feeding. Virtually all stroke patients experience some recovery of neurologic function, often as long as 12 months after their stroke. It is important to be aware of a patient's neurologic impairments and frequently reevaluate the patient's abilities as recovery and rehabilitation continue.

The person who has had a stroke should be evaluated initially for gag reflex, difficulty swallowing, paralysis of the muscles of the face,

*Further information on Alzheimer's disease and other forms of dementia may be obtained from Alzheimer's Disease and Related Disorders Association (ADRDA), 360 N. Michigan Avenue, Suite 601, Chicago, Illinois 60601.

sensory impairments (including diminished temperature sensation and impairment of vision), difficulty with communication, and difficulty performing hand-to-mouth movements, since impairment of any of these will lead to a serious feeding problem (15). In addition, it is important to be aware that some stroke patients may have persistent dizziness and nausea. Others may be too weak to sit upright or may have muscle spasms or contractures that prevent them from sitting or lying normally.

Aspiration of saliva or food is a constant concern in the stroke patient with a poor gag reflex or with difficulty swallowing. If the gag reflex is absent, a feeding tube may be necessary. If there is ever any question about a patient's gag reflex, feeding should not be attempted unless there is equipment and trained personnel available for immediate suctioning, should this be necessary (16).

Treatment of persons who have had a stroke usually includes one or more of the following: aspirin, Persantine (dipyridamole), and Coumadin (warfarin). Coumadin is an anticoagulant that acts by blocking the action of vitamin K. Coumadin is one drug whose activity is affected greatly by other medications and diet. Any person who takes Coumadin should be instructed to avoid sudden changes in the amounts of food or alcohol consumed (17). Also the patient should avoid eating large quantities of foods rich in vitamin K (see Table 17-4, p. 257).

PARKINSON'S DISEASE

Parkinsonism occurs in the latter part of life; most frequently in late middle age. It is an incurable, progressive degenerative condition involving the central nervous system. It is characterized by slowness of movement (bradykinesia), difficulty initiating movement (akinesia), involuntary tremulous motion, and muscle weakness. The slowness, rigidity, and tremors create feeding problems. In addition, most patients with Parkinson's disease suffer a moderate inability to suck, close lips, bite, chew, and swallow. They exhibit poor grasp, poor hand-mouth coordination, and poor control over the trunk and arms (18).

Feeding Disabilities

For those with Parkinson's disease, meals are laborious, greatly prolonged, and intensely frustrating. A positive mealtime attitude and an attractive meal presentation can go a long way toward overcoming physical difficulties with feeding. Specific recommendations about feeding devices to aid the person with Parkinson's disease continue independent feeding are discussed later in this chapter.

Food/Medication Interaction

Parkinson's disease affects the mature brain as a result of a deficiency of the neurotransmitter dopamine. This deficiency cannot be restored directly since dopamine is destroyed by peripheral tissue and does not cross the blood-brain barrier. Instead, a precursor that can enter the brain and produce dopamine is given. Levodopa (Larodopa) is an amino acid that can effect dramatic relief of symptoms. Since levodopa is absorbed and transported by the same mechanisms that transport other amino acids, its action may be compromised by a high protein intake. It has been suggested that patients taking levodopa restrict their daily dietary intake to 0.5 g protein/kg of body weight. This is below the recommended (RDA) intake of 0.8 g protein/kg. If the protein sources are of high biological value (meat, poultry, fish, eggs, cheese, milk), this recommendation should be adequate (19). Others suggest keeping the protein intake at no more than the 0.8 g/kg recommended (20). In any event, for the person with Parkinson's disease, protein intake should not be liberal since this will interfere with levodopa therapy.

The conversion of levodopa to dopamine depends on the presence of vitamin B_6 (pyridoxine). Excessive B_6 causes an increase in peripheral dopamine production and lesser dopamine formation in the brain, reversing the therapeutic effects of levodopa. Vitamin supplements containing B_6 should not be given, and patients should be counseled not to eat large amounts of foods high in pyridoxine (see Table 17–5, p. 258). A diet low in B_6 is not recommended either since levodopa therapy itself may induce a vitamin B_6 deficiency (19). There is no clinical evidence that restriction of B_6 has a positive effect on the treatment of Parkinson's disease.

Currently, many patients are being given Sinemet (levodopa/ carbidopa) as an antiparkinson agent. This medication has fewer side effects, and pyridoxine does not interfere with its action (21). Table 12–1 gives the nutritional considerations for some of the medications used to treat Parkinson's disease.

Parkinson's disease is aggravated by obesity. Weight loss will help the patient regain some motor function (20). It is common for patients with Parkinson's disease to be underweight. This can occur for many reasons: medication side effect; lack of time or ability to eat; disinterest in an unappealing diet. Both obesity and significant underweight can adversely affect treatment.

Table 12-1 Food and Medication Interaction in Parkinson's Disease

Drug	Generic name	Dietary significance	Possible problems
Artane	Trihexyphenidyl HCl	Take with food	Dry mouth, constipation, nausea, vomiting
Benadryl	Diphenhydramine HCl	No alcohol	Gastrointestinal distress: nausea, anorexia, vomiting, diarrhea, constipation
Cogentin	Benztropine mesylate	No alcohol	Dry mouth, possible swallowing difficulty, depressed appetite, bloating, constipation, nausea
Larodopa	Levodopa	Take with food; limit foods high in protein; limit foods high in B_6; no coffee	Gastrointestinal distress: anorexia, dry mouth, difficulty swallowing, gas, nausea, vomiting, constipation
Sinemet	Levodopa/carbidopa	Take with food	Possible weight gain, edema, gas, nausea, vomiting
Tremin	Trihexyphenidyl	See Artane	See Artane

It should also be noted that a small sample of geriatric patients have presented with an abnormal increase in appetite. The increased appetite subsided after Parkinson's was diagnosed and treatment became effective. This evidence suggests that an unexplained increase in appetite in older patients may be a symptom of undetected Parkinson's disease (22).

FEEDING THE PERSON WITH A MOVEMENT DISORDER

Many stroke patients have paralysis or weakness of one or both arms, as well as muscles around the face, mouth, tongue, and other areas. Most patients with Parkinson's disease have a tremor, as well as stiffness of muscles of the hands, arms, legs, and face. Patients with advanced dementia may have incoordination or unsteady movements of the hands and arms. All three of these types of patients have a *move-

ment disorder—be it an inability to move, an extra movement such as a tremor, or an impairment of the ability to move normally such as with weakness or clumsiness.

All persons with a movement disorder will have some impairment of the ability to feed themselves. For an older person, the inability to feed oneself can be a devastating blow. It marks a loss of independence and a loss of normal life-style and can lead to withdrawal and depression.

Whenever possible, every effort should be made to let the patient continue to eat independently by using feeding devices. Cups with double handles, weighted bases, and covers with spouts make it easier to get liquids to the mouth. Extra-long straws secured to the cup with a straw holder eliminate picking up the liquid-filled cup. Liquids are frequently avoided by older patients when they become difficult to manage. Dishes with rims are easy to find and far more attractive than metal plate guards. These dishes allow the patient to scoop food against the plate edge. Utensils with built-up or loop handles are useful if grasp is weak or fingers do not flex completely. Standard utensils may be adapted by slipping a foam rubber curler over the handle. The rough surface of the curler increases friction and aids in holding. A universal cuff, consisting of a band with a pocket to insert an ordinary utensil and Velcro fastener to secure around the handle, may also be used. A bib should never be used unless absolutely necessary, as this serves only to emphasize the patient's inability to cope with the neurologic disease and adds to his frustration and embarrassment (18,23). Table 4–2, p. 75, lists suppliers of feeding aids.

Meal Consistency

With advanced Parkinson's disease or advanced dementia or after certain strokes, chewing and swallowing may be difficult. A semisoft, soft, or pureed diet may be required. Making a pureed diet appealing and appetizing poses quite a challenge. However, with a little imagination the caregiver can suggest and/or prepare inviting meals.

For the person with a movement disorder, meals go slowly. It is important to allow adequate time for chewing and swallowing. If rushed or treated with impatience, the older person may indicate he is finished long before he is actually satisfied. Serving small, frequent meals is better than three large meals. Patients will eat more and be less frustrated if someone has taken the time to prepare some of the food in advance: cut meat into very small pieces, butter bread and cut in quarters, serve vegetables with a sauce so they are easier to pick up and swallow. With some innovative menu planning, many patients can be kept for a long period of time on a soft or semisoft diet without resorting to pureed food. Table 12–2 offers many ideas that are worth suggesting to the patient. Food selected for a soft diet should be similar to regular food cooked soft or tender but not pureed. This diet promotes ease in eating.

For the patient who is able to chew but has some difficulty with the muscles around the mouth, it is best to give foods with more texture (24). This will make it easier for the patient to manipulate the food in the mouth and will make it easier to swallow. For example, toast should be served instead of bread, and baked potatoes instead of mashed, if possible.

Table 12–2 Food Suggestions for a Soft Diet

Main Dish Ideas	Fruits
Any tender meat, fish, poultry*	Chunky apple sauce
Chopped meat in cream sauce	Poached pears
Chopped egg in cream sauce	Ripe banana
Omelet or scrambled egg	Cooked peeled fresh fruits
Soft vegetable in cheese sauce	Canned fruit
Rice in cream or cheese sauce	
Spaghetti sauce with chopped meat over small shaped pasta	*Desserts*
Noodle pudding	Pudding
Soufflé	Custard
Cooked cereal	Ice cream
Cottage cheese	Yogurt and fruit sauce
Groats (kasha) with gravy	Pudding cake
Cornmeal mush	Junket
	Gelatin
Vegetable Ideas	Sherbet
Mashed potatoes	Soft cake
Mashed sweet potatoes	
Mashed squash	*Liquids*
Mashed potatoes with chopped spinach	All allowed (except when restricted by physician)
Creamed vegetables	
Vegetables pureed with diced vegetables (e.g., carrot or turnip purée with baby peas)	
Avocado	
Creamed cauliflower	
Asparagus tips	
Creamed spinach	

*Cut in small pieces or shredded and served with sauce or gravy is most acceptable.

For the older patient with difficulty in chewing or swallowing, the diet must be modified in texture. Foods are pureed so that they may be ingested with reasonable comfort. A pureed diet need not resemble baby food. There is no reason to restrict seasoning or flavoring unless specifically ordered, and it should be remembered that almost any food can be blenderized. Patients should be encouraged to modify the texture of food they have traditionally enjoyed. Even blueberry pie can be pureed retaining its sweet, rich flavor (25).

Though all pureed foods must be smooth, the thickness can vary depending on the swallowing ability of the patient. Purees can be thickened with instant potato flakes, infant cereals, and whole-grain bread crumbs. The latter will add fiber to the diet and aid in handling constipation. Not only thickness but color should be considered so that a pureed meal has visual appeal.

Pureed cauliflower, turkey breast, and mashed potatoes are nutritionally acceptable but visually unappealing (25). Veal, chicken, and chopped beef puree well but often turn an unappetizing gray. A sprinkle of paprika or a spoonful of steak sauce can restore a more traditional meat color (25).

Pureed or blenderized food has a stronger taste than when served in its original form. Sweets increase in intensity and may need the sweetness reduced by the addition of milk, unflavored bread crumbs, yogurt, or tart fruit (25).

Cooking juice and can liquids (e.g., canned vegetable liquid) should be saved as they provide good liquifiers. Other handy liquifiers for thick purees are cream soup, sour cream, clear soup, and tomato juice. Even rice and spaghetti water add a fuller taste to a blenderized meal. Many prepared meals and entrees blenderize well and may be used. Canned Chinese food, prepared spaghetti combinations, frozen stuffed peppers, lasagna, and fish dinners with sauce make tasty purees (25). Convenience foods cannot be used by patients on a low-sodium diet since most are quite high in sodium. To flavor low-sodium purees, one can try some of the following suggestions: mixed herbs, low-sodium salad dressing, low-sodium broth or bouillon, curry, tarragon, dill, dash or cayenne, lemon or lime juice, mustard, or saltless seasoning mixtures.

A few foods simply cannot be pureed with good results. Salad greens and peas tend to be bitter, ham becomes excessively salty, bacon tastes like pureed rubber bands, and steak and roast beef often remain stringy (25). Experimentation is the best way to determine whether pureeing adversely affects taste or smell. So many foods, however, puree well that it is worth encouraging the patient or caregiver to keep trying.

If a patient has such impairment that he cannot suck through a straw, it is best for liquids to be given in a transparent cup. This will lead to less spillage (16).

Bedridden patients and patients with impaired movement often are constipated. This is partly because some of the drugs given to control the condition worsen the constipation, as do inactivity, the consistency of the diet, and the lack of saliva to moisten food. Stool softeners and an increase in dietary fiber along with the consumption of 4–8 glasses of fluid a day is the best treatment (20).

Patient aid:

The Parkinson's Patient: What You and Your Family Should Know
(English or Spanish version)

available from:

National Parkinson Institute
1501 N.W. 9th Ave.
Bob Hope Road
Miami, Florida 33136

REFERENCES

1. King, D.W., Pushpavaj, N., O'Toole, K., Morbidity and mortality in the aged, *Hosp. Pract.*, p. 97, Feb. 1982.

2. Watson, G., *Nutrition and Your Mind.* New York: Harper & Row, 1972.

3. Goodwin, J.S., Goodwin, J.M., Garry, P.J., Association between nutritional status and cognitive functioning in a healthy elderly population, *JAMA* 249:2917, 1983.

4. Schorah, C.J., et al., Clinical effects of vitamin C in elderly in-patients with low blood vitamin C levels, *Lancet* 1:403, 1979.

5. Brocklehurst, J.C., et al., The clinical features of chronic vitamin deficiency: A therapeutic trial in geriatric hospital patients, *Gerontol. Clin.* 10:309, 1968.

6. Wurtman, J.J., The involvement of brain serotonin in excessive carbohydrate snacking by obese carbohydrate cravers, *J. Am. Diet. Assoc.* 84:1004, 1984.

7. Low, C., Nutrition and neurologic function, *Nutrition & M.D.* 4:3, 1984.

8. Hardin, W.B., Neurologic aspects, in: Franz A. Steinberg, ed., *Care of the Geriatric Patient*. St. Louis: C.V. Mosby Co., 1983.

9. Baschmann, M.B.T., Brain structure and its implication in metabolism in aging: A review, *Am. J. Clin. Nutr.* 36:759, 1982.

10. Locke, S., Neurological Disorders of the elderly, in William Reichel, ed., *Clinical Aspects of Aging*. Baltimore: Williams & Wilkins, 1983.

11. Hutton, J.T., Senility reconsidered, *JAMA* 245:1025, 1981.

12. Coyle, J.T., Price, D.L., DeLong, M.R., Alzheimer's disease: A disorder of cortical cholinergic innervation, *Science* 219:1184, 1983.

13. Thal, L.J., Current concepts of the pathogenesis of senile dementia of the Alzheimer type, *Geriatr. Med. Today* 3:86, 1984.

14. Nangeroni, J.B., Pierce, P.S., Development of a geriatric diet through behavioral observation of feeding behaviors of regressed and demented patients, *J. Nutr. Elderly* 3(2):25, 1983.

15. Tilton, C.N., Maloof, M., Diagnosing the problem in stroke, *Am. J. Nurs.* 82:596, 1982.

16. Hynak-Hankinson, M.T., et al., Dysphagia evaluation and treatment: The team approach, Part II, *Nutr. Support Serv.* 4(6):30, 1984.

17. Mancall, E.L., Covington, T.R., Alanso, R.J., Therapy of neurologic disorders in the elderly, *Hosp. Pract.*, p. 106E, Oct. 1984.

18. Klinger, J.L., *Mealtime Manual for People With Disabilities and the Aging*. Camden, N.J.: Campbell Soup Co., 1978.

19. Gillespie, N.G., et al., Diets affecting treatment of parkinsonism with levodopa, *J. Am. Diet. Assoc.* 62:525, 1973.

20. Selvey, N.P., Diet for patients receiving levodopa therapy for parkinsonism: questions and answers, *JAMA* 236:1169, Sept. 6, 1976.

21. Moore, A.O., Powers, D.E., *Food Medication Interactions*. Tempe, Arizona, (P.O. Box 26464), 1981.

22. Rosenberg, P., et al., Increased appetite (bulimia) in Parkinson's disease, *J. Am. Geriatr. Soc.* 25:277, June 1977.

23. *Resource Kit on Food, Nutrition and the Disabled Nutrition Information Service*, Ryerson Polytechnical Institute, Toronto, 1981.

24. Nutritional therapy of the stroke patient, *Nutrition & M.D.* 6(4):5, 1980.

25. Thompson, E.S., Thanks, but no spare ribs! *Nutr. Today* 16:23, May/June 1981.

Chapter 13

NUTRITIONAL ANEMIAS

Anemia is a reduction in the oxygen-transporting capacity of the blood, which, in turn, reduces the supply of oxygen to body tissues. This is indicated by a hematocrit or hemoglobin level that is below normal. In many men, the hemoglobin concentration declines in old age. This reduction is probably due to lessened androgen production. Women do not show a similar decline (1) (see Table 13-1). Blacks, in general, have lower hemoglobin values than whites, even when matches for economic status. This difference ranges from 0.3g/dl to 1g/dl and persists in the elderly (2).

Although aging per se is never the cause of anemia, a reduced hematocrit is not uncommonly found in older adults because of the increased incidence of underlying pathologic conditions leading to anemia. Gastritis may lead to malabsorption of nutrients needed for blood formation. After a total gastrectomy, all patients become deficient in vitamin B_{12} within a few years. After a partial gastrectomy, 14 to 60% have depressed vitamin B_{12} levels and 2 to 6% have megaloblastoid changes in the marrow (3). Iron and folic acid deficiency may also occur after partial gastrectomy. Anemia due to copper deficiency has been reported in patients who have had extensive bowel surgery and received hyperalimentation without appropriate copper replacement (4).

Anemia may develop as a result of bleeding from hemorrhoids, hiatus hernia, diverticulitis, carcinoma, or ulcers. Disorders often seen in

Table 13–1 Average Hemoglobin Levels in Older Adults

Age	Men	Women
45–64	14.9 g/dl	13.6 g/dl
65–74	14.7 g/dl	13.6 g/dl

Source: Fulwood, R., et al., *Hematological and Nutritional Biochemistry Refrence Data for Persons 6 Months–74 Years of Age: United States 1976–80* (Vital and Health Statistics Series 11 No. 232), Public Health Service, D.H.H.S. Publication (PHS) 83-1682, Government Printing Office, Washington, D.C., 1982.

the elderly such as autoimmune hemolytic diseases, chronic inflammatory diseases, intestinal parasitosis, and renal disease can result in anemia. The use of antiinflammatory drugs such as aspirin and indomethacin (Indocin), antiarrhythmics such as quinidine and procainamide (Pronestyl), antihypertensives such as alpha-methyldopa (Aldomet), and antibiotics such as penicillins and, sometimes, cephalosporins can cause anemia (5).

Some drugs—chloramphenicol (Chloromycetin), nitrofurantoin (Macrodantin), primaquine, and sulfa compounds—cause hemolysis in persons with glucose-6-phosphate dehydrogenase deficiency (6). Prosthetic cardiac valves or even severely diseased unreplaced cardiac valves can cause hemolysis by mechanical means.

A variety of nutrients is needed for the production of red blood cells: iron, folic acid, vitamin B_{12}, protein, pyridoxine, ascorbic acid, copper, and vitamin E. A deficiency of any of these can result in anemia, but nutritional anemias are most commonly due to a lack of iron, folic acid, and/or vitamin B_{12}. A deficiency of iron causes microcytic anemia while a deficiency of folic acid and/or vitamin B_{12} causes macrocytic anemia.

MICROCYTIC ANEMIA

The majority of persons with microcytic red blood cells have iron deficiency usually caused by bleeding (thalassemia and anemia from a chronic disease are other causes). As the body does not lose iron normally, and the diets of most Americans usually contain enough iron to prevent deficiency, men and postmenopausal women develop iron deficiency essentially only because of apparent or occult bleeding. Iron deficiency anemia rarely remains stable; it becomes worse as time passes.

Elevated total iron-binding capacity (TIBC) and decreased serum iron (SI) with saturation of the TIBC less than 16% are typical findings (7).

Treatment of iron deficiency anemia in older adults rests on remedying the underlying cause, be it a disease or drug used. In addition, iron replacement is needed to restore normal hemoglobin levels. Dietary treatment of iron deficiency is a slow process when attempted without supplemental iron. The RDA of iron for adult men and postmenopausal women is 10 mg/day. The usual diet in the United States provides 6 mg of iron for each 1000 kcal consumed. Older adults should be made aware of which foods are rich in iron and encouraged to use these foods (see Table 13-2). Food is a more pleasurable way to obtain needed iron than pills.

The heme form of iron in meat is better absorbed than the iron in vegetables. Eating meat or fish with other iron-containing foods will increase the amount of iron that is absorbed. Foods rich in vitamin C such as citrus fruits, cabbage, and potatoes will enhance iron absorption, as does sorbitol. Fiber, antacids, and tea interfere with iron absorption (8).

Supplemental iron in the form of ferrous salts is the most readily utilizable source of iron. Ferrous sulfate (20% elemental iron), ferrous gluconate (11.6% elemental iron), ferrous fumarate (33% elemental iron), or ferrocholinate (12% elemental iron), given in doses that provide about 200 mg of elemental iron daily, will be adequate for most persons with iron deficiency anemia. Side effects such as constipation and gastric irritation may occur in some individuals. Taking iron with meals or decreasing the daily dose to 110–120 mg of elemental iron may relieve such symptoms. Enteric-coated tablets may be unsatisfactory for patients with achlorhydria, those who have had surgical short-circuiting procedures, or those with rapid transit times. Iron absorption decreases progressively along the gastrointestinal tract, and the enteric coating may not be dissolved in time to allow adequate absorption. For these persons, a liquid iron supplement is preferable (9).

It is important to keep in mind that many so-called iron-enriched foods have added iron that is not in the form of ferrous salts. As nonferrous iron supplements may be poorly absorbed, these foods should not be relied on alone to replenish an iron-deficient patient.

Persons with iron deficiency may have unusual dietary cravings called *pica*. Eating large amounts of ice—pagophagia—appears to result from iron deficiency (10). Eating clay—geophagia—can interfere with iron absorption and may result in significant iron deficiency (11). A recent report describes a 74-year-old black woman with recurrent iron deficiency anemia linked to magnesium carbonate pica. This substance sold for gymnastic and industrial use had been suggested as a laxative by a neighborhood pharmacist (12).

Table 13–2   Food Sources of Iron

Food	Portion	Iron (mg)
Apple	1 medium	0.5
Apricots, dried	4 halves	0.8
Avocado	½	1.3
Bean sprouts	½ cup	0.5
Beef	3 oz	2.7
Blueberries	⅝ cup	1.0
Bread, white	1 slice	0.6
Bread, whole wheat	1 slice	0.8
Carnation Instant Breakfast	1 envelope	4.5
Chicken, fried	¼	1.8
Chickpeas	½ cup	3.0
Corn muffins	1	0.6
Egg	1	1.1
Enriched pasta	½ cup	2.0
General Mills Kix	1 oz	8.1
General Mills Golden Grahams	1 oz	4.5
Grape-Nuts	1 oz	0.5
Green beans	½ cup	0.4
Kellogg's Product 19	1 oz	18
Kellogg's Special K	1 oz	4.5
Kidney beans	½ cup	2.2
Lentils	½ cup	2.1
Liver	3 oz	8.0
Molasses	1 tbsp	0.9
Nabisco Instant Cream of Wheat	1 oz	8.1
Peanuts, roasted	1 tbsp	0.5
Potato	1 small	0.5
Prunes	4	1.5
Prune juice	½ cup	5.2
Quaker Life	1 oz	8.1
Quaker Corn Bran	1 oz	8.1
Raisins	1 tbsp	0.4
Shredded wheat	1 biscuit	0.9
Split peas, dried	½ cup	1.5
Spinach	½ cup	2.0
Rice	½ cup	0.7
Tofu	½ cup	2.0
Turkey	3 oz	1.5
Walnuts	1 tbsp	0.2

MACROCYTIC ANEMIA

A deficiency of either folic acid and/or vitamin B_{12} can cause a macrocytic anemia. Vitamin B_{12} is needed in minute amounts: the RDA for adults is 3 mcg. Macrocytic anemia that is attributable to B_{12} deficiency (for example, pernicious anemia) is almost always due to a lack of gastric intrinsic factor, which is needed for B_{12} absorption. The major dietary source of vitamin B_{12} is animal products. However, even strict vegetarians who eat no animal products rarely develop this problem (see Table 13–3).

The incidence of pernicious anemia is age-related (13). The frequency increases with age, so that while the incidence is 1 out of 5000 persons aged 30–40 years, the number affected increases to 1 per 200 in those aged 60–70. Persons with thyroid disorders or diabetes have an increased incidence.

Lifelong therapy with vitamin B_{12} injections is needed for persons with pernicious anemia. A loading dose of 1 mg is given intramuscularly 5 or 6 times in the first month and thereafter 1 mg per month is given (14).

Table 13–3 Food Sources of Vitamin B_{12}

Food	Amount	Micrograms
Beef liver	3½ oz	80.0
Chicken liver	3½ oz	24.1
Clams, canned	½ cup	20.0
Raw oysters	3½ oz	18.0
Liverwurst	2 slices	9.2
Crabmeat, canned	3½ oz	8.5
Sardines	3½ oz	8.3
Salmon, canned	3½ oz	7.5
Product 19, Kellogg's	1 cup	6.0
Tuna fish	3½ oz	3.0
Morningstar Farms Sausages	3	2.4
Beef steak	3 oz	2.2
Hamburger	3 oz	1.8
Veal, lean	3½ oz	1.8
Haddock	3½ oz	1.7
Lamb	3½ oz	1.6
Kix, Kellogg's	1½ cup	1.5
Yogurt	8 oz	1.3
Flounder	3½ oz	1.2
Milk	8 oz	1.0
Ham	3½ oz	0.8
Cottage cheese	½ cup	0.7
Egg	1	0.6
Carnation Breakfast Bar	1	0.6
Buttermilk	8 oz	0.5
Swiss cheese	1 oz	0.5
Bleu cheese	1 oz	0.4
Camembert cheese*	1 oz	0.4
Cheddar cheese	1 oz	0.3

*As cheese ripens, the amount of B vitamins increases.

Deficiency of vitamin B_{12} can lead to severe neurologic effects as well as anemia. That is why it is essential that pernicious anemia not be treated with folic acid, which will correct the anemia of vitamin B_{12} deficiency but will not help the neurologic symptoms. Daily folic acid intake of 0.4 mg, the RDA for the vitamin, will not mask pernicious anemia (15).

Diets in the United States are estimated to contain from 200 to 250 mcg of folic acid daily, about one-half the RDA for adults. Body stores of folic acid last only a few months, and dietary deprivation for as short a time as 5 months can cause anemia. Many alcoholics and narcotics abusers often suffer from folic acid deficiency because they eat little food. In addition, alcoholics have reduced absorption and disturbed metabolism of the vitamin. Elderly persons who eat a limited diet such as tea and toast with few raw foods may become deficient in folic acid. Anticonvulsant drugs, glutethimide (Doriden), and barbiturates can cause deficiency, as can large amounts of aspirin such as is commonly used for rheumatoid arthritis. Folic acid antagonists, such as metho-

Table 13–4 Food Sources of Folic Acid

Food	Amount	mg
Product 19, Kellogg's	1 cup	0.40
Brewers' yeast	1 tbsp	0.31
Orange juice	1 cup	0.16
Romaine lettuce, chopped	1 cup	0.10
Brussels sprouts	3 large	0.10
Carnation Breakfast Bar	1	0.10
Crispix, Kellogg's	¾ cup	0.10
Cocoa Krispies	1 cup	0.10
Beets	2 medium	0.09
Sweet potato	1 medium	0.08
Asparagus	5 to 6 spears	0.06
Orange	1 medium	0.06
Wheat germ	¼ cup	0.05
Cantaloupe, diced	1 cup	0.05
Grapefruit juice	½ cup	0.05
Milk, regular	1 cup	0.04
Red pepper	1 medium	0.04
Avocado	½ medium	0.04
Yogurt	8 oz	0.03
Beer	12 oz	0.03
Cucumber	1 small	0.03
Cabbage	½ cup	0.02
Potato	1 medium	0.02
Strawberries	1 cup	0.02
Whole-wheat bread	1 slice	0.02

trexate used in the treatment of psoriasis and leukemia, can also result in deficiency. Gluten-sensitive enteropathy (sprue) may interfere with the absorption of folic acid and can occur in the elderly even without the usual accompanying diarrhea.

Folic acid is present in many foods (see Table 13–4). It is readily absorbed from bananas, lima beans, liver, and brewer's yeast. Its availability is somewhat lower in orange juice, romaine lettuce, egg yolk, cabbage, and wheat germ. Folic acid is easily destroyed by long cooking, especially of finely divided foods such as rice and beans.

The usual therapeutic dose of folic acid is 1.0 mg daily. The Food and Drug Administration limits the amount of folic acid that may be included in over-the-counter supplements to 0.4 mg to protect against the possibility of folate oversupplementation masking pernicious anemia. A daily supplement of 0.4 mg of folic acid, which is the RDA, may be desirable for older adults as they are vulnerable to deficiency.

REFERENCES

1. Conley, C.L., Anemia: Accurate diagnosis and appropriate therapy, *Hosp. Pract.*, p. 57, Sept. 1984.

2. Lynch, S.R., et al., Iron status of elderly Americans, *Am. J. Clin. Nutr.* 36:1032, 1982.

3. Williams, W.J., et al., *Hematology.* New York: McGraw-Hill Book Co., 1972, p. 270.

4. Dunlop, W.M., et al., Anemia and neutropenia caused by copper deficiency, *Ann. Internal Med.* 80:470, 1974.

5. Leonard, J.R., Levy, G., Gastrointestinal blood loss during prolonged aspirin administration, *N. Engl. J. Med.* 289:1020, 1973.

6. Adler, S.S., Anemia in the aged: Causes and considerations, *Geriatrics* 35:49, 1980.

7. Bainton, D.F., Finch, C.A., The diagnosis of iron deficiency, *Am. J. Med.* 37:62, 1964.

8. Russell, R.M., Naccarto, D.V., Current perspectives on trace elements, *Drug Ther.* 7(10):115, 1982.

9. Stuckey, W.J., Common anemias: A practical guide to diagnosis and management, *Geriatrics* 38:42, 1983.

10. Reynolds, R.D., et al., Pagophagia and iron deficiency anemia, *Ann. Intern. Med.* 68:435, 1968.

11. Mengel, C.E., et al., Geophagia with iron deficiency and hypokalemia—Cachexia africana, *Arch. Intern. Med.* 114:470, 1964.

12. Leming, P.D., et al., Magnesium carbonate pica: An unusual case of iron deficiency, *Ann. Int. Med.* 94(5):660, 1981.

13. Reynolds, E.H., Neurological agents of folate and vitamin B$_{12}$ metabolism, *Clin. Haematol.* 5:661, 1976.

14. Schilling, R.F., Pernicious anemia (questions and answers), *JAMA* 253(1):94, 1985.

15. Herbert, V., et al., Symposium: Folic acid deficiency: A review, *Am. J. Clin. Nutr.* 23:841, 1970.

Chapter 14

INFECTIOUS DISEASE

As the proportion of our population over 65 increases, our knowledge of infectious diseases in the older adult needs to increase. Infection may cause as many as 30% of all deaths in the elderly and up to one-third of all reversible dementia (1). Though infectious disease is prevalent, its presentation in the elderly is often atypical. Confusion, poor immune response, absence of fever, hyopthermic reactions, sluggish function of the automatic nervous system, and the use of drugs, particularly aspirin and steroids, may make detection and treatment of infection difficult (2).

The elderly are more susceptible to infections than younger persons. Elderly people may have a chronic condition or disease that puts them at increased risk (2). When this is coupled with the clustering that occurs in a nursing home or senior citizen center, infection is often difficult to prevent, and spread of infection may be difficult to control (3). Approximately 50% of the older patients in a nursing home will develop an infection within the first year after admission, with the incidence of infection increased in the 70-to-90-year-old group (4).

Immunization status should be ascertained and noted at the time of admission to a long-term care facility so appropriate primary series or booster doses can be given as necessary. The incidence of tetanus is the highest in persons over 60 with about three-fourths of the cases resulting in death. Though most cases are from injuries that occur in the home to ambulatory older adults, institutionalized older adults with cutaneous ulcers and gangrene should be considered at risk (5). The U.S. Public Health Service recommends that all persons over age 65 receive an annual flu vaccine and pneumococcal vaccine every 5 years. Pneumonia is all too common in older patients. It may be accompanied by dehydration and mental confusion and may result in death (1,2).

One study reported an infection rate of 16.2% among 532 nursing home residents, citing infected decubitus ulcers, conjunctivitis, urinary tract infection (UTI), and lower-respiratory-tract infections as the most common (6). UTI are second only to respiratory infections as the cause of febrile illness in patients over 65 (7). In many cases, though UTI infection is present, fever is absent, thereby making detection difficult (8). Diminished fever response to infection may not be unusual for the older patient. Twenty-nine percent of older patients with bacteremia were afebrile (temperature of less than 100° F) on clinical evaluation (2).

Infection control for the independent living and homebound older adult is also obviously important. Proper food sanitation techniques to prevent food-borne illness and infection control education for the caregiver are essential to prevent disease transmission.

Infection or sepsis is closely related to undernutrition. As nutritional status declines, the infection rate rises. The incidence of pulmonary infection and pneumonia increases as a function of weight loss. Nutritional deficiencies adversely affect the integrity of the skin, leading to poor wound healing and skin infections. These are significantly more common among those who are nonambulatory, fecally incontinent, or diabetic (6). Poor diet may be a cause of disruption of the integrity of the mucous membrances and thus allows bacteria ready access to the body. Medications that dry out the nose and mouth further reduce the patient's ability to withstand infection. Those elderly who are poorly nourished, refuse to eat, suffer from cancer, or are chronically ill will show depressed immune response. Furthermore, an active infection predisposes the patient to other infections creating a cycle of illness that requires aggressive therapy.

Active infectious disease, even without the presence of poor nutrition, will affect nutritional status. Frequently the symptoms of the infection—anorexia, fever, nausea, vomiting, coughing, dyspnea, and diarrhea—compromise food intake and absorption, which directly affect recovery (9).

Owing to the effect of infection on nutritional status, there is an *increased* need for nutrients and fluid in elderly persons with infection. For centuries starvation was an accepted method for treating an infection or fever. Protein was withheld because it was mistakenly believed that it promoted fever. Although modern medicine has discarded these antiquated practices, feeding the sick is still often greatly influenced by cultural or traditional beliefs (9). The elderly in some cases will adhere to traditional beliefs and practices very strongly. Using chicken soup and herb teas or avoiding milk and juice is a common practice. Relatives will bring in special foods, or those elderly living at home may limit certain foods in an attempt at self-treatment. Much of these dietary manipulations are harmless and may have a placebo effect. However, it is important to determine and note the nature of self-prescribed diet manipulation because in certain cases this may lead to a food-drug interaction or a limitation of fluids that could result in serious consequences.

NUTRITIONAL DEFICIENCY

Nutritional deficiencies result in decreased immune function and in increased susceptibility to infection. This interaction occurs most often in the poor, the hospitalized patient, the surgical patient, and the ambulatory elderly (9). The elderly may simultaneously fit into many or all of these groups, compounding their risk of susceptibility and the duration and severity of infectious disease (10). In managing infection in the older patient, it is imperative to consider the patient's own immune defenses and to realize that recovery depends on these defenses (2). The patient's nutritional state, which to a great extent will mirror the functional state of the host-defense response, must be preserved to maintain immune function and contribute to host resistance.

The impact of malnutrition on infection can be seen very clearly in a number of usual clinical situations. Intestinal parastic infections, common to many cultural groups, can both induce malnutrition and exacerbate existing undernutrition by maldigestion, malabsorption, competition for nutrients, gastrointestinal nutrient losses, and catabolic nutrient losses. Older individuals from Southeast Asia, Africa, Mexico, and the Caribbean may be host to many parasitic pathogens that remain subclinical as long as the host-defense mechanism is intact (10).

Hospitalized patients undergoing surgery and/or receiving intravenous alimentation are at great risk for infection. Not only is it possible to rapidly induce malnutrition by this method of nutritional support, but in addition, the surgical site and intravenous line reduce the integrity of the protective skin barrier. Proper nutritional support is certainly possible for such patients. Many hospitals have specialized enteral and parenteral nutritional support teams for just such a situation. All too often, it is presumed that the patient's problems have been solved at the successful completion of pharmacologic or surgical treatment. At this point, even though the infection may be resolved, the patient may be in negative nutrient balance and may require aggressive nutrition intervention to eliminate the risk of a recurrent or new infection and to restore immune function (9).

Nutritional rehabilitation of any patient found to be poorly nourished will significantly reduce complications due to infection. Identifying the nutritionally stressed older patient is not always easy. To help in this task, a catabolic stress index was developed by Dr. Bruce Bistrain.

The metabolically stressed patient excretes increased amounts of urinary nitrogen as a result of increased breakdown of proteins throughout the body. For any given nitrogen and energy intake, the stressed patient excretes more nitrogen than the unstressed patient.

$$\text{Stress index} = \text{UUN} - (1/2 \text{ N intake} + 3 \text{ g})$$

Score:
Less than 0 = No significant stress
   0–5   = Moderate stress
More than 5 = Severe stress

The stress index equals the 24-hour urine urea nitrogen (UUN), which reflects the amount of digested protein, whether exogenous or endogenous, minus half the nitrogen intake (1/2 N intake) plus 3 g of nitrogen (3 g). The equation assumes that 50% of the nitrogen consumed is utilized and 3 g of nitrogen, known as the obligatory nitrogen loss, is excreted even if the patient consumes no protein. The score indicates the patient's degree of metabolic stress. The stress index is useful for identifying catabolic stress in a patient in whom stress is not suspected (11). For example, an older woman is admitted for knee replacement surgery, which by itself would not be considered especially stressful. The stress index might show that the woman was in fact catabolic owing to an undetected underlying infection, markedly increasing her risk for surgery at that time.

NUTRITIONAL REQUIREMENTS IN INFECTIOUS DISEASE

The goal of nutritional support in infectious disease should be improved nutritional status. In cases of severe infection, this is probably unrealistic. In these situations, therapy should focus on preventing further depletion.

Nutrient Needs

Specific recommendations for nutrient needs during infection are lacking. Serum vitamin A and C levels are diminished along with blood levels of zinc and iron. Fever increases the need for B-complex vitamins as more are used as the metabolic rate increases along with body temperature. Vomiting, sweating, and diarrhea cause loss of electrolytes and water (12). Supplementation with a daily, multivitamin-mineral compound should be adequate to meet needs.

Administration of therapeutic doses in excess of the normal RDA adult requirement are unnecessary. Furthermore, evidence has demonstrated that large nutrient doses may be deleterious to recovery. Vitamin C, in particular, is often promoted for its prophylactic effect. However, some research has suggested that daily supplementation in excess of 2000 mg for more than 2 weeks will reduce the antimicrobial activity of leukocytes (13). Until metabolic function during infection is more clearly understood, very large doses of nutrients should not be encouraged since they may produce an adverse effect on cellular function. Five hundred milligrams of vitamin C given daily to healthy people over the age of 70 did enhance the cell-mediated immune response, suggesting a nontoxic, inexpensive, easy-to-administer method to improve immune competence (14).

In certain instances, a nutrient deficiency may protect the individual against infectious organisms. Iron depletion is part of the body's response to infection (10). It has been suggested that this compensatory mechanism is the body's attempt to reduce the amount of free iron available for the infectious organisms for growth and replication. Septic patients should not be given supplemental iron beyond daily maintenance needs. If a major iron deficit is evident by a low hematocrit or hemoglobin, the physician should order administration of packed red cells (15).

It should not be forgotten that aspirin, either alone or as found in many over-the-counter preparation may induce a deficiency of vitamin C and may also lead to iron deficiency (see Chapter 17).

Elderly clients frequently take vitamin-mineral supplements, which they may increase during episodes of infection. It is important that the caregiver determine what and how much the client is taking to prevent potential interference with treatment.

Energy Needs

The body's response to infection is associated with an increase in basal metabolic rate (BMR). The BMR increases from 20% to 60% above normal in patients with infection. To estimate the resting metabolic expenditure (RME) for stressed patients, clinicians rely on the Harris and Benedict equation developed in 1919. This equation predicts BMR based on an individual's sex, weight, height, and age. It was customary to adjust the BMR values upward by 10% to arrive at the RME (16). To-

Table 14–1   Calculation for Determining Resting Metabolic Expenditure (RME)

RME (men) = (66.47 + 13.75W + 5.0H − 6.76A) × (activity factor) × (injury
         factor)
RME (women) = (65.10 + 9.56W + 1.85H − 4.68A) × (activity factor) × (injury
         factor)
where W = weight in kilograms; H = height in centimeters; A = age in years

Activity factor	Injury factor*			
Confined to bed = 1.2	Surgery		Trauma	
Ambulatory = 1.3	Minor	= 1.1	Skeletal	= 1.35
	Major	= 1.2	Head injury with	
	Infection		steroid therapy	= 1.6
	Mild	= 1.2	Blunt	= 1.35
	Moderate	= 1.4	Burns	
	Severe	= 1.8	40% BSA†	= 1.5
			100% BSA	= 1.95

*The injury factor should be tapered as metabolic responses return to normal, non-stressed levels.
†Body surface area.

day, however, this adjustment is not necessary since more current work on the Harris and Benedict equation has demonstrated consistent 10–15% overestimation in energy needs (17). Table 14–1 provides an equation that may be used to calculate daily calorie needs based on the Harris and Benedict equation with consideration of the degree of stress and an activity factor.

FEEDING CONSIDERATIONS IN INFECTIOUS DISEASE

Fever

The catabolic response to infection begins with the onset of fever. If the infection is severe and prolonged, there will be muscle wasting and weight loss as lean body mass is catabolized for energy. The nutritional goal is to keep the patient in nitrogen balance. This will be difficult during the acute phase of an infection owing to anorexia, vomiting, diarrhea, and possible gastrointestinal malabsorption. After 3–4 days, negative nitrogen balance begins to stabilize, and with nutritional support, positive balance can be achieved. Seventy to ninety grams of protein a day is recommended with some suggesting intakes of 2.0 g protein/kg of body weight (15,16). A diet planned to provide over 100 g of protein would be difficult for most elderly patients to eat and should not be given. The use of high-protein beverages to supplement small frequent feedings is a wiser approach and will generally supply sufficient protein within the range of 70 to 90 g daily.

If milk is tolerated, the following protein-fortified milk drink can be used to increase both protein and calorie intake.

	Calories	Protein(g)
1 8-oz glass of milk	160	9
3 tbsp nonfat dry milk	45	4.5
1 tbsp chocolate syrup	49	0.5
	254	14.0

Two glasses of protein-fortified milk a day add approximately 500 kcal and 28 g of protein to the patient's intake. Other flavorings such as maple, vanilla, coffee, strawberry, or banana may be used if desired. For those who are lactose intolerant, Lact-Aid fluid or treated milk may be used. Yogurt can also be used if the person prefers to eat the snack rather than drink it.

Bland, easily digested food of soft or regular consistency should be offered frequently. Small feedings at intervals of 2 to 3 hours are ideal. Fluid diets should be avoided as they are overly filling out of proportion to their caloric and nutrient content. For some patients, liquid diets increase abdominal distention and discomfort. Most older patients experience less nausea and anorexia eating solid foods.

Feeding a feverish patient may be difficult because of lethargy, nausea, flatulence (gas), and a cottony sensation that may be present in the mouth. In cases of high fever, flatulence and bloating may cause severe discomfort, which may be relieved only after vomiting. The bloating is due to immotility of the bowel. Until it subsides, it is best to restrict carbohydrate foods and milk. All sugars and especially lactose (milk sugar) will ferment in a poorly motile bowel and will thus cause additional gas. Some patients need fat restriction as well. Fruit juice and high-protein foods such as low-fat cheese and hard-cooked eggs may be well tolerated by those who wish to eat. High-protein liquid supplements may also be offered. Supplying ample fluids is essential to replace losses and promote urination to help clear body wastes. A minimum of 10 cups (2500 ml) daily is recommended.

Vomiting

Infectious illness modifies the motility of the gastrointestinal tract. Motility is reduced and nausea and vomiting result, which will cause a loss of large amounts of water and hydrochloric acid from the stomach along with losses of sodium, magnesium, and chloride. The older patient may then be left mildly dehydrated and at risk for alkalosis. When gut motility is increased, diarrhea results, interfering with the absorption of nutrients. Depending on the severity of the diarrhea, losses of fluid and sodium may be substantial. The patient may rapidly become dehydrated and be at risk for acidosis.

After vomiting, the patient should be allowed to rinse the mouth but not swallow since swallowing might precipitate a gag response and initiate further vomiting. After an hour without vomiting, a small amount of water should be offered. If the water is tolerated, the patient may sip water or suck on crushed ice. Gradually, over the next 2 to 4 hours, one may introduce other fluids, dry crackers, dry toast, and dry unsweetened cereal without milk. Small shredded wheat and bran cereals are too high in fiber to be fed at this time whereas other varieties of refined dry cereals, like cornflakes, may have a shape that requires them to be eaten with a spoon. Minus milk, these cereals will not be well received. The size and shape of many other cereals, such as Kix, Cheerios, and Chex, let them easily be eaten as finger foods.

When the patient has not vomited for 4 to 6 hours, small meals at regular intervals may be started. For the next 24 to 36 hours, it is best to offer foods of the patient's choice that are high in carbohydrate and low in fat. Bananas, applesauce, canned fruit, breads, cereals, rice, and pasta are good choices. Fluid replacement is necessary, but milk should be avoided as it may cause discomfort.

Diarrhea

Diarrhea may be precipitated by many causes: foodborne infection, bacterial infection, drugs, malabsorption syndromes, metabolic disease, alcoholism, cancer, and laxative abuse. The reaction to grief often results in gastrointestinal disruption and diarrhea. Diarrhea that lasts longer than 2 days requires medical assessment. Often cancer, cirrhosis, uremia, or other conditions may be the underlying cause. A physician must evaluate the patient to rule out a serious disorder.

Traditionally, the management of diarrhea was bowel rest, fasting the patient for 24 to 48 hours. This course of treatment leaves the patient low in fluid and nutrients and is not currently regarded as a good approach. Dietary management of diarrhea should be aggressive. Losses of fluid and electrolytes must be replaced to prevent dehydration, alkalosis or acidosis, and possible associated weakness. Potassium replacement, in particular, is important. Fruit juice that is high in potassium such as orange, grapefruit, pineapple, and tomato juice should be offered as part of the patient's fluid replacement. When diarrhea is prolonged, as in liver disease or intestinal parasitosis, nutritional deficiencies may develop and tissue protein losses can be severe, leading to depressed serum proteins. Vitamin B_{12}, folic acid, niacin, and iron deficiencies have also been observed.

An elderly patient with diarrhea should never be allowed to go without food and liquids for longer than 12 hours. Ideally, fluid replacement should be started immediately. During the initial phase, the patient should be allowed to sip water. This should be followed by clear fluids, full fluids, and finally a regular diet low in fat, fiber, and milk. This diet progression should take no more than 72 hours. See Table 14–2 for food suggestions to offer when a patient needs a clear-fluid or full-fluid diet. It has been noted that the duration and severity of diarrhea does not change whether the patient is fasted or fed. A patient given ample nutrients and fluids is better able to recover from the infection that is causing the diarrhea and at the least will have sufficient nutrient reserves when the disruption is resolved.

Even though milk and milk foods are listed under "Full Fluid" in Table 14–2, these choices should be withheld until the patient is free of diarrhea for 24 hours. Lactose (milk sugar) may precipitate further diarrhea. An occasional patient may temporarily become lactose intolerant because of damage to the absorptive mucosa. If so, milk should be withheld for 1–3 weeks to allow the mucosa to heal. (For further information on lactose intolerance, see Chapter 6.) Other fluids to avoid are: bouillon, which is too high in sodium and will draw fluids into the intestines; herbal teas, which may contain cathartics such as senna, buckthorn bark, dockroot, and aloe leaves; and soy isolate formulas.

Table 14–2 Food Suggestions for a Patient Needing a Clear-Fluid or Full-Fluid Diet

Clear fluid	Full fluid
Broth	All clear fluids
Strained fruit juice	Strained vegetable soups
Fruit ades	Strained cream soups
Plain gelatin	Milk
Ginger ale	Milk drinks
Seltzer	Ices
Mineral water	Plain sherbet
Very weak tea	Plain ice cream
Water	Pudding
Ice pops (low in sugar)	Custards
	Cooked refined cereals
	Vegetable juices

Fluid replacement is critical during illness. Elderly patients readily become dehydrated from fever, infection, or diarrhea (18). Healthy aged individuals experience a reduction in the normal thirst mechanism, which would otherwise restore fluid losses form such stresses (19). Therefore, thirst, by itself, is not a reliable index of fluid replacement.

Older individuals must be encouraged to replace lost fluids even though they may not perceive thirst. A daily intake of 50 ml of fluid/kg of body weight should be adequate to maintain fluid balance. Oral electrolyte replacement solutions should be offered throughout the active phase of diarrhea. Some patients tolerate these solutions better when they are diluted with equal amounts of water or frozen into popsicles. If the patient finds the smell objectionable, serve the drink over crushed ice, in a capped container, sipped through a straw.

Fluids Used as Acidifiers

Drinking cranberry juice is often suggested to prevent or control urinary tract infections. This dietary misinformation stems from an old reference reporting the value of 12 oz of cranberry juice daily in relieving the symptoms of chronic kidney inflammation in a 66-year-old woman. Subsequent research has not supported this recommendation (20,21). Even though cranberry juice contains a precursor of hippuric acid, which has strong antibacterial action in the urine, most patients cannot drink enough to affect urinary pH. Amounts well in excess of 1 qt daily led to only transient changes in urinary pH. Cranberry juice is usually sold as cranberry cocktail, which is approximately one-third cranberry juice mixed with sugar and water. One quart of cranberry cocktail averages 580 kcal. Medications such as K-Phos (potassium acid phosphate) and Uracid (dl-methionine) or vitamin C (2-4 g daily) provide a more consistent and sustained lowering of urinary pH.

REFERENCES

1. Smith, I.M., Infectious diseases in the elderly patient, *Geriatrics* 35:51, Feb. 1980.
2. Finkelstein, M.S., Unusual features of infections in the aging, *Geriatrics* 37:65, April 1982.
3. Avorn, J., Nursing-home infections—The context, *JAMA* 305(13):759, Sept. 24, 1981.
4. Schneider, E.L., Infectious diseases in the elderly, *Ann. Intern. Med.* 98(3):395, 1983.

5. Sherman, F.T., Tetanus and the institutionalized elderly (letter), *JAMA* 244(19):2159, Nov. 14, 1980.

6. Garibaldi, R.A., et al., Infections among patients in nursing homes, *JAMA* 305(13):731, Sept. 24, 1981.

7. Mayer, T.R., UTI in the elderly: How to select treatment, *Geriatrics* 35:67, March 1980.

8. Romano, J.M., Kaye, D., UTI in the elderly: Common yet atypical, *Geriatrics* 36:113, June 1981.

9. Keusch, G.T., Interaction of infections and nutrition: Clinical implications, *Clin. Nutr.* 2(2):5, March/April 1983.

10. Solomons, N.W., Nutrition and parasitic disease, *Clin. Nutr.* 2(2):16, March/April 1983.

11. Clark, N.G., Identifying the stressed patient, *R.D.* 3(4):4, 1983.

12. Davis, J.M., Nutrition in sepsis, in: *Surgical Nutrition*, Vol 3, Contemporary Issues in Clinical Nutrition, M.F. Yarborough, and P.W. Curreri, eds. N.Y.: Churchill, Livingston, Inc. 1981.

13. Vitamin C and phagocyte formation, *Nutr. Rev.* 36:183, June 1978.

14. Kennes, B., et al., Effect of vitamin C supplements on cell-mediated immunity in old people, *Gerontology* 29(5):305, 1983.

15. Duncan, J.L., Bistrain, B.R., Blackburn, G.L., Septic stress, nutritional management of the patient, *J. Med. Consult.* 22(11):235, Nov. 1982.

16. Long, C.L., Energy and protein requirements in stress and trauma, Part I, *Crit. Care Nurs. Currents* 2(1):1, Jan.-March 1984.

17. Heymsfield, S., et al., Overestimate of energy expenditure by widely used equation, *Am. J. Clin. Nutr.* 34(4): 681, 1984.

18. Leaf, A., Dehydration in the elderly, *N. Engl. J. Med.* 311(12):791, Sept. 20, 1984.

19. Phillips, P.A., Reduced thirst after water deprivation in healthy elderly men, *N. Engl. J. Med.* 311(12):753, Sept. 20, 1984.

20. Kinney, A.B., Blount, M., Effect of cranberry juice on urinary pH, *Nurs. Res.* 28(5):287, Sept.-Oct. 1979.

21. Kahn, H.D., et al., Effect of cranberry juice on urine, *J. Am. Diet. Assoc.* 51:251, Sept. 1967.

Chapter 15

SKIN

AGING SKIN

The skin of an elderly person provides a great deal of information. It gives clues about internal disease, provides signs of past environmental effects, and reflects the "natural," inherited, aging tendencies of the individual. A farmworker at age 50 will have a complexion that is strikingly different from that of an office worker of the same age, and an office worker from Texas will have a complexion very different from someone with the same occupation living in Northern Alaska. On the other hand, two elderly persons may both complain of severe itching (pruritus) while one is suffering from uremia and the other from biliary obstruction. Also, two persons of the same age, each with similar degrees of sun exposure and identical health, may look quite different in terms of wrinkling and pigmentation changes, because of different inherited rates of skin aging.

Skin Manifestations of Malnutrition

For reasons of economics, physical infirmity, underlying disease, and life-style, many elderly persons are malnourished. Virtually all the classic vitamin deficiency diseases have skin manifestations, and deficiencies in other nutrients may also alter the skin, nails, or hair (1).

Cracks in the corners of the mouth are often cited as a classic sign of nutrient deficiency. However, the great majority of cases in the elderly are due to alterations in dental occlusion (2). If the bite is malaligned, from atrophy of the gums or ill-fitting dentures, there is an increased overlap of the lips at the corners of the mouth. This allows for accumulation of food and saliva, which in turn leads to irritation and infection with fungus or bacteria, or both, leading to cracking and soreness of the skin.

Deficiencies of protein, fat, or carbohydrate can lead to scaling, dry skin, poor wound healing, and loss of papillae of the tongue. Also, these deficiencies may lead to altered immune status, which in turn can result in unusual skin infections or infestation. Shingles (herpes zoster), a virus-induced skin rash, most commonly occurs in the elderly and only in those with impaired immunity to the virus (2). Norwegian scabies, an infestation by large numbers of scabies mites, is occasionally seen in the elderly. This infestation affects only those with neurologic or immunologic abnormalities.

Of the classic vitamin deficiency diseases, only a few are still seen in this country, and these are seen only rarely. Thiamin deficiency, seen primarily in alcoholics, leads to beriberi. The skin manifestations of beriberi are edema, especially of the face and hands, with or without a weeping rash (3). The long-term use of isoniazid (INH) for antituberculous therapy may lead to a functional deficiency of pyridoxine (vitamin B_6). Occasionally, pyridoxine deficiency can lead to a diffuse reddening and scaling of the central face, neck, and groin (4).

Recurrent aphthous stomatitis (canker sores) have been attributed to deficiencies of vitamin B_{12}, folic acid, or iron (5). An early sign of iron deficiency may be a spooned shape of the fingernails (koilonychia). There also may be a diffuse thinning of the hair, even before anemia from the iron deficiency occurs.

Obesity

Often overweight causes an irritation of opposing folds of skin due to friction or sweating. Occlusion of skin between body folds allows for the buildup of moisture in an area of darkness, which promotes fungus growth. Skinfolds may also block sweat ducts, which can lead to an intensely itchy heat rash. Obesity is often associated with poor blood and lymph drainage from the lower extremities, which allows for skin infections that are slow to heal (3).

Diabetes

Persons with diabetes frequently develop one or more characteristic skin conditions. Most common is diabetic dermopathy. This broad term refers to the fragile nature of diabetic skin and its poor ability to heal. Hyperpigmentation and atrophied areas may indicate undiagnosed diabetes (3). An elderly person with these skin lesions should have fasting blood sugar checked. Another indication of the fragility of the skin in diabetics is the frequent occurrence of large blisters after little or no trauma (6). These blisters, if not properly treated, may lead to deeper cutaneous ulceration. Diabetics have an increased tendency toward skin infections, which tend to be more severe than similar infections in non-diabetics.

Skin ulcerations occur because of the frequency of skin infections and because diabetic neuropathy often renders the individual unaware of serious trauma to the extremities. It has recently been suggested that the administration of continuous subcutaneous insulin and normalization of the blood sugar enhances the healing of diabetic foot ulcerations (7).

Skin Problems From Nutrient Supplements

Many individuals follow self-prescribed nutrient supplementation regimens. Others may be given large nutrient doses for therapeutic uses. These practices may lead to skin changes. Topical vitamin E has been used in an attempt to minimize wrinkling and other aging changes in the skin. Using vitamin E oil can cause contact or irritant dermatitis with redness, itching, and scaling (8). Megadoses of vitamins can also lead to skin changes. Vitamin A overdose leads to scaling of the skin and hair loss. Recently, it has been noted that megadoses of pyridoxine (vitamin B_6) are toxic and may cause a blistering eruption of the skin (8). Oral niacin is still used for the treatment of hyperlipidemia. This may, after prolonged use, cause fishlike scales over large parts of the body (9).

Dietary Intervention in Skin Disease

Chronic skin diseases have been attributed to substances in the diet, and a wide range of different diets have been studied as being potentially beneficial in many different skin diseases. Unfortunately, at present, meaningful dietary intervention is possible in only a small number of cases.

Acne rosacea is a common, chronic skin condition involving the face of older persons; it is the acne vulgaris of the elderly. In rosacea, a common finding is dilated blood vessels in the face, which may be aggravated by alcoholic beverages, hot drinks, and spicy foods.

Herpes labialis (fever blisters or cold sores) is common in the elderly, with some individuals experiencing frequent and recurrent attacks. One study has shown that oral vitamin C and bioflavonoids may be useful for shortening duration of attacks. Two hundred milligrams of each, vitamin C and bioflavinoid, should be taken 3 times daily for 3 days beginning with the first sign of the fever blister (10).

Dermatitis herpetiformis is an uncommon skin condition in which very itchy blisters form on many parts of the body. Most treatments for this disease are toxic. However, it has been shown that the dose of medication needed to control dermatitis herpetiformis can be reduced or even eliminated if the patient follows a gluten-free diet (11). The diet must be adhered to for several months before full benefit is realized and then must be followed indefinitely or there will be a recurrence of the skin disease.

Exfoliative dermatitis is an uncommon skin ailment, but one that requires hospitalization because essentially all of the skin on the body rapidly scales off. There is ongoing loss of the constituents of the skin as well as water, which is usually held inside the body by intact skin. In this state the person is much more susceptible to infection. Close monitoring of nutritional and metabolic parameters is needed. Water loss and iron deficiency anemia are problems (12). It is also important to remember that in these individuals whose skin is turning over very rapidly, folate deficiency must be anticipated and looked for.

Skin cancer is the most common form of cancer in the United States. It has been shown that persons developing skin cancer have lower serum levels of vitamin A, and it has been suggested that vitamin A may be protective against skin cancer (13). In addition, a great deal of work has been done with nutritional factors predisposing and/or preventing malignant melanoma, a deadly form of skin cancer (14). However, most of this work is inconclusive.

DECUBITUS ULCERS

Nontraumatic, chronic skin ulcers usually result from inadequate oxygen and nutrients to epithelial and supportive tissue, which gradually leads to their breakdown, necrosis, and sloughing. The ulcer is like an iceberg, the largest part being under the surface (15). These decubiti or pressure sores develop after prolonged sitting or lying.

Pressure sores are a significant complicating factor in the management of the long-term patient. Surveys show that in general hospitals, 3–5% of all patients develop pressure sores during hospitalization. The patients most likely to develop them are those who are elderly, have alterations of mental status, are incontinent, are bed- or wheelchair-bound, or are unable to ambulate without assistance (16).

In a study of 50 patients with bedsores, age was found to be a less significant factor than the underlying condition. Underlying conditions were most often stroke, multiple sclerosis, fracture of the hip, or senile dementia (17).

One in three pressure sores develops within the first week of hospitalization, and over two-thirds appear within the first 2 weeks (18). The amount of pressure and the time needed to produce a decubitus ulcer vary with the condition of the patient. Changes in the subcutaneous tissue, congestion of capillaries, and reddening of skin can occur after only 2 hours of pressure on an area (19). An elderly woman with a fractured hip, if left on her back, is likely to have a sacral blister within 12 hours. Persistent pressure will eventually cause a pressure sore in any person, regardless of health, but if there is adequate blood pressure and vascular supply, the amount of damage is reduced.

Many factors contribute to the development of pressure sores—friction from improper bedding or unmade beds, moisture from perspiration or incontinence, poor skin condition, use of large quantities of sedative medication, radiation therapy, barbiturate sensitivity (which can cause blisters), sensory loss, and physical handicaps (such as paraplegia) that prevent self-changing of posture. Nutritional status may enhance a patient's susceptibility to pressure sores.

Nutritional Factors in Etiology

Body weight has a major influence on the development of pressure sores. Obesity can either increase or decrease susceptibility. Adipose tissue is poorly vascularized, so when subjected to sustained pressure, it is more vulnerable to breakdown than is lean tissue. Furthermore, fat is not as resilient as other tissue; thus, it is more subject to shearing forces. In addition, extreme obesity can interfere with movement and encourage moisture collection in skinfolds. On the other hand, small amounts of fat tend to cushion the body against pressure and have a protective function. Experts believe that obesity after age 75 may be helpful in protecting against injury to the skin from pressure (20).

In addition to subcutaneous fat, muscle tissue can act as a cushion to prevent decubitus ulcers. A severely underweight person has atrophied muscles that are an inadequate cushion for the bone. A thick layer of active muscle prevents bony joints from sticking out against the body surface and cutting off the blood supply.

Protein deficiency delays wound healing. Serum albumin levels are normally 3.5–4.5 g/dl. Reduction of this level, sometimes to as low as 1.6 g/dl is more closely correlated with the formation of pressure sores than is weight loss. The presence of hypoalbuminemia reflects general debility and increased susceptibility to tissue breakdown and may be the difference between a superficial, easily healed pressure sore and one that is deep and resists treatment.

Tissue vitality, which is the capacity of the tissue to resist infection and heal itself, is more closely related to nitrogen (protein) balance than to body weight (19). Protein deficiency may be aggravated as protein-containing fluids seep out of sores onto dressings. Resultant negative nitrogen balance predisposes the patient to edema in which elasticity, resiliency, and vitality of the skin are decreased. Edema slows the rate of diffusion of oxygen and metabolites between capillaries and cells as the rate of diffusion decreases in proportion to the distance from the capillary to the cell.

Anemia increases the risk for skin breakdown. Not all anemias are due to nutritional factors: occult bleeding, hemoglobinopathies, effects of drugs, or chronic disease may cause anemia. Many anemias, however, are caused by deficiencies of such nutrients as iron, vitamin B_{12}, folate, protein, copper, riboflavin (vitamin B_2), and ascorbic acid (vitamin C). Low hemoglobin levels result in lowered oxygen content, leading to death of tissues subjected to pressure. When chronic infection is present, red blood cell formation is inhibited, and the blood cell life-span is shortened, further aggravating the situation.

In a study of patients with pressure sores it was found that over 45% had anemia (defined as a hemoglobin of less than 12 g/dl for females and less than 14 g/dl for males) compared with an incidence of 26% in a control population. An interesting finding of this study was that 50% of those with pressure sores had been maintained on tube feedings (21).

Hyperglycemia or elevated blood glucose levels make tissues unhealthy. When there is skin damage, infection and widespread tissue death are likely. Long-standing hyperglycemia is associated with vascular disease, which impairs the ability of the skin to both maintain its integrity and heal itself once damaged.

When the body loses water, the skin becomes dry, inelastic, and fragile. Older patients are more susceptible to dehydration than are younger ones. A high intake of protein can cause dehydration because of diuresis due to increased urea production.

Atherosclerosis, or thickening of blood vessel walls, reduces arterial blood flow and may predispose a patient to pressure sores (22). In addition, a patient with peripheral atherosclerosis is likely to also have heart disease and be prone to pressure sores on the basis of decreased cardiac output, leading to reduced blood flow and oxygen delivery to the skin.

Loss of appetite and reduced intake of food result in nutritional deficiencies and weight loss. In a well-nourished person, pressure sores heal quickly when treated locally and with frequent turning to relieve pressure. However, the healing process can be depressed by caloric and nutritional deficiencies. Anorexia is found in a large proportion of patients who are bedridden, depressed, or alcoholic. Pain, heart failure, excess smoking, and some medications such as D-penicillamine, excess digitalis, methimazole, lithium carbonate, and captopril may also cause a loss of appetite (23). Confusion and paralysis limit food intake as the patient may need spoon feeding or use of a nasogastric tube. Malnutrition itself aggravates anorexia since it impairs gastrointestinal function and promotes apathy.

Nutritional Considerations

A high-carbohydrate, high-protein, moderately low-fat diet with adequate calories should be prescribed for patients at risk for developing pressure sores or for those who already have them. Establishment of decubitus awareness programs in long-term care facilities has been recommended. Personnel from all disciplines are involved in these programs, which focus on physical prevention of decubitus ulcers as well as on close monitoring of patients' nutritional intake. Nurse's aides turn and position patients every 2 hours, lubricate the skin, and encourage intake of fluids. Protein-and-vitamin-rich food intake is also encouraged. Breakfast is planned to include 2 eggs daily, 4 oz of orange juice, and cereal cooked in nonfat dry milk. An additional 4 oz of orange juice is served at lunch, and intake of 64 oz of liquid daily is encouraged (24) (see Table 15–1).

Both sufficient calories and adequate protein are essential to promote normal wound healing. Chronic invalids and the elderly may have a low protein intake because of lack of money, reduced chewing ability, lack of storage and preparation facilities, or even because of a lack of energy to prepare foods.

On a protein-free diet, the daily loss of protein is about 20 g, but even under basal conditions, an intake of this amount would not be sufficient to replace the natural loss. Fever and infection destroy body pro-

Table 15–1   Diet Modifications for Persons at Risk of Developing
Decubitus Ulcers

Diet

Protein 75–80 g
       2½ cups milk
       6–8 oz of meat or alternate
Calories 1800–2200 or as needed to maintain optimum weight
Fluids 64 oz

Nutrient supplements

Vitamin C 100 mg
    Citrus juice and/or supplement
Zinc 15 mg
    Zinc-rich foods and/or supplement
Iron
    Supplement, if indicated by reduced hemoglobin

---

tein, and more is lost as protein-containing pus or exudate drain. With trauma and resultant negative nitrogen balance, 90–100 g of protein can be lost daily. Loss of body protein results in deficiency in synthesis of tissue and blood proteins, leukocytes, enzymes, hormones, and antibodies. This can cause a delay in the healing process as well as increased susceptibility to infection.

The patient who has lost weight and cannot restore normal weight should have a diet that provides no less than 2500–3500 kcal daily. A diet made up of 100 g of protein, 500 g of carbohydrate, and 75 g of fat might be appropriate. If there is infection of if the patient has had surgery recently, the daily caloric intake should be as much as 4000–4500, divided among 150 g of protein, 600 g of carbohydrate and 150 g of fat.

There is no significant difference in the digestibility or use of egg albumin, protein hydrolysate, or amino acid mixtures that have an egg protein profile. The patient is more likely to eat and enjoy whole protein foods, the cost of which is much less than for hydrolysates or amino acid mixtures. Therefore, unless there are problems with digestion, it is best to use common protein foods. Protein intake can be increased, if necessary, by the use of dry skim milk or amino acid mixtures, such as Casec (Mead Johnson) mixed into regular food. Start by adding small amounts and increase gradually to 60 g daily. High-protein supplementation can result in high-nitrogen loads that might not be tolerated in patients with renal or hepatic insufficiency.

No matter how well a diet is planned, the foods must be eaten for the patient to benefit. To encourage the consumption of larger amounts of calories and protein, six small feedings should be given daily. These can be supplemented with tube feedings and intravenous feedings, if necessary. Intravenous hyperalimentation can be utilized to achieve weight gain, positive nitrogen balance, and improved wound healing when adequate nutrition is impossible by other means. In a study of 80 patients with pressure sores, 70% on oral intake needed additional commercial meal replacements and vitamin/mineral supplements. Thirty-four percent required enteral or parenteral nutritional support (15).

Pyridoxine (vitamin B_6) and small amounts of thyroid extract and small doses of insulin have also been suggested as useful in improving appetite (25).

Four to eight glasses of fluid is the recommended daily intake. Whenever possible, liquids with caloric value should be given—fruit juice, fruit ades, milk, soft drinks, and high-calorie liquid supplements. A glass of crushed ice available to the patient throughout the day can increase fluid intake, as can the use of ice pops as snacks.

Supplements

Vitamin C functions in collagen formation, and adequate body stores of the vitamin are needed for normal wound healing. The body loses ascorbic acid during stress and bacterial infections and when wounds are present. There are significant losses after surgery. The stress of hospitalization, smoking, and common drugs such as aspirin, barbiturates, hydrocortisone, and diphenylhydantoin (Dilantin, an anticonvulsant) increase the need for vitamin C. Clinical studies show that healing of decubitus ulcers in patients who are not deficient in vitamin C can be significantly accelerated with supplements above the recommended dietary allowance (26,27). Supplements of 250 mg of ascorbic acid given orally two or three times daily are suggested.

Lack of thiamin (vitamin B_1) decreases collagen synthesis, impairs the formation of mature collagen, and decreases tensile strength of the excised wound (28). In addition the B vitamins—thiamin (vitamin B_1), niacin, riboflavin (vitamin B_2), folate, vitamin B_{12}, and pyridoxine (vitamin B_6)—are needed to maintain a normal blood supply. Some anemias are due to a deficiency of these vitamins, which are also needed for energy metabolism. A supplement at the recommended dietary allowance level is suggested.

Vitamin E functions as an antioxidant and may reduce the amount of peroxides generated in a wound that inhibit fibroblast development and thus depress wound healing. Vitamin K is needed for blood clotting, and its supply may be reduced in a patient taking antibiotics. Supplements of these vitamins may be useful if there is a possibility of deficiency.

An iron supplement of the recommended dietary allowance is indicated if there is iron deficiency anemia and the hemoglobin is below 12 g/dl. If there is an open wound, iron supplements are probably not sufficient to restore a lowered hemoglobin, and transfusions can be used to achieve and maintain a hemoglobin level of 12.5 g/dl.

A zinc deficiency is reported to be common among institutionalized people because their diets are usually low in animal products and other foods high in zinc (see Table 15-2). According to recent studies, zinc deficiency wounds are common in the average hospital, and patients benefit from zinc supplementation (30). Between 15 and 20% of normal body stores of zinc are held in the skin, which is the basis for the use of zinc ointments on pressure sores. However, zinc ointments are useful also because they form a moisture-proof barrier that both protects the skin from irritants and prevents excessive moisture loss from the wound.

Table 15-2   Sources of Zinc

Food	Amount	Zinc (mg)
Breads		
Bagel	1	0.5
Hamburger or hot dog roll	1	0.2
Rye	1 slice	0.4
White	1 slice	0.2
Whole wheat	1 slice	0.5
Cereal, pasta, rice		
40% Bran Flakes	1 oz	1.0
Corn flakes	1 oz	0.7
Granola	1 oz	0.6
Macaroni	1 cup	0.7
Oatmeal	½ cup	0.6
Puffed Oats	1 oz	0.8
Puffed Wheat	1 oz	0.7
Rice, brown	½ cup	0.6
Rice, white	½ cup	0.3
Shredded wheat	1 oz	0.8
Wheat germ	1 tbsp	0.9
Dairy		
Cheddar cheese	1 oz	1.0
Cottage cheese	½ cup	0.5
Ice cream	½ cup	0.3
Milk	1 cup	0.9
Yogurt	1 cup	0.9

Table 15–2   (*Cont.*)

Food	Amount	Zinc (mg)
Fruits		
Peaches	1 fresh	0.2
Banana	1 fresh	0.3
Vegetables		
Beans, boiled	1 cup	1.8
Broccoli, cooked	⅔ cup	0.4
Cabbage, boiled	½ cup	0.3
Cabbage, raw	½ cup	0.15
Carrot	1 medium	0.3
Chickpeas	½ cup	1.0
Corn	½ cup	0.4
Green beans	½ cup	0.2
Lettuce	1 cup	0.2
Lentils	½ cup	1.0
Lima beans	1 cup	1.7
Onions, chopped	½ cup	0.3
Peas	½ cup	0.6
Spinach	½ cup	0.6
Meat		
Beef	3 oz	4.9
Beef, ground	3 oz	3.8
Braunschweiger (liver sausage)	1 oz	0.8
Bologna	1 slice	0.5
Frankfurter, beef	1	0.9
Frankfurter, pork	1	0.7
Ham	3 oz	3.4
Lamb	3 oz	4.2
Liver, calf	3 oz	5.2
Pork, loin	3 oz	2.6
Veal	3 oz	3.6
Fish		
Clams, hardshell, raw	4–5	1.1
Clams, softshell	3 oz	1.4
Crab	½ cup	3.3
Fish	3 oz	0.9
Lobster	½ cup	1.5
Oysters, Atlantic	1 oz	25.0
Oysters, Pacific	1 oz	3.0
Salmon, canned	½ cup	1.0
Shrimp	½ cup	1.3
Tuna	½ cup	0.9

Table 15–2   (*Cont.*) Sources of Zinc

Food	Amount	Zinc (mg)
Poultry and eggs		
Chicken		
Drumstick & skin	1	1.4
Drumstick, no skin	1	1.3
Breast & skin	½	0.9
Breast, no skin	½	0.7
Egg	1	0.5
Turkey		
Light	3 oz	1.8
Dark	3 oz	3.7
Miscellaneous		
Corn chips	1 oz	0.4
Doughnut	1	0.2
Graham crackers	2 (1 large)	0.2
Peanuts	1 tbsp	0.3
Peanut butter	1 tbsp	0.5

Zinc supplements not only increase the rate of wound healing but also improve the appetite, so that food intake begins to reach the high-calorie and high-protein intakes needed for healing (31). Zinc sulfate is commonly given three times daily in doses of 200 mg in persons with poorly healing wounds. This supplement yields 50 mg of zinc. Recent evidence indicates that the calcium absorption in adult men with low calcium intakes can be inhibited by daily supplements of 150 mg of zinc. This does not occur with calcium intakes of at least 800 mg (the Recommended Dietary Allowance). (32).

REFERENCES

1. Kenneth, H., Nutrition, aging and the skin, *Geriatrics* 39(2):69, Feb. 1984.
2. Domonkos, A.N., Arnold, H.L., Odom, R.L., eds. *Andrew's Diseases of the Skin*, 7th ed. Philadelphia: W.B. Saunders, 1982.
3. Rook, A., Wilkinson, D.S., *Textbook of Dermatology*, 3rd ed. Boston: Blackwell Scientific Publications, 1979.
4. Vilter, R., et al., The effects of vitamin B_6 deficiency induced by desoxypyridoxine in human beings, *J. Lab. Clin. Med.* 42:335, 1953.
5. Wray, D., et al., Recurrent aphthae: Treatment with vitamin B_{12}, folic acid, and iron, *Br. Med. J.* 2:490, 1975.

6. Bernstein, J.B., Cutaneous lesions associated with diabetes millitus, *Prac. Cardiol.* 9(9):101, 1983.

7. Rubenstein, A., Pierce, C.E., Bloomgarten, Z., Rapid healing of diabetic foot ulcers with continuous subcutaneous insulin infusion, *Am. J. Med.* 75:161, 1983.

8. Baer, R.L., Stillman, M.A., Cutaneous skin changes probably due to pyridoxine abuse, *J. Am. Acad. Dermatol.* 10:527, 1984.

9. Ruiter, M., Meyler, L., Skin changes after therapeutic administration of nicotinic acid in large doses, *Dermatologyica* 120:139, 1960.

10. Terezhalmy, G.T., Bottomley, W.K., Pellen, G.B., The use of a water-soluble bioflavonid-ascorbic acid complex in the treatment of recurrent herpes labialis, *Oral Surg. Oral Med. Oral Pathol.* 45:56, 1978.

11. Fry, L., et al., Clearance of skin lesions in dermatitis herpetiformis after gluten withdrawal, *Lancet* 1:288, 1973.

12. Freedberg, I., Baden, H., The metabolic response to exfoliation, *J. Invest. Dermatol.* 38:277, 1962.

13. Moriarty, M., et al., A comparative study of a number of nutritional and immunological indices in patients with skin cancer, *Irish J. Med. Sci.* 152:242, 1983.

14. Wagner, R.F., Di Sorbo, D.M., Nathanson, L., Nutrition and melanoma, *Int. J. Dermatol.* 23:453, 1984.

15. Myers, S.A., Karamatso, J., Nutritional care of the patient with pressure sores, *Nutr. Support Serv.* 3(7):47, 1983.

16. Reuler, J.B., Cooney, T.G., The pressure sore: Pathophysiology and principles of management, *Ann. Intern. Med.* 94(5): 661, 1981.

17. Moolten, S.E., Bedsores in the chronically ill patient, *Arch. Phys. Med. Rehab.* 53(9):430, 1972.

18. Agate, J.N., Pressure sores, in: *Textbook of Geriatric Medicine and Gerontology.* Edinburgh: Churchill Livingstone, 1978, pp. 640.

19. Kosiak, M., Etiology of decubitus ulcers, *Arch. Phys. Med. Rehabil.* 42(1):19, 1961.

20. Bailey, B.N., *Bedsores.* London: Edward Arnold Ltd., 1967, p. 1.

21. Michocki, R.J., Lamy, P.P., The problem of pressure sores in a nursing home population: Statistical data, *J. Am. Geriatr. Soc.* 24(7):323, 1976.

22. Berecek, K.M., Etiology of decubitis ulcers, *Nurs. Clin. North Am.* 10(1):164, 1975.

23. Miller, D.R., Kennedy, S.K., Drug-induced taste dysfunction, *U.S. Pharmacist* 6(2):20, 1981.

24. Luros, E.A., Rational approach to geriatric nutrition, *Diet. Currents* 8(6):Nov.-Dec. 1981.

25. Moolten, S.E., Bedsores: An update, *Hosp. Med.*, 18(8):64A, Aug. 1982.

26. Ringsdorf, W., Cheraskin, E., Vitamin C and human wound healing, *Oral Surg.* 53(3):231, 1982.

27. Burr, R.G., Rapan, K.T., Leukocyte ascorbic acid and pressure sores in paraplegia, *Br. J. Nutr.* 28(20):275, 1972.

28. Thiamin and wound repair, *Nutr. Rev.* 40:316, 1982.

29. Cohen, D.K., Hypogensia, anorexia and altered zinc metabolism following thermal burns, *JAMA* 223(8):914, 1973.

30. Greger, J.L., Dietary intake and nutritional status in regard to zinc of institutionalized aged, *J. Gerontol.* 32(5):549, 1977.

31. Pories, W.J., Acceleration of wound healing in man with zinc sulfate given by mouth, *Lancet* 1:121, 1967.

32. Spencer, H., et al., Effect of the calcium intake on the inhibitory action of zinc on calcium absorption, *Am. J. Clin. Nutr.* 35(4):829, 1982.

Chapter 16

RESPIRATORY DISEASE

Respiratory diseases are quite common in the elderly. This is in part because, as a person ages, many changes occur that predispose to the development of respiratory infections and other lung disease. The tissues of the lung become more stiff. Changes in the vertebrae occur leading to a posture that overdistends the lungs. There is a reduction in the power of the intercostal muscles and diaphragm so that the elderly person has a decreased ability to breathe deeply and cough forcibly. Cardiac disease is prevalent among the elderly; thus so is congestive heart failure, which often leads to fluid accumulation in the lungs and to decreased ability to exchange oxygen and carbon dioxide.

Perhaps as important in the elderly as any of the above is chronic obstructive pulmonary disease (COPD). COPD is a chronic, progressive disease, usually the consequence of cigarette smoking. It leads to chronic bronchitis and emphysema, which, along with pneumonia, are the major respiratory diseases of elderly persons.

Many, if not all, elderly persons with emphysema or chronic bronchitis shows signs of malnutrition, and nutritional considerations should be an important part of any comprehensive treatment plan (1). Unfortunately, the ambulatory patient with respiratory disease is usually not given diet instructions.

VENTILATOR-DEPENDENT PATIENTS

When a patient's respiratory function deteriorates to the point that he must be placed on a ventilator, both medical and nutritional problems become increasingly complex. In some cases, respiratory failure may be precipitated by starvation; it has been shown that malnutrition interferes with the functions of lung tissue (2). Therefore, correction of malnutrition should be a basic goal of therapy for ventilator-dependent patients.

Such correction may not be as simple as it sounds since the protocols for managing ventilator-dependent patients often do not focus on nutritional needs (3,4). Most respiratory failure patients are admitted to the hospital on an emergency basis, making a complete nutritional assessment impossible. Some patients are already exhibiting signs of progressive malnutrition, which may have precipitated the crisis. Furthermore, patients in critical care units often have NPO as their diet order. These inherent system problems make the delivery of quality nutritional care difficult but not impossible.

It is self-defeating to provide patients with sophisticated breathing apparatus while slow starvation causes cannibalization of the respiratory muscles (4,5). When adequate calories and nitrogen are not provided, the patient enters a state of catabolism. The respiratory muscles will be broken down in an attempt to provide fuel and amino acids for the body (5). Weakness of the respiratory muscles as a result of protein-calorie malnutrition interferes with breathing patterns and gas exchanges, leading to pneumonia, other infections, and collapse of the lungs (6) (see Figure 16–1).

Nutritional Considerations

There are no published studies that prove a conclusive relationship between malnutrition and pulmonary failure (6). Those working in the field, however, based on their clinical experience and observation, have made some recommendations for nutritional management of the ventilator-dependent patient (3,4,5,6).

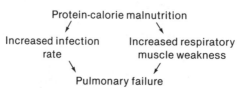

Figure 16–1 Effect of protein-calorie malnutrition on respiratory muscles.

PROTEIN

If the purpose of nutritional support is to preserve lean body mass, 1.2–1.8 g protein/kg body weight should be given. This will approximate 200–300 mg of nitrogen/kg. If lean body tissue must be restored, 1.6–2.5 g protein/kg should be given (250–400 mg nitrogen/kg) (see Table 16–1). Overenthusiastic administration of protein is unwise since it can lead to unnecessary metabolic demands (5,7).

CALORIES

Ventilator-dependent patients may have metabolic requirements as much as 30% above normal (4). If the patient's nutritional status is adequate, an energy intake of 1.0–1.2 times the normal requirement should be given. If the patient is nutritionally depleted, energy requirements increase to 1.4–1.6 times normal (3,7) (see Table 16–1).

Diets high in carbohydrate have been associated with increases in CO_2 production leading to hypercapnia (excess of CO_2 in the blood). For patients with marginal respiratory function there is a risk of respiratory dysfunction if large amount of glucose are given (3,7). On the other hand, septic, catabolic patients may not be able to adequately metabolize fat. Providing excessive lipid to these patients may delay weaning from the ventilator (3). It has been recommended that ventilator-dependent patients be given 50% of nonprotein calories as glucose and 50% as fat (5,7).

Commercial enteral liquid feedings having glucose as the major source of energy could lead to increased CO_2 production, as discussed previously. These feedings are thus inappropriate for the ventilator-dependent patient. Many older adults, especially if malnourished, have lactase deficiency, making milk-based feedings a poor choice. Low-residue, lactose-free, enteral liquid diets with a fat content of 20–50%

Table 16–1 Calorie and Protein Recommendations for Respirator-Dependent Patients

Nutritional status	Age (yr)	Recommended calories/day*		Recommended grams of protein/day*	
		Male	Female	Male	Female
Normal	51–75	2400–2880	1800–2160	67–100	53–79
	76+	2050–2460	1600–1920	67–100	53–79
Depleted	51–75	3360–3840	2520–2880	90–140	70–110
	76+	2870–3280	2240–2560	90–140	70–110

*Based on *Recommended Dietary Allowances*, 9th ed., 1980.

Table 16-2 Enteral Liquid Feedings that Contain a Balance of Fat and Carbohydrate Energy Suitable for the Respirator-Dependent Patient

Product	Percent of energy	
	Lipid	Carbohydrate
Pulmocare	55.2	28.1
Nutri-1000	46.7	38.2
Isocal	37.0	50.0
Magnacal	36.0	50.0
Nutri-Aid	31.6	54.0
Ensure	31.5	54.5
Precision Isotonic	28.1	59.9
Flexical Standard	30.0	61.0
ViPep	22.0	68.0

Adapted from Dietel, M., Rice, T.W., Williams, V.P., Nutritional management of ventilator-dependent patients, *Nutr. Support Serv.* 3:9, Feb. 1983.

are the best choices (3). Table 16-2 lists some acceptable lactose-free feedings.

VITAMINS AND MINERALS

Adequate vitamin and mineral intake must be emphasized (5). A common metabolic problem among respirator patients is hypophosphatemia, and unless corrected, it will weaken respiratory muscles and delay weaning from the ventilator (4,6). Iron serves an important role in maintaining immunocompetence and in oxygen delivery to the tissues. Anemic patients may lack normal levels of oxygen in the blood. Hemoglobin concentration should be monitored and, in most instances, maintained between 12 and 14 g/dl. Attention should be paid to the patient's acid-base status. Both acidosis and alkalosis interfere with the ability of hemoglobin to transfer oxygen at the tissue level (6).

FLUID

There is a good deal of disagreement concerning what constitutes proper fluid management for the ventilator-dependent patient. Regardless of the protocol followed, maintenance of fluid balance is important to avoid extreme decreases below normal in the body's circulating fluids (hypovolemia) and to avoid fluid overload, which itself can interfere with oxygen exchange in the lungs (6).

Feeding Methods and Problems

The enteral route is always the preferred feeding method even for a patient on a ventilator. Many patients can still chew and swallow in the usual manner despite a nasotracheal or tracheostomy tube being in place (3). Older patients, however, may find it unappealing or may be too anxious to eat when intubated. Therefore, enteral feeding, via a feeding tube, is most commonly used (4). When proper precautions are taken with tube placement, volume delivered, and elevation of the head of the bed, aspiration is unlikely to occur (3,5).

As with other tube-fed patients, diarrhea may be a problem for the ventilator-dependent patient. The problem can often be resolved by diluting feedings to isotonic or hypotonic concentrations, using elemental feedings if serum albumin is below 3.0 g/dl or switching from a magnesium-based antacid (e.g., Mylanta) to an aluminum-based variety (e.g., Amphogel). Be aware, however, that aluminum-based antacids bind phosphate, and prolonged use will contribute to hypophosphatemia. In some patients, severe gastric distention is a problem and may require medical intervention. Mylicon (simethicone) drops added to the feeding solution have been shown to be effective (4). Reglan (metoclopromide) has recently been introduced and also is very effective in aiding in emptying of the stomach.

Total parenteral nutrition (TPN) is used when the gastrointestinal tract is nonfunctional. There is a high risk of complications when using TPN with older patients, and these complication may adversely affect pulmonary status; however, when no other feeding method is available, it must be initiated (6). For transient gastrointestinal dysfunction lasting no more than 7–10 days, peripheral parenteral nutrition (PPN) is a logical choice with gradual transfer to enteral feeding as gastrointestinal function improves (5).

Adequate nutrition may be the deciding factor in whether a patient can be taken off the ventilator. Over 90% of patients whose calorie and nitrogen losses were repleted were successfully weaned from the ventilator as compared to 55% who were given minimal nitrogen and calorie replacement (5).

As the patient is weaned from the ventilator, the transition to oral feeding follows. Anorexia and early satiety are common problems among patients being weaned from respirators. These patients are often anxious, and may be receiving medication that causes anorexia. Parenteral or enteral feedings may be discontinued once the patient is able to eat 60% of a regular diet (4). However, intake must be continually monitored to prevent the patient from becoming nutritionally depleted once again.

In some older patients with end-stage chronic obstructive pulmonary disease, weaning is not possible and long-term mechanical ventilation is a necessity. For these patients, nutritional adequacy may be a criterion for determining eligibility for ventilator care at home (7,8).

COPD (CHRONIC OBSTRUCTIVE PULMONARY DISEASE)

Chronic Bronchitis

The patient with chronic bronchitis has been called the "blue bloater." This is because patients with this type of COPD are usually slightly cyanotic (blue), and for reasons that are not entirely clear, these patients are almost always obese and edematous (bloater). The obesity is an important factor perpetuating this condition. Obese individuals have decreased flexibility of the chest wall and have upward displacement of the diaphragm by contents of the abdomen. This leads to restriction of respiration and the patient continues to be cyanotic, lethargic, and prone to repeated respiratory infections, which, in turn, may cause permanent lung damage. Also, an important point to remember is that even though a "blue bloater" appears *overnourished*, he may not be *well nourished* (2). His diet may be high in carbohydrates, which will lead to increased production of carbon dioxide in the body and will add to his cyanosis. He may be taking in very little protein, and his body may be catabolizing its own muscle tissue, including respiratory muscles, in order to obtain necessary amino acids.

Chronic Emphysema

In contrast to the blue boater is the patient with chronic emphysema, known as the "pink puffer." He is not cyanotic but must exert great effort to exchange adequate amounts of air in his overinflated, saccular lungs (so he is constantly huffing and puffing). Pink puffers are usually normal or underweight. Those with longstanding emphysema are underweight. This is because "pink puffers" find eating difficult and tiring. With advanced emphysema, breathing requires frequent and extensive movements because the lungs have lost most of their elastic material and so air must not only be drawn into the lungs, it must be pushed out. Most people develop a style of breathing that includes an upright hunched-over posture and exhaling through pursed lips. Most activity, including the act of eating, requires extra breathing effort. The patient eats inadequate amounts of food because eating is tiring. It is clear that the undernourished person with severe emphysema can develop a vicious cycle of poor protein intake leading to catabolism of muscle, leading to worsening ventilatory function and increased work of breathing, which may lead to even less food intake. In addition, this patient may be taking several medications that may cause anorexia or nausea, further compounding the problem.

Dietary Intervention for COPD

An important part of the treatment should include weight loss for "blue bloaters" and weight gain or maintenance for "pink puffers."

Excessive carbohydrate will lead to the production of excessive carbon dioxide, which is undesirable in a person with compromised respiratory function (9). However, the brain and red blood cells require glucose for energy so that if there is insufficient carbohydrate for this, some of the body's muscle protein will be broken down and converted to glucose. Accordingly, carbohydrate calories should be 25–40% of the daily energy intake.

A sufficient but not excessive amount of protein should be provided so as not to exceed the body's need for protein. Excess protein is converted to carbohydrate, which in turn would lead to increased carbon dioxide production. A protein intake of 12–20% of total calories is suggested. Protein intake should be maintained at a minimum of 0.8 g/kg of ideal body weight per day (2).

Fats are a concentrated source of calories and are used as an alternate energy source when carbohydrate must be limited. Thirty-five to fifty percent of the day's calories should be provided as fat (3).

Patient aid:

Nutrition and Chronic Respiratory Disease

available from:

Cindy Brown, M.S., R.D.
St. Peter's Community Hospital
2475 Broadway
Helena, Montana 59601

REFERENCES

1. Hunter, A.M.B., et al., The nutritional status of patients with chronic obstructive pulmonary disease, *Am. Rev. Respir. Dis.* 124:376, 1981.

2. Brandstetter, D.E., et al., Nutritional requirements in chronic obstructive lung disease, *Resident Staff Physician* 30(1):18, 1984.

3. Dietel, M., Rice, T.W., Williams, V.P., Nutritional management of ventilator-dependent patients, *Nutr. Support Serv.* 3:9, Feb. 1983.

4. Leong, E.T., Beno, M.C., Libby, G.F., Nutritional care of the ventilator-dependent patient: Role of the dietitian, *Nutr. Support Serv.* 3:24, July 1983.

5. Harris, S.W., Nutritional therapy for the respirator-dependent patient, *Nutr. Support Serv.* 2:42, Aug. 1982.

6. Horovitz, J.H., Nutrition in postoperative respiratory failure, in: *Surgical Nutrition*, M.F. Yarborough, P.W. Curreri, eds. New York: Churchill Livingston, Inc., 1981.

7. Weissman, C., Askanazi, J., Nutrition and respiration, *Clin. Consult. Nutr. Support*, 2:6, April 1982.

8. Maguire, M., Miller, T.V., Young, P., Teaching patients' families to provide ventilator care at home, *Dimensions Crit. Care Nurs.* 1:244, July-Aug. 1982.

9. Feurer, I.D., Hain, W.F., Mullen, J.L., Nutritional regimens and carbon dioxide production, *Hosp. Physician*, 20(1):42, Jan. 1984.

Chapter 17

NUTRITIONAL CONSIDERATIONS WITH DRUG USE

Older adults comprise 11% of the population, yet they use 25% of all prescribed and over-the-counter drugs (1). These include insulin, oral hypoglycemic agents, inhibitors of gastric acid secretion, diuretics, sedative-hypnotics, and also aspirin, acetaminophen, laxatives, antacids, and alcohol-containing tonics. A consistent increase in the average number of different drug categories used is found as age increases (2).

The average older person has one or more chronic diseases and takes from three to seven different medications at any given time (1). The amount of money spent by older adults in this country on drugs is measured in billions of dollars annually. Older adults, as a group, take significantly more medication than any other age group.

Clearly, this population is receiving a great deal of medication, which is important for several reasons. Older adults are at increased risk for adverse drug reactions, which occur seven times more frequently in adults over age 65 than in those under age 29. It has been estimated that 25% of all patients over the age of 80 experience some form of abnormal drug reaction (3). In addition, inadequate nutritional status increases the risk for harmful interactions between drugs and food.

There is always the potential for a food and drug interaction. Drugs may have an effect on food that is eaten, or food that is eaten may alter the action of drugs that are taken. These drug-nutrient interactions are an important consideration when caring for the elderly who, because of body changes, the prevalence of poor nutrition, and the possibility of dehydration, may be more sensitive to these effects.

THE IMPACT OF DRUGS ON NUTRITIONAL STATUS

A great many drugs commonly taken by mature adults may act to cause, or worsen, malnutrition or specific deficiency states. Drugs may disturb taste perception, alter appetite, or interfere with nutrient absorption or nutrient excretion. Caregivers must be aware of the nutritional actions of specific drugs when evaluating a patient for nutritional problems. See Table 17–1 for a listing of drugs that may have an impact on nutritional status.

One nutritional problem not found in Table 17–1 is intestinal obstruction. Partial gastrointestinal obstruction has occurred in elderly persons who, because of poor eyesight, confusion, or other reasons, have accidentally swallowed the desiccant material in a pill bottle. This material is added to many bottles of medication in order to absorb moisture in the air and help slow the decomposition of the drug. Most desiccants are encapsulated in material that will dissolve if swallowed.

Table 17–1   Drug-Nutrient Interactions

Drug	Effect on nutrition
Antacids	
Aluminum hydroxide (Maalox)	Decreases absorption of phosphate, vitamin A; inactivates thiamin; deficiency of calcium and vitamin D
Calcium carbonate (Tums, Titrilac)	Decreases absorption of fatty acids; nausea
Anticoagulant	
Coumarin (Coumadin)	Vitamin E enhances action; vitamin K reduces effectiveness, limit food high in vitamin K; limit alcohol, caffeine, green tea; silicon additives in cooking oils inhibit absorption
Anticonvulsants	
Barbiturates (phenobarbital)	Decreases absorption of vitamin B_{12} and thiamin; deficiency of folate, vitamins D and K
Hydantoin (Dilantin)	Decreases serum folate, pyridoxine, calcium, vitamin B_{12} and D; increases excretion of vitamin C; increases copper; do not take with foods enhanced with monosodium glutamate (MSG)

Table 17-1   (Cont.)

Drug	Effect on nutrition
Antidepressants	
Tricyclic (Elavil)	Increases food intake (large amounts may suppress intake)
Monoamine oxidase inhibitors (Parnate, Nardil)	Interacts with tyramine in food causing headaches, hypertensive crises, diarrhea
Antiinflammatory agents	
Colchicine	Decreases absorption of vitamin B_{12}, carotene, fat, lactose, sodium, potassium, protein, cholesterol
Glucocorticoids (prednisone)	Decreases absorption of calcium and phosphorus; increases food intake and salt retention
Zomepirac (Zomax)	Nausea, anorexia, flatulence
Antihypertensives	
Hydralazine (Apresoline)	Anorexia, vomiting, nausea, diarrhea, constipation
Captopril (Capoten)	Decreases taste, anorexia, nausea, vomiting, diarrhea
Methyldopa (Aldomet)	Increases need for vitamin B_{12} and folate; diarrhea, constipation, nausea, vomiting, flatulence, dry mouth
Antimetabolites	
5-Fluorouracil (Efudex)	Diarrhea, altered taste, sore mouth; decreases protein absorption; increases need for thiamin
Methotrexate	Decreases absorption of vitamin B_{12} and folate; nausea, vomiting, diarrhea
Antimicrobials	
Ampicillin	Do not take with fruit juice; nausea, vomiting, diarrhea
Chloramphenicol	Increases need for riboflavin, vitamin B_{12}, and pyridoxine
Erythromycin (Erythrocin or E-Mycin)	Do not take with fruit juice; diarrhea, nausea, vomiting
Isoniazid (INH)	Decreases absorption of vitamin B_{12}; pyridoxine deficiency; secondary niacin deficiency; dry mouth
Lincomycin (Lincocin)	Diarrhea, nausea, vomiting
Methenamine (Mandelamine)	Maintain adequate fluid intake

Table 17–1   (Cont.) Drug-Nutrient Interactions

Drug	Effect on nutrition
Metronidazole (Flagyl)	Dry mouth, nausea, vomiting, unpleasant taste
Neomycin	Decreases absorption of fat, carotene, protein, vitamins, A, D, K, B_{12}, potassium, sodium, calcium, iron
Nitrofurantoin (Fura-dantin)	Maintain adequate protein; nausea, vomiting, diarrhea
Sulfamethoxazole and trimethoprim (Septra, Bactrim)	Decreases absorption of folate; decreases bacterial synthesis of folate, vitamin K, and B vitamins; increases urinary excretion of vitamin C
Sulfisoxazole (Gan-trisin)	Decreases absorption of folate; decreases bacterial synthesis of folate, vitamin K, and B vitamins; increases urinary excretion of vitamin C
Tetracycline	Nausea, vomiting, diarrhea; decreases absorption of fat, protein, calcium, iron, magnesium, zinc; decreases bacterial synthesis of vitamin K; do not take with milk or foods high in iron
Antipyretics	
Acetaminophen (Ty-lenol)	Carbohydrates retard absorption
Acetylsalicyclic acid (aspirin)	Decreases serum folate; increases excretion of vitamin C, thiamin, potassium, amino acids, glucose; nausea, gastritis
Indomethacin (Indocin)	Anorexia, nausea, vomiting, diarrhea, flatulence
Phenylbutazone (Buta-zolidin)	Decreases absorption of folate; increases excretion of protein; constipation, nausea, vomiting
Hypercholesterolemic Drug	
Cholestyramine (Ques-tran, Cuemid)	Decreases absorption of fats, vitamins A, D, E, K, B_{12}, folate; constipation
Laxatives	
Bisocodyl (Dulcolax)	Do not take with milk since this may cause disintegration of the enteric coating
Dioctyl-sodium sulfo-succinate (Colace)	Take with milk or juice; increases absorption of cholesterol and vitamin A; alters absorption of water and electrolytes; nausea, vomiting, diarrhea, bitter taste
Mineral oil	Decreases absorption of vitamins A, D, E, and K
Phenolphthalein (Ex-Lax)	Decreases absorption of vitamins A, D, E, and K

Table 17-1   *(Cont.)*

Drug	Effect on nutrition
Miscellaneous	
Diazepam (Valium)	Constipation, nausea, salivary changes
Digitalis (Lanoxin, Digoxin)	Increases excretion of potassium, magnesium, calcium; nausea, vomiting, anorexia, diarrhea; incompatible with protein hydrolysates; *caution with herbal teas*
Griseofulvin (Fulvican)	Altered taste, dry mouth
Levodopa (Larodopa)	Anorexia, nausea, vomiting, dry mouth, constipation; increases need for vitamins B_{12}, C, pyridoxine; increases excretion of sodium, potassium; *limit foods rich in pyridoxine*
Levothyroxine sodium (Synthroid)	*Do not take with goitrogenic foods,* i.e., Brussels sprouts, cabbage, mustard greens, cauliflower, spinach, kale, rutabaga, soybeans, turnips
Lithium carbonate (Lithane, Lithotabs, Lithonate)	*Not compatible with decreased salt diet*
Iron salts (Feosol, Fergon)	When taken with whole grains, absorption is decreased; when taken with vitamin C, absorption is increased
Penicillamine	Loss of taste; increased requirement for pyridoxine; increased excretion of zinc, iron, copper, pyridoxine; anorexia, nausea, vomiting, diarrhea
Potassium chloride (K-Ciel, Kaochlor, K-Lor, K-Lyte-Cl, Slow-K)	Decreases absorption of vitamin B_{12}; diarrhea, nausea, vomiting
Cimetidine (Tagamet)	Bitter taste, diarrhea, constipation
Thiazide diuretics (Diuril, Hydroduiril)	Increases excretion of sodium, potassium, chloride, magnesium, zinc, riboflavin; anorexia, nausea, vomiting, diarrhea, constipation

However, some desiccants are packaged in insoluble material, and these, if swallowed, may cause obstruction of the gastrointestinal tract (4).

THE EFFECTS OF NUTRIENTS ON DRUG ACTIVITY

There are several ways in which foods may alter the action of a drug. Food may affect the absorption, metabolism, and excretion of a drug.

Certain nutrients themselves have druglike activity and may potentiate or antagonize the action of a drug. Also, some nutrients are capable of behaving like a drug in certain instances when another drug is being taken.

When food and drugs are mixed, the absorption of the drug may be enhanced, unaffected, or diminished. It is widely known that fat-soluble vitamins are best absorbed when taken with a meal that is rich in fat. Similarly Fulvicin (griseofulnin), a drug used to treat fungal infections, is best absorbed when taken during a meal that is rich in fat. Alternatively, some drugs are very poorly absorbed if taken with certain foods. For example, tetracycline, a commonly used antibiotic, cannot be absorbed if taken at the same time as calcium- or iron-containing foods. Similarly, food may delay the absorption of Digoxin (digitalis), Lasix (furosemide), Pro-Banthine (propantheline bromide). Other drugs such as Ampicillin and penicilin G are inactivated by acids and thus cannot be taken with acidic foods such as citrus juices (5). See Tables 17–2 and 17–3 for a more complete listing of drugs best taken with meals and those best taken on an empty stomach.

Some foods, especially when eaten in large quantities, may have effects similar to those of drugs. In addition, certain foods directly antagonize the effects of a drug. For instance, Coumadin (warfarin), a commonly used anticoagulant, acts by inhibiting the action of vitamin K. When large amounts of vitamin E are taken, there is inhibition of the absorption of vitamin K. Thus, if a person is taking Coumadin and then begins taking vitamin E, there will be an enhancement of the effect of Coumadin. Alternatively, if a person taking Coumadin eats a large

Table 17–2   Drugs That Should Be Taken with Meals

Aldactone	Fulvicin	Ornade
Aldoril	Furadantin	Parnate
Apresoline	Grifulvin	Phenobarbital
Aspirin	Hydrodiuril	Pondimin
Butazolidin	Indocin	Prednisone
Colace	Inderal	Premarin
Darvon Compound	Isoniazid	Questran
Dilantin	Kaochlor, K-Ciel,	Sinemet
Diuril	K-Lor, K-Lyte-Cl,	Sinequan
Dramamine	Slow-K	Tagamet
Elavil	Larodopa (levodopa)	Tandearil
Empirin Compound	Lithotabs, Lithonate,	Thorazine
with Codeine	Lithane†	Triavil
Feosol*	Mandelamine	Valium
Fer-In-Sol*	Mellaril	Zyloprim
Flagyl	Oretic	

*Do not take with milk; use a fruit juice high in vitamin C.
†Take with milk.

Table 17–3 Drugs That Should Be Taken on an Empty Stomach

Achromycin*†	Efudex	Mylanta
Aminophylline,	Epsom salts‡	Penicillamine
Theophylline,	Erythromycin*	Penicillin*
Slo-Phyllin	Fleet	Pronestyl
Ampicillin	Gantrisin	Quinidex
Castor oil‡	Gavison	Quinidine
Chloramphenicol	Gelusil	Septra
Cuprimine	Isoniazid (INH)	Somophyllin
Demeclocycline	Levodopa (Larodopa)	Tetracycline†
(Declomycin)*†	Librax	Theodur, Theolair
Doxycycline	Lincomycin	Tylenol*†
(Vibramycin)	(Lincocin)	

*Fruit juice, vegetable juice, soda, and wine are all acidic drinks and will reduce the effectiveness of antibiotics.

†Avoid milk and dairy products; they reduce effectiveness.

‡Take with juice.

quantity of food that is rich in vitamin K, there will be reversal of the effect of the Coumadin. See Table 17–4 for a listing of foods that are rich in vitamin K. Similarly, the action of levodopa, used in Parkinson's disease, is inhibited by pyridoxine. Table 17–5 lists foods that are rich in

Table 17–4 Foods Rich in Vitamin K

Food	Amount	mcg
Turnip greens, cooked	⅔ cup	650
Lettuce	¼ head	129
Cabbage, cooked	⅔ cup	125
Beef liver	3 oz	110
Broccoli, cooked	½ cup	100
Spinach, cooked	½ cup	80
Pork liver	3 oz	30
Peas, cooked	⅔ cup	19
Ham	3 oz	18
Green beans, cooked	¾ cup	14
Cheese	1 oz	14
Egg	1	11
Ground beef, raw	4 oz	10.5
Milk	1 cup	10
Chicken liver	3 oz	8
Peach	1 medium	8
Butter	1 tbsp	6
Tomato	1 small	5
Banana	1 medium	3
Applesauce	⅓ cup	2
Corn oil	1 tbsp	2
Bread	1 slice	1

Table 17–5   Foods Rich in Vitamin B$_6$ (Pyridoxine)

Food	Amount	mg
Most, Kellogg's	1 cup	2.0
Tuna, canned	3½ oz	0.90
Liver	3 oz	0.84
Chicken	3½ oz	0.70
Corn flakes	1 cup	0.70
Banana	1 medium	0.61
Kix, General Mills	1½ cups	0.50
Avocado	½ medium	0.46
Pork	3 oz	0.45
Beef	3 oz	0.44
Halibut	3 oz	0.43
Brussels sprouts, cooked	4 large	0.40
Carnation Instant Breakfast	1 envelope	0.40
Egg yolk	1	0.30
Corn, canned	½ cup	0.30
Sunflower seeds	2 tbsp	0.22
Brewer's yeast	1 tbsp	0.20
Cottage cheese, creamed	½ cup	0.20
Asparagus, cooked	½ cup	0.20
Summer squash, cooked	½ cup	0.20
Wheat germ	2 tbsp	0.15
Frankfurter	1	0.14
Lima beans, cooked	½ cup	0.12
Cantaloupe	¼ melon	0.12
Peanut butter	2 tbsp	0.11
Tomato	1 medium	0.10
Yogurt	8 oz	0.10
Spoon Size Shredded Wheat	1 cup	0.10
Peanuts	2 tbsp	0.10

Table 17–6   Foods High in Tyramine (or Other Sympathomimetic Amines)

Aged cheese	Beer	Pineapple
(Stilton,	Bologna	Raisins
Cheddar,	Broad beans	Salami
Gruyere,	Canned figs	Sausage
Camembert,	Chianti wines	Sherry
Brie,	Chicken liver	Sour cream
Ermantaler)	Chocolate	Soy sauce
Avocado	Coffee	Yeast extract
Bananas	Cola drinks	Yogurt
Beef Liver	Pickled herring	

pyridoxine and should be eaten in moderation by someone taking levodopa.

When a person is given an antidepressant medication that is a monoamine oxidase inhibitor (MAOI), foods that are rich in tyramine are then able to act like drugs in the body. Foods that are rich in tyramine are ordinarily tolerated well by anyone. However, in the presence of an MAOI, tyramine-rich foods can cause extremely high blood pressure, headaches, diarrhea, and other derangements that may be fatal. Therefore, it is essential that persons taking MAOI completely avoid foods that are rich in tyramine (6,7). These foods are listed in Table 17–6.

See Table 17–1 for a listing of other actions that food may have on certain drugs.

OVER-THE-COUNTER MEDICATION

Many potent medications are available in this country without prescription. It is therefore extremely important to ask all patients about the use of over-the-counter medications. It has been shown that older adults use a great deal of nonprescription medications and may use such preparations regularly for years (8).

The two major concerns, nutritionally, about over-the-counter medications are the content of alcohol and the content of sugar of many of the products available (see Tables 17–7 and 17–8). The issue of alcohol intake in the form of non-prescription medications is discussed in Chapter 5. It is important for the older diabetic to be aware of the fact

Table 17–7   Alcohol in Pharmaceuticals

Drug	Percent alcohol
Acetaminophen elixir	6.5–10.5
Benadryl elixir	12–14
Benylin cough syrup	5
Breacol (mentholated)	20
Breacol (regular formula)	10
Broncho-Tussin	40
Cascara Sagrada Aromatic Fluid Extract	18
Chlortrimetron	7
Comtrex Nighttime Multisymptom	25
Co-Tylenol Liquid Cough Formula	7
Dexamethasone elixir	3.8–5.7
Digoxin elixir	9–11
Dimetapp elixir	2.3

Table 17-7   (*Cont.*) Alcohol in Pharmaceuticals

Drug	Percent alcohol
Diphenhydramine HCl elixir	12–15
Dramamine liquid	5
Dristan Cough Formula Syrup	12
Eldertonic	15
Feosol elixir	5
Genvitol	5
Geralix liquid	12
Geriatric elixir	12
Geri-Pen elixir	5
Geritol	12
Gerix elixir	20
Kaochlor 10% liquid	5
Lomotil liquid	15
Lufyllin-GG elixir	17
Mellaril solution	4.2
Nembutal elixir	18
Neo-Synephrine	8
Novahistine DMX	10
NyQuil	25
Oxtriphylline elixir	18–22
Periactin syrup	5
Peri-Colace syrup	10
Pertussin 8-Hour Cough Formula	9.5
Pertussin Night-Time Cold Medicine	25
Phenobarbital elixir	12–15
Potassium Gluconate elixir	5
Prolixin elixir	14
Quibron elixir	15
Reserpoid elixir	14
Robitussin	3.5
Romilar CF	10
Secobarbital elixir	10–14
Seconal elixir	12
Stannitol elixir	23
Symptom, 1,2,3 and Multi	5
Tedral elixir	15
Theolixir	20
Triaminic Expectorant	5
Tylenol liquid	7
Valerian	68
Vicks Day-Care	7.5
Vicks Formula 44	10
Viro-med	16.63

Adapted from: Dukes, G.E., Kuhn, J.G., and Evens, R.P., Alcohol in Pharmaceutical Products, *American Family Physician*, 16:97, September 1977.

Table 17–8   Alcohol-Drug Interaction

Drug classification	Potential reaction if alcohol is taken	Drugs in this classification
Analgesics	Stomach irritation GI bleeding Liver damage Increased risk of hemorrhage Increased central nervous system depression Possible respiratory arrest	Aspirin (acetylsalicylic acid) Alka-Seltzer Bufferin Excedrin Codeine Datril Darvon Demerol Morphine Norgesic Tylenol
Antihistaminics	Increased central nervous system depression Drowsiness	Allerest Benadryl Contac Dimetapp Dramamine Dristan Periactin
Hypertensive agents	Increased drug effect Possible hypotension Possible intoxication	Aldomet Catapres Combipres Diuril Dyazide Enduron Lasix
Anticoagulants	Increased or decreased effect	Coumadin Dicumarol
Oral antidiabetic	Decreased antidiabetic effect Flushing Severe headache Pounding heartbeat Dizziness Shortness of breath Sweating Initial rise in blood pressure Weakness Nausea and vomiting	Diabinese Dymelor Orinase
Antialcohol	Flushing Severe headache Pounding heartbeat Dizziness Shortness of breath Sweating	Antabuse

Table 17–8 (*Cont.*) Alcohol-Drug Interaction

Drug classification	Potential reaction if alcohol is taken	Drugs in this classification
	Initial rise in blood pressure Weakness Nausea and vomiting Confusion Unconsciousness "Disulfiram reaction"	

Antiinfectives	Reaction similar to that seen with antialcohol medication	Amcill
		  (ampicillin)
		Chloromycetin
		  (chloramphenicol)
		Flagyl
		Gantrisin
		Grisactin
		Grifulvin

Antiarthritis drugs	Reaction similar to that seen with antialcohol medication	Butazolidin (phenylbutazone)
Sedatives and tranquilizers	Increased sedative effect Increased central nervous system depression Possible fatal reaction Serious depression of brain function	Compazine Dalmane Librium Mellaril Miltown Nembutal Valium Seconal Phenobarbital
Antidepressants	Extreme increase in blood pressure Excessive sedation Incoordination Stomach upset Possible fatal reaction	Aventyl Elavil Marplan Norpramin Novane Sinequan
Cardiovascular agents	Increased absorption with possible hypotension Cardiac arrhythmias	Nitroglycerine Lanoxin Digoxin Digitoxin

that many nonprescription drugs have large amounts of sugar; therefore, they contribute calories and may make diabetic control difficult. Table 17–9 lists a number of presently available products of a variety of types that contain minimal amounts of sugar and thus are acceptable for use by a diabetic person.

Table 17-9   Nonprescription Medications with Little or No Sugar Content

Cough medicine	Colrex expectorant, Sorbituss syrup, Hytuss tablets, Queltuss tablets, Coramine solution, Dimetapp elixir, Dimetane expectorant—DC
Decongestants	Afrin spray, Neosynephrin spray (avoid pills)
Analgesics	Use acetaminophen, as aspirin may lower blood sugar
Antidiarrheals	Pepto-Bismol, Kaopectate
Laxatives	Phospho-Soda, Konsyl, Agoral (all enemas and suppositories are acceptable)
Antacids	Di-Gel, Gelusil, Maalox, Mylanta, Riopan, Mylicon drops
Antinausea agents	Dramamine
Vitamins	Califerol Drops, Geriplex—FS Liquid, Homicebrin

COMPLIANCE WITH MEDICATION

More than half of all older patients do not take their medications as prescribed (9). It has been shown that the elderly person who is most likely to be a poor complier with medication is one who has been a compliance problem in the past, is taking multiple medications, has a poor mental status, lives alone, has a fixed income, or has visual difficulties (1).

There are several different approaches to the problem of poor compliance with medication. First, and probably most important, is good, thorough communication with the patient about the need, use, and possible side effects of the medication. There are booklets available that emphasize the importance of good compliance (see Patient Aid, p. 264). These resources offer suggestions about how to keep track of multiple medications. Compartmentalized drug containers, available at the pharmacy, can be set up to help the older person keep track of daily medications.

A new product designed to improve compliance is the *Med Tymer** which is a special medicine bottlecap that contains a timer and sounds an alarm when medications are to be taken. The pharmacist is able to dispense these, set appropriately for each medication that needs to be taken.

*Boston Medical Research, Inc., Suite L-10, 160 Commonwealth Avenue, Boston, Massachusetts 02116.

Patient aid:

Using Your Medication Wisely:
A Guide for the Elderly

available from:

DHEW Publication No. (ADM) 80-705
National Institute on Drug Abuse
5600 Fishers Lane
Rockville, Maryland 20857

REFERENCES

1. Tideiksaar, R., Drug noncompliance in the elderly, *Hosp. Physican*, 20(3):92, March 1984.

2. Hale, W.E., et al., Drug use in a geriatric population, *J. Am. Geriatr. Soc.* 27(8):374, 1979.

3. Lamy, P.P., What the physician should keep in mind when prescribing drugs for an elderly patient, *Geriatrics* 32:37, 1977.

4. Muhletaler, C., et al., The pill bottle desiccant, a cause of partial gastrointestinal obstruction, *JAMA* 243:1921, 1980.

5. Block, C.D., Popovich, N.C., Black, M.C., Drug interaction in the G.I. tract, *Am. J. Nurs.* 77(9):1426, 1977.

6. Giovannitti, C., and Schwinghammer, T., Food and drugs—Managing the right mix for your patient, *Nursing 81* 11(7):26, 1981.

7. Horowitz, O., et al., Monoamine oxidase inhibitors, tyramine, and cheese, *JAMA* 188:90, 1964.

8. Gunby, P., Elderly may over-mix prescription, non-prescription drugs, *Arch. Intern. Med.* 142:1607, 1982.

9. Polk, I.J., Drug compliance in the elderly, *JAMA* 248:1239, 1982.

Part III

PSYCHOSOCIAL FACTORS THAT AFFECT NUTRITIONAL INTAKE

Chapter 18

PSYCHOSOCIAL FACTORS AND SOCIETAL SYSTEMS THAT AFFECT NUTRITIONAL CARE

by Elaine B. Jacks, M.S., R.N.
Director, Multidisciplinary Center on Aging
Adelphi University
Garden City, New York

To be an older adult today is a unique experience and one without past precedent. As life-span increases, an individual may be considered "old" for 30 years or more. For some this period will be the longest segment of their lives.

Each individual brings to old age all the cultural attitudes and beliefs that have resulted from a lifetime of interaction with a specific group. A person's heritage includes a value system, a world view, and normative structure. How each individual integrates these elements results in his unique personality. It has long been understood that lifestyle, attitudes, and behavior affect food intake. Food preferences are cumulative beginning with the era and region of early socialization. Added to this are the results of life's experiences and the current status of the individual.

Owing to the diversity of age, heritage, race, education, economic status, and health, it is impossible to lump "older adults" into a homogeneous group and form generalizations. Yet, if effective health care and nutritional guidance are to be offered to our aging population, caregivers must understand the impact of psychosocial factors on food intake and nutritional status. Table 18-1 list some of the psychosocial factors that effect the nutritional status of older adults. These factors may have created the existing health problem or may be a complicating factor.

Table 18-1 Psychosocial Factors Influencing Nutritional Status of Older Adults

Social status
Cultural food habits
Economic status
Socialization
Emotional instability
Life change stressors (e.g., loss of spouse, relocation, retirement)
Religious food habits
Regional food preferences
Personal taste preferences and food taboos
Dependent/independent living arrangements
Adaptation to unfamiliar surroundings (e.g., nursing home, living with adult children)
Educational level
Marital status
Folk health belief system
Lack of food preparation skills
Family abuse and/or neglect

ECONOMIC STATUS

Those older individuals at greatest risk of nutritional problems are those who are economically deprived. Income is reduced at retirement, and often this lowered income is not adequate to meet basic needs. Women and minority groups are overrepresented in the poor and near-poor income groups, estimated to number 5.5 million, or one-fourth of all persons aged 65 or older (1). In 1981 the Bureau of Labor Statistics estimated three hypothetical annual budgets for a retired couple living in an urban area. The estimated average annual cost, excluding personal income taxes, of the lower budget for an urban retired couple was $7,226. The intermediate and higher budgets were $10,226 and $15,078, respectively. Medical care at all three budget levels showed the largest increase, rising 15% above the reported 1979–1980 period. At the lower budget this means $1085, or 15% of the couple's annual income, was spent on medical care. An additional $2,183, or 30%, was spent on food. Thirty-two percent was spent on housing, leaving only 23% of the annual income to cover all other expenses (2). Even at this lower income budget the couple is living substantially above the poverty line, set at $4,400 (3).

EDUCATIONAL STATUS

Older Americans received most of their formal education and consumer education when the products, services, and market system were considerably less complex than today (4). A substantial number of older adults have had limited schooling (less than 5 years). This has led to the erroneous assumption that nutrition education materials and programs must be oversimplified to be effective. What the aged lack in physical capabilities and education they make up for in "life experience." Anyone who has survived for six, seven, or eight decades has accumulated a body of practical knowledge and experience that serves as the basis for new learning. Nutrition educators need to encourage the older adult to rely heavily on what they already know to help them find workable solutions to existing problems.

When developing education programs for older adults, particular attention should be paid to the age composition of the group. The pace of discussion and the topics selected that are of interest to those in their 40s and 50s will differ drastically from the delivery and choice of topics for participants in their 70s. And those in their 70s, who are often reasonably healthy and living independently, want to learn far different information than the 80-year-old living in a nursing home or attending a geriatric day care program. All these groups need and benefit from nutrition education sessions. When asked what consumer information older individuals most want to learn, food and nutrition was listed fourth in a group of 13 items. Medical services, utilities, and taxes were ranked more important (4). This observation shows that once basic needs are addressed, people are interested in their health and well-being.

Research has also demonstrated that though it is difficult to make dietary changes at all ages, older adults can and will make these changes when they perceive them as beneficial (5,6). Medical and social reasons were given most often as reasons to change food habits (6).

Very few of the currently available audiovisual consumer education materials were developed with the older learner in mind (4). The development of appropriate models for older individuals with differing needs is the new challenge on the horizon.

An emergent curriculum model is a more useful tool for personalizing nutrition information for the present-day heterogeneous older population. The emergent curriculum model enables the learner to assist in curriculum construction. This model does not start with a predetermined curriculum based on assumptions but evolves as the participants of the group engage in open dialogue. They discuss their needs and areas of misinformation that need clarification. Nutrition topics emerge from this dialogue, and the end product is a learning unique to the needs of the group. This learning model is not threatening to those with less formal education and at the same time is broadening for those who have a substantial background of knowledge. Contributions by group members can help to reinforce self-esteem. Evaluation of this model is based on whether or not the experience satisfied informational needs of the participants rather than on what specific information was learned. The emergent curriculum considers the humanistic value of self-benefit as an important key to measure success (7).

MALE VS. FEMALE ACCOMMODATION TO AGING

Social scientists have identified some observed differences in food-related behaviors between men and women in later life. Though much of this information is observational, it can be of value in helping the caregiver to interpret sociological factors that may have an impact on nutritional status.

In response to the changes associated with aging, many women display high levels of psychological stress. Loneliness is prevalent among older women, and they tend to display higher levels of anxiety, depression, and sensitivity (8). Frequently they may become preoccupied with health, often developing hypochondria. Whether the dysfunctions or malfunctions they report are real, imagined, or exaggerated, they will influence food selection and rejection. Digestive upsets, constipation, "poor" blood, and fatigue are often attributed to and/or "treated" by certain foods.

Even though older women usually report their retirement as "voluntary" rather than "mandatory," sociological data show that women enjoy retirement less than men and take a longer time to adjust to it (8). Older women spend less money on weekly groceries than men and this amount decreases proportionately as income increases. Thus, having adequate funds to purchase food does not automatically ensure an adequate intake (9). Older women are more likely to prepare food for themselves than older men, and when they do, the variety of food used is greater (10).

Older men are less likely to respond to aging by becoming psychologically stressed. Among older, working-class men, aging brings about an acceptable disengagement, a lessened involvement with friends and organizations. Most working-class men report that they enjoy retirement. They are the "rocking-chair people" who find more pleasure passively observing society than actively entering into it. Older men are willing to spend more money on weekly groceries than older women, regardless of their earnings. They eat out more frequently, making this one of their major social events (9). Older men may lack interest in or skill for food preparation. If they are forced to prepare their meals, their food choices are more limited than those of older women (10).

For both older men and older women, those who remain the most socially active show the greatest variety in food use and consumption

(9). This supports the assumption that for older adults socialization may be the most important factor in rekindling interest in eating. Continued socialization is as important to maintaining adequate nutritional status as the availability of adequate food.

SOCIAL ISOLATION

While poor nutrition is the result of improper food selection, improper food selection may be caused by a social problem rather than a health problem. Many older adults find themselves socially isolated.

Neighborhoods in transition may interrupt eating habits, particularly for the low-income urban dweller. Nutritional crises can be precipitated when store owners vacate, leaving aged residents in familiar but suddenly hostile neighborhoods. Where will the Jewish widow get her meat after the kosher butcher closes his store? The Italian neighborhood that integrates a wave of Puerto Rican immigration leaves little that is familiar to the aged Italians who remain. When customary foods are no longer available and the person feels culturally isolated, food choices may be reduced as a response to both loneliness and unavailability of familiar products. There is no replacement for the faithful corner druggist, the helpful neighbor, or the favorite fruit stand. The familiarity of places, people, and artifacts enhances stability and security as one ages.

A change in living situations and a change in social activities are ranked among life changes that are considered major life stressors. Loss of spouse, loss of other family members, change in health, financial problems, loss of a close friend, change in living conditions, and change in personal habits are among other stresses listed on a life change units scale. If a number of these life stressors are clustered wtihin a reasonable time frame, as may be the case with many older individuals, illness or death may result (11). Life changes, particularly those that result in isolation from society, may serve as predictors of future health.

There are more residentially isolated older women than older men. This is because women live longer than men, and in many cases their spouses have predeceased them. In addition, the unequal sex distribution among the aged leaves fewer chances for the older woman to remarry. Some older individuals choose to live alone. They have been "loners" all their lives, and though they may experience loneliness, they are socially adjusted (12). A small number of older women may feel a sense of freedom living alone for the first time, free of the obligations to a spouse or children. They choose to live independently rather than seek a roommate or live with family. Even though socially adjusted and capable of caring for themselves, isolates may suffer from poor nutrition because they are not motivated to shop, cook, and eat by themselves (9).

Desolates are those who live alone, though not by choice (12). These people come to live alone because of a scattering and/or death of relatives and friends. Each loss of a companion necessitates a rearrangement of life-style. If the losses are many or rapid in succession, there are no substitutes with whom the person can form meaningful relationships. The emotional upset due to lack of a support system may manifest itself as actual pain, physical complaints, or constant recapitulation of the past. Grief may be a constant companion of the desolate aged, and they may exhibit eccentric behavior. Subgroups of the aged population most at risk for desolation are women and blacks, 75 years old and over (13).

Studies have shown that as age increases, the number of persons in a household decreases, the amount spent on weekly groceries decreases, and the frequency of meals eaten alone increases (9). When social support structures can be provided, this has been positively correlated with a higher intake of specific nutrients—vitamin A, thiamin, calcium, phosphorus, and magnesium. Important predictors of nutrient levels were social support systems such as marriage, close attachment to neighbors, and religious involvement. Social support systems that place the older individual in an uncomfortable dependency position may have a negative consequence on dietary intake. Support groups should offer cooperative associations that foster a feeling of independence and contribution among those aged members who participate (14).

On occasion, aged individuals caught in a neighborhood decline or left in a socially isolating position may be uprooted and forced to live with adult children and/or grandchildren. Antagonism for "old-country" or "old-fashioned" ways on the part of the children or grandchildren often results in withdrawal and exaggerated emphasis on the old ways on the part of the elderly family member. It can be speculated that much of the behavior that ultimately leads to confinement of the aged in a long-term care facility is related to conflicts over food and eating. Assisting families to understand, tolerate, and support the defensive use of food by the aged may reduce the need for institutional care (13).

Abuse and neglect of elderly persons, through the withholding of food, can be a manifestation of family abuse toward older family members. There is increasing information on the abuse and neglect of elderly persons, and the evidence seems to indicate that it is a social problem of greater magnitude than once realized. Table 18–2 lists characteristics of those families most at risk for family-mediated abuse or neglect of older members.

Table 18–2 Groups at High Risk for Family-Mediated Abuse or Neglect

Elderly persons living at home whose care needs exceed or soon will exceed the family's ability to meet them.

Elderly persons whose primary caretakers are expressing frustration in dealing with care needs.

Elderly persons whose primary caretakers are demonstrating signs of stress.

Elderly persons in families with a norm of family violence (past or present evidence of child or spouse abuse).

Elderly persons who abuse drugs or alcohol or who live with family members who abuse drugs or alcohol, or who have episodes of loss of control.

Elderly persons whose primary caretaker is under severe external stress (loss of job, illness, family problems).

Source: O'Malley, T.A., et al., Identifying and preventing family-mediated abuse and neglect of elderly persons, *Ann. Intern. Med.* 98:998, 1983.

Caregivers must be alert to the following manifestations of abuse or neglect: recurring or unexplained injuries; nontreatment of medical problems; poor hygiene; malnutrition; dehydration; depression, withdrawal, or fearfulness; imposed social or physical isolation; and oversedation or misuse of medications (15).

DISORDERED BEHAVIORS

A wide range of disordered behavior is seen in old age. Organic as well as functional disorders occur that can affect a person's health and nutritional status. The main differentiating factor is orientation. If the person is oriented to time, place and person, he probably does not have much organic damage. Depression, paranoia, or delusions in the elderly are not different from those at any age and are usually amenable to treatment (16).

The psychotic elderly may refuse to eat because of delusions that the food is poisoned or crawling with insects or because of voices that instruct them not to eat. Hoarding of food or other priceless objects is not uncommon. Hoarded food may not always be eaten. Some may insist on having these items ever-present, carrying them from place to place in shopping bags (13).

Many factors such as impaired hearing, pain, constipation, hypotension, electrolyte imbalance, and an elevated temperature can lead to a faulty perception of the environment and precipitate an inappropriate response or disordered behavior in an older individual (16). Undernutrition is a major contributing factor in the symptoms of confusion often seen in depressive disease.

Undernutrition coupled with depression creates a self-sustaining downward spiral. Depression often causes anorexia and subsequent weight loss. This food deprivation can accentuate the symptoms of depression leading to an even lessened food intake and deepening depression. If neglected, this vicious cycle can lead to apathy, isolation, malnutrition, neglect of physical health, enhanced depression symptomatology, and eventually death (17).

In 1973 in Minnesota, 38 people over age 65 died of starvation that was not secondary to any condition such as cancer or alcoholism that might result in malnutrition. These deaths were psychologically induced by the downward spiral of depression and faulty nutrition, serving as a grim example of the ultimate effect of neglected depression in the elderly (17).

The older client with anorexia, insomnia, and feelings of worthlessness and despair may not always be suffering from depression (18). The problem may be grief. Grief can be a constant companion to the elderly. Even people who have successfully "rolled with the punches" throughout life may find that old age is accompanied by too many losses too quickly to be overcome. Allowing the client to vent his feelings of loss and helping him to reestablish a social support system is vital.

Overnutrition can also be a direct result of depression or grief. Eating is a way to cope with feelings of loneliness, helplessness, and anxiety (17). It is a way to obtain comfort. Some eat excessively to induce sleep. Even the improvished aged can become overweight. These people are in a paradoxical situation. They are overweight and undernourished at the same time. They purchase "comforting" foods (cakes, candy, dessert, alcohol) that are high in calories but low in nutrients, leaving them deficient in protein, vitamins, and minerals.

FOOD AS A POSITIVE SOCIAL FACTOR

Eating is one of life's most pleasurable, recurring experiences and should remain so throughout life. Research has demonstrated that the quality of the diet is improved when the meal is shared with others rather than eaten alone (19).

The federal program that targets senior citizens for food and nutrition services is the Title III Nutrition Program, funded through the Older Americans Act. It consists of the congregate meals and the home-delivered meal programs.

The congregate-meals program, in line with the legislative intention to provide nutritionally sound meals and to reduce the isolation of

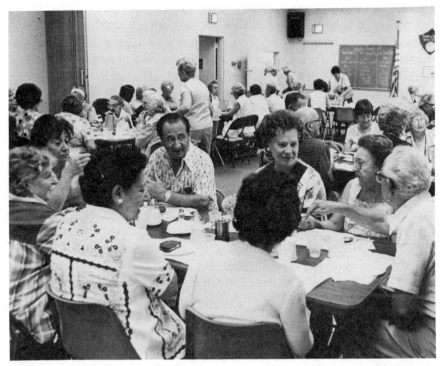

Enjoying lunch in a congregate-meal setting.

old age, offers one hot meal per day along with activities and support services at meal sites. Most typically the noon meal is offered to participants 60 years old and to their spouses of any age. Projects funded by the federal government must provide one hot meal per day at least 5 days per week. Local programs may offer a similar service as infrequently as once a week or as often as 6 days a week depending on the scope and resources available to the local projects.

The home-delivered-meals component of the federal program targets the frail and less mobile elderly by providing one meal a day, delivered directly to their residence. Delivery of meals to the homes of the handicapped and aged was one of the earliest types of feeding programs to be established. "Meals on Wheels" began in England in 1939, and Philadelphia organized the first United States program in 1954. Currently, besides the federally funded service, "Meals on Wheels" programs are run by state, county, and privately funded organizations. Home-delivered meals may be adapted for modified diets, and in some instances they are suited to religious or ethnic preferences (20).

Home-delivered meals meet nutritional as well as social needs. Many meals recipients have no visitors except the volunteer deliverer who comes daily or five times a week. The volunteer provides social contact and often becomes friends with the recipient (21). In the case of temporary disability, the positive social contact resulting from the home-delivered meal may interest the person in joining the congregate-meals program at a local site when able. In the case of chronic disability, home-delivered meals may enable the individual to continue living independently and forestall institutionalization.

Many programs attempt to serve more than one meal daily. They deliver a hot lunch and leave a light supper that is cold or needs only simple heating. Other programs deliver a hot dinner and leave sandwiches for the following day's lunch. In the late 1970s in order to close the significant service gaps that exist in congregate-dining and home-delivered meals programs, NASA (National Aeronautics and Space Administration) was asked to use its food technology to develop a convenient, economical, shelf-stable meal system for the homebound elderly (22). These early demonstration programs proved successful, and today private companies are offering shelf-stable meals for delivery to homebound elderly or as a substitute for congregate meals when a service gap exists (23).

A number of innovative local programs have emerged to meet the needs of the older population. Elderly luncheon clubs have been started that group together five or six older adults who may or may not be participants in home-delivered meal programs, who rarely get out of their apartments/homes, and who have few social contacts. The "club" meets together one or more days per week to share a luncheon meal in the apartment/home of a luncheon club leader. the leader acts as a host/hostess for the group. Bulk meals are delivered to the home of the group leader through the delivery system already in place for home-delivered meals (24). Delivering to one site for multiple meals saves time, but more important, it provides the extended social contact that is not normally available to participants of the home delivery system. New York City restauranteurs, food suppliers, and food retailers have set up a unique, charitable organization called "Citymeals-on-Wheels." This program has supplied free holiday dinners and donated surplus food, day-old baked goods, and numerous other commodities to provide thousands of additional meals to the elderly in the city (25).

For the older individual who enters a long-term care facility, this life-style change is often devastating and results in behaviors such as depression, anger, and refusal to eat. Female residents who are dissatisfied with their lives also have poor appetites. They show lower-than-normal calorie and nutrient intakes for all nutrients except vitamin C (26). The social function of eating must be addressed as a major intervention program in enhancing the quality of life for residents. Dining-room service as opposed to bedside service increases the amount of food eaten and helps to orient the resident to time and place. Even severely regressed residents show improvement by being in the company of less impaired residents (27). Other benefits observed are less meal skipping, more socialization, and fewer complaints about meal service when central dining service is offered. Some innovative caregivers have taken this concept of resident involvement even further by offering kitchen tours, establishing food committees, featuring theme dinners, and occasional in-house restaurant menus where residents have a choice of selections (28,29). Food demonstrations and tasting parties have been successfully used as a recreational activity to foster reminiscence, a sense of continuity, and well-being (30).

CULTURAL, RELIGIOUS, AND REGIONAL FOOD PRACTICES

People define food culturally not on the basis of the nutritional value of particular items. Food habits are learned; therefore, they are a way for a particular culture to exert a standardizing influence on the behavior of an individual in the group so that the group comes to have common eating patterns. Food habits are established early in life and are resistant to change. The place of culture and culturally congruent foods in the lives of older adults is significant. Most older individuals believe that people have a better chance of maintaining health or regaining health if they eat culturally familiar foods (31). Cultural origins and socioeconomic status appear to be better indicators of persistent dietary habits in the elderly than educational background (32).

Little work has been done to identify food preferences among aged members of specific cultural groups. Understanding the interplay of traditional food behavior, folk healing practices, and religious prohibitions on food intake is vital to ensure optimum health care. Food is frequently used to send health messages, and the astute caregiver must be able to translate these messages to effectively serve a culturally similar aged population.

A gradient of dietary importance has been established to explain the inflexibility of food habits. The gradient consists of the "core diet," which includes regular staple foods universal to a group; the "secondary" core, foods used widely but not universally; and "peripheral foods," those foods used most infrequently. The greatest resistance to change has been encountered in the "core diet," which includes cultural foods (32). When applied to a generational model, the first or oldest generation is least likely to change (31,32,33,34,35).

Although it is impossible to discuss each cultural, religious, or regional subgroup of older individuals in the United States, the following examples can be used to demonstrate the importance of maintaining ties to one's heritage and the obligation of the health care community to recognize this and develop a health care delivery system that does not presuppose acculturation. If acculturation is assumed, compliance with medical and nutritional therapies will be far below that which is anticipated.

Regional Food Preferences

The United States has long been divided into geographic areas that are identified with certain foods. Presentation of and encouragement of the use of "down-home" foods may foster reminiscences, which are considered psychologically important in the adjustment to the final stage of life (12). A large proportion of today's aged were raised in a culture of poverty because of their rural or immigrant origins. Many may still be existing at an economic level far below the standard. Foods associated with status—bakery items and convenience foods—may be preferred to foods, like beans, identified with the poverty of their childhood or early adulthood.

"Soul food" considered traditional fare of Southern blacks, may be savored and enjoyed by a 70-year-old because of its group association but disliked by his 45-year-old son because it reminds him of an environment he is trying to forget. For the older man his attitudes, behaviors, and preferences for food reflect the atmosphere prevalent in his formative years. His son's perception of what is culturally appropriate has changed to reflect the times through which he has lived (36). This once again points out the generational differences and the lesser degree of change seen in older individuals.

Health Belief Systems That Affect Food Intake

Generational differences in health ideas and beliefs and the reliance by older individuals on folk healing and other self-help measures may have a direct bearing on the adherence to specific dietary modifications. An older individual is more likely to seek out a folk healer. The reasons for this are numerous: shared language; referral by a friend or relative; potential familiarity with the procedures to be used; sensitivity to the person's cultural beliefs; and careful explanations of the healing experience (34). Modern health care delivery can provide all these same needs given a basic understanding of the client's cultural background and the time and language skills necessary to carefully explain the necessary treatment or diet modification.

Older Puerto Ricans and other Spanish-speaking groups may adhere to the hot-cold theory of disease. Health is conceived as a state of balance; illness is the result of an imbalance. Foods, herbs, and medications are classified as hot or cold. The are used therapeutically in varying combinations to restore the body's natural balance. Cold-classified illnesses are treated with ''hot'' medications and foods, while hot illnesses are treated with ''cool'' substances. Many chronic disorders are attributed to a chill or eating excessive amounts of cold-classified foods. Arthritis is cold-classified; therefore, people with arthritis will not eat orange juice, bananas, raisins, and other cold-classified foods. If an elderly arthritic patient is prescribed a diurectic for high blood pressure and told to eat potassium-rich foods (bananas, orange juice, raisins, dried fruit), he generally will not comply. The hot-cold classification influences the way a client adheres to the therapeutic regimens for hypertension, colds, ulcers, constipation, and gastrointestinal problems, as well as arthritis (33,37).

Religious Food Practices

Religious beliefs are strong in this country among the older segment of the population. Food taboos, fasting periods, and holidays are important religious observances that give structure and meaning to one's existence. An elderly Catholic may still insist on ''meatless'' Fridays even though this practice is no longer required by the church.

In many areas of the United States, older Jewish people make up a large ethnic community. Social events often revolve around the synagogue, which may have senior groups and a feeding program. Health professionals working with elderly Jews have an obligation to understand the profound effect their religion has on their daily life and food habits. Nutritional information must be interpreted with a knowledge of the practice of *kashruth*, the Jewish Dietary Laws. They are observed to varying degrees by members of the Jewish faith. What is fit and proper to eat is *kosher*. Holiness is the fundamental reason for the Jewish Dietary Laws; the hygienic value of the laws is considered incidental. The separation of milk and meat is emphasized so that the two may not be prepared, cooked, or eaten together. This separation leads to a classification of foods. They are ''milchig'' (milk and/or dairy products), ''fleishig'' (meat, fowl, and products made from them), and ''pareve'' (fruits, vegetables, grains, fish, and eggs). ''Pareve'' foods may be eaten with either ''milchig'' or ''fleishig'' because they are considered neutral.

To ''keep kosher'' means the person follows the Jewish Dietary Laws and has set up his kitchen and eating pattern to conform with kashruth. This means meals are either labeled dairy (containing no meat foods) or meat (containing no dairy foods). To classify meals takes some planning. In most cases, dairy meals are served at breakfast and lunch, and a meat meal is served at dinner. Separate sets of dishes and cooking utensils must be maintained, one for meat preparation and one for dairy. This equipment is stored separately and washed separately. Although it may appear to be a complicated process to maintain a kosher home, in practice this manner of food preparation and eating becomes a way of life, and the complexities of the process rarely pose problems (38).

REFERENCES

1. *Statistical Reports on Older Americans:5.Characteristics of the Black Elderly—1980*, U.S. Department of Health and Human Services, DHHS Publication No. (OHDS) 80-20057, Super. of Doc. Wash., D.C. April 1980.

2. Three Budgets for a Retired Couple, Autumn 1981, U.S. Department of Labor, Bureau of Statistics, *News*, USDL 82-266, 1982.

3. Talbot, D.M., Assessing needs of the rural elderly, *J. Gerontol. Nurs.* 11(3):39, 1985.

4. Burton, J.R., Hennon, C.B., Consumer education for the elderly, *J. Home Econ.* 73:24, Summer 1981.

5. Wong, H., Krondl, M., Williams, J.I., Long-term effect of a nutrition intervention program for the elderly, *J. Nutr. Elderly* 2(1):31, Fall 1982.

6. Parham, E.S., Nutrition education for the elderly, *J. Home Econ.* 72(1):24, Spring 1980.

7. Ludman, E.K., The emergent curriculum: A tool for nutrition education for the elderly, *J. Nutr. Elderly* 2(3):17, Spring 1983.

8. Atchley, R.C., Selected social and psychological differences between men and women in later life, *J. Gerontol.* 31(2):204, 1976.

9. Brown, E.L., Factors influencing food choices and intake, *Geriatrics* 31:89, 1976.

10. Krondl, M., et al., Food use and preceived food meanings of the elderly, *J. Am. Diet. Assoc.* 80:523, June 1982.

11. Rahe, R.H., McKean, J.D., Arthur, R.J., A longitudinal study of life-change and illness patterns, *J. Psychosom. Res.* 10:355, 1967.

12. Troll, L.E., Eating and aging, *J. Am. Diet. Assoc.* 59:456, 1971.

13. Weinberg, J., Psychologic implications of the nutritional needs of the elderly, *J. Am. Diet. Assoc.* 60:293, 1972.

14. McIntosh, W.A., Shifflett, P.A., Influence of social support systems on dietary intake of the elderly, *J. Nutr. Elderly* 4:5, Fall 1984.

15. O'Malley, T., et al., Identifying and preventing family-mediated abuse and neglect of elderly persons, *Ann. Intern. Med.* 98:998, 1983.

16. Schwab, M., Caring for the aged, *Am. J. Nurs.* 73:2049, Dec. 1973.

17. Garetz, F.K., Breaking the dangerous cycle of depression and faulty nutrition, *Geriatrics* 33:73, June 1976.

18. Grief versus depression in elderly patients, *JAMA* 241:1558, April 13, 1979.

19. Grotkowski, M.I., Sims, L.S., Nutritional knowledge, attitudes and dietary practices of the elderly, *J. Am. Diet. Assoc.* 72:499, May 1978.

20. McCeney, E., Meals on Wheels for kosher clients in central Maryland, *J. Nutr. Elderly* 5(1):57, Fall 1985.

21. Hanson, G., Considering "social nutrition" in assessing geriatric nutrition, *Geriatrics* 35:49, March 1978.

22. Rhodes, L., NASA food technology, a method for meeting the nutritional needs of the elderly, *Gerontologist* 17(4):333, Aug. 1977.

23. Chason, M., Nourishment and independence for the elderly with home delivered shelf stable meals featuring retort pouch entrees, *J. Nutr. Elderly* 3(3):67, 1984.

24. Balsam, A.L., Duffy, M., Elderly luncheon clubs: Bridging the gap between congregate and home delivered meals, *J. Nutr. Elderly*, 2(4):31, Summer 1983.

25. Greene, G., Citymeals-on-Wheels, *J. Nutr. Elderly* 2(4):27, Summer 1983.

26. Harrill, I., Erbes, C., Schwartz, C., Observations on food acceptance by elderly women, *Gerontologist* 16(4):349, 1976.

27. Rankin, G., The therapeutic value of a dining room program in a geriatric setting, *J. Gerontol. Nurs.* 1(3):5, July/Aug. 1975.

28. "Restaurants" in nursing homes liven up meals, *Restaurants Institutions* 89(3):32, Aug. 1, 1981.

29. Horowitz, R.G., A creative dining experience in long term care, *J. Nutr. Elderly* 3(4):39, Summer 1984.

30. Lefkowitz, L., Food demonstration as a social activity in a nursing home, *J. Nutr. Elderly* 2(2):31, Winter 1982.

31. Newman, J.M., Ludman, E.K., Chinese elderly: Food habits and beliefs, *J. Nutr. Elderly* 4(2):3, Winter 1984.

32. Nalbandian, A., Bergan, J.G., Brown, P.T., Three generations of Armenians: Food habits and dietary status, *J. Am. Diet. Assoc.* 79:694, Dec. 1981.

33. Harwood, A., The hot-cold theory of disease, *JAMA* 216(7):1153, May 17, 1971.

34. Snyder, P., Health service implications of folk healing among older Asian Americans and Hawaiians in Honolulu, *Gerontologist* 24(5):471, 1984.

35. Netland, P.A., Brownstein, H., Acculturation and the diet of Asian-American elderly, *J. Nutr. Elderly* 3(3):37, Spring 1984.

36. Baily, F.E., Walker, M.L., Socio-economic factors and their effects on the nutrition and dietary habits of the black aged, *J. Gerontol. Nurs.* 8(4):203, April 1982.

37. Smith, L.K., Mexican-American views of Anglo medical and dietetic practices, *J. Am. Diet. Assoc.* 74:463, April 1979.

38. Natow, A.B., Heslin, J., Understanding the cultural food practices of elderly observant Jews, *J. Nutr. Elderly* 2(1):49, Fall 1982.

Appendix A

PROGRESSIVE HOSPITAL DIET

The regular hospital diet, sometimes referred to as the "normal," "house," "standard," or "general" diet, is intended for the patient whose condition does not require therapeutic modification. This regular diet may be modified in terms of items allowed, methods of preparation, and consistency for patients who cannot tolerate a regular diet. These modifications of the regular diet are often referred to as the progressive hospital diet, because they are ordered by the physician progressively for pre- and postoperative patients, patients with acute infections, patients with certain gastrointestinal conditions, debilitated patients who have feeding and swallowing problems, and after myocardial infarction.

Soft diets follow a normal meal pattern, are soft in consistency, easy to chew, made up of easily digested food, and contain no harsh fiber or richly seasoned foods. Acceptable foods are those moderately low in cellulose and connective tissue.

Full-liquid diets provide nutritional support for the patient who is acutely ill, unable to chew and/or swallow solid or semisolid foods. This diet is made up of foods that liquefy at room or body temperature. Foods allowed in this diet are free of cellulose and irritating condiments (e.g., mustard, ketchup) or spices (e.g., black pepper, chili powder). The caloric density and iron content of this diet may be inadequate for long-term use. Also, the cholesterol content is high because of the

Progressive Hospital Diet

	Regular	Soft	Full liquid	Clear liquid
Characteristics	All foods easy to digest; individual intolerances, food habits, ethnic values, and food preferences considered	Normal diet modified to have limited fiber; primarily liquids and semisolid foods (soft-cooked low-fiber foods often used instead of purees)	Foods fluid at room temperature	Only clear fluids A temporary diet No gas-producing or irritating foods Can provide only 400–600 kcal/day
Adequacy	Complete	Complete iron intake may be inadequate	To be adequate requires careful planning If used longer than 48 hours, should use ↑protein, ↑calorie supplements	Inadequate ↓Protein ↓Minerals ↓Vitamins ↓Calories
Use	All patients not requiring therapeutic diets	Between full fluid and regular Between acute illness and convalescence Acute infection Chewing difficulties GI disorders	Post op Acute infections During fevers Acute GI problems Intolerance to solids	Acute illness Immediate post op To relieve thirst To prevent dehydration To reduce fecal matter To prevent stimulation of the GI tract Prior to certain tests

Foods	All of the basic four	All liquids	All clear fluids	Water
		Fine and strained cereals	All forms of milk	Chopped ice
		Well-cooked spaghetti, macaroni, and noodles	Strained soups	Tea
		Tender cooked and pureed vegetables	Fruits and vegetable juices containing pulp	Coffee
		Potatoes, boiled, mashed, creamed, or baked without skin	Eggnogs*	Fat-free clear broth
		Cooked fruits (no skin or seeds)	Plain ice cream and sherbert	Boullion and consomme
		Ripe bananas	Junket and plain gelatin	Soda
		Ground meat, fish, poultry	Soft custards	Synthetic fruit juice
		Eggs	Pureed vegetables and meat for soup only	Ginger ale
		Mild cheese	Cereal gruels	Plain gelatin
		Enriched white and whole-wheat bread and crackers		Fruit juices without pulp
		Ices, ice cream		Fruit ices
		Gelatin, junket, pudding, custard		

*Because of the danger of *Salmonella* infection from raw egg, a commercial eggnog preparation is recommended.

285

amount of milk offered. Monotony in this diet is the main barrier to patient acceptance. Planning six or more feedings a day may encourage a more adequate intake by the patient.

If full liquids are used for more than a few days, then the patient must also receive a nutritionally complete oral supplement (e.g., Sustacal) since the full-liquid diet usually provides no more than 40 g of protein/day.

Clear-liquid diets provide no more than 600 kcal/day, largely from carbohydrates. The protein in this diet, largely as gelatin, is limited in amount and quality. Most clear-liquid diets provide only about 5 g protein/day. Clear liquids are usually given immediately postoperatively or in the acute stages of infection, particularly of the gastrointestinal tract. The primary objectives of this diet are to prevent dehydration, relieve thirst, and minimize stimulation to the gastrointestinal tract. Clear-liquid diets should be used only for limited periods of time, generally no more than 24–36 hours. Fluids should be offered throughout the day as tolerated by the patient.

Appendix B

DIABETIC EXCHANGE LISTS FOR MEAL PLANNING

One of the most important aspects of diabetes management is dietary care. The Food Exchanges are lists of foods grouped by similar values of carbohydrates, proteins, and fats so that they can be substituted in your daily meal plans. Foods have been divided into six categories: milks, vegetables, fruits, breads, meats, and fats. Foods in any one group can be substituted or exchanged with other foods within the same group.

BREAD EXCHANGES

One exchange of bread contains 15 g of carbohydrate, 2 g of protein, and 70 kcal.

Bread

White (including French and Italian)	1 slice	English muffin, small	½
		Plain roll, bread	1
Whole wheat	1 slice	Frankfurter roll	½
Rye or pumpernickel	1 slice	Hamburger bun	½
Raisin	1 slice	Dried bread crumbs	3 tbsp
Bagel, small	½	Tortilla, 6″	1

Cereal

Bran flakes	½ cup
Other ready-to-eat unsweetened cereal	¾ cup
Puffed cereal (unfrosted)	1 cup
Cereal (cooked)	½ cup
Grits (cooked)	½ cup
Rice or barley (cooked)	½ cup
Pasta (cooked), noodles, spaghetti, macaroni	½ cup
Popcorn (popped, no fat added)	3 cups
Cornmeal (dry)	2 tbsp
Flour	2½ tbsp
Wheat germ	¼ cup

Crackers

Arrowroot	3
Graham, 2½″ sq.	2
Matzoh, 4″ × 6″	½ cup
Oyster	20
Pretzels, 3⅛″ long × ⅛″ dia.	25
Rye wafers, 2″ × 3½″	3
Saltines	6
Soda, 2½″ sq	4

Dried beans, peas, and lentils

Beans, peas, lentils (dried and cooked)	½ cup
Baked beans, no pork (canned)	¼ cup

Starchy vegetables

Corn	⅓ cup

Prepared foods

Biscuit, 2″ diameter (omit 1 fat exchange)	1
Corn bread, 2″ × 2″ × 1″ (omit 1 fat exchange)	1
Corn muffin, 2″ diameter (omit 1 fat exchange)	1
Crackers, round butter type (omit 1 fat exchange)	5
Muffin, plain small (omit 1 fat exchange)	1
Potatoes, French fried, length 2″ to 3½″ (omit 2 fat exchanges)	8
Potato or corn chips (omit 2 fat exchanges)	15
Pancake, 5″ × ½″ (omit 1 fat exchange)	1
Waffle, 5″ × ½″ (omit 1 fat exchange)	1

VEGETABLE EXCHANGES

One exchange of vegetables contains about 5 g of carbohydrate, 2 g of protein, and 25 kcal. One exchange is ½ cup.

Asparagus	Cucumbers	Greens (*cont.*)	Sauerkraut
Bean sprouts	Eggplant	Mustard	String beans
Beets	Green pepper	Spinach	(green or yellow)
Broccoli	Greens	Turnip	Summer squash
Brussels sprouts	Beet	Mushrooms	Tomatoes
Cabbage	Chards	Okra	Tomato juice
Carrots	Collards	Onions	Turnips
Cauliflower	Dandelion	Rhubarb	Vegetable juice cocktail
Celery	Kale	Rutabaga	Zucchini

The following raw vegetables may be used as desired:

Chicory	Lettuce
Chinese cabbage	Parsley
Endive	Radishes
Escarole	Watercress

Starchy vegetables are found in the bread exchange list.

FRUIT EXCHANGES

One exchange of fruit contains 10 g of carbohydrate and 40 kcal.

Apple	1 small	Grape juice	¼ cup
Apple juice	⅓	Mango	½ small
Applesauce		Melon	
(unsweetened)	½ cup	Cantaloupe	¼ small
Apricots, fresh	2 medium	Honeydew	⅛ medium
Apricots, dried	4 halves	Watermelon	1 cup
Banana	½ small	Nectarine	1 small
Berries		Orange	1 small
Blackberries	½ cup	Orange juice	½ cup
Blueberries	½ cup	Papaya	¾ cup
Raspberries	½ cup	Peach	1 medium
Strawberries	¾ cup	Pear	1 small
Cherries	10 large	Persimmon, native	1 medium
Cider	⅓ cup	Pineapple	½ cup
Dates	2	Pineapple juice	⅓ cup
Figs, fresh	1	Plums	2 medium
Figs, dried	1	Prunes	2 medium
Grapefruit	½	Prune juice	¼ cup
Grapefruit juice	½ cup	Raisins	2 tbsp
Grapes	12	Tangerine	1 medium

Cranberries may be used as desired if no sugar is added.

MEAT EXCHANGES

Lean Meat

One exchange of lean meat (1 oz) contains 7 g of protein, 3 g of fat, and 55 kcal.

Beef	Baby beef (very lean), chipped beef, chuck, flank steak, tenderloin, plate ribs, plate skirt steak, round (bottom top), all cuts rump, spare ribs, tripe	1 oz

Lamb	Leg, rib, sirloin, loin (roast and chops), shank, shoulder	1 oz
Pork	Leg (whole rump, center shank), ham smoked (center slices)	1 oz
Veal	Leg, loin, rib, shank, shoulder, cutlets	1 oz
Poultry	Meat without skin of chicken, turkey, Cornish hen, guinea hen, pheasant	1 oz
Fish	Any fresh or frozen	1 oz
	Canned salmon, tuna, mackerel, crab, and lobster	¼ cup
	Clams, oysters, scallops, shrimp	5, or 1 oz
	Sardines, drained	3

Cheeses containing less than 5% butterfat	1 oz
Cottage cheese, dry and 2% butterfat	¼ cup
Dried beans and peas (omit 1 bread exchange)	½ cup

Medium-Fat Meat

For each exchange of medium-fat meat omit ½ fat exchange.

| Beef | Ground (15% fat), corned beef (canned), rib eye, round (ground commercial) | 1 oz |
| Pork | Loin (all cuts tenderloin), shoulder arm (picnic), shoulder blade, Boston butt, Canadian bacon, boiled ham | 1 oz |

Liver, heart, kidney, and sweetbreads (these are high in cholesterol)	1 oz
Cottage cheese, creamed	¼ cup
Cheese: Mozzarella, Ricotta, farmer's cheese, Neufchatel, Parmesan	3 tbsp
Egg (high in cholesterol)	1
Peanut butter (omit 2 additional fat exchanges)	2 tbsp

High-Fat Meat

For each exchange of high-fat meat omit 1 fat exchange.

Beef	Brisket, corned beef (brisket), ground beef (more than 20% fat), Hamburger (commercial), chuck (ground commercial), roasts (rib), steaks (club and rib)	1 oz
Lamb	Breast	1 oz
Pork	Spare ribs, loin (back ribs), pork (ground), country-style ham, deviled ham	1 oz
Veal	Breast	1 oz

Poultry	Capon, duck (domestic), goose	1 oz
Cheese	Cheddar types	1 oz
Cold cuts		4½″ × ⅛″ slice
Frankfurter		1 small

MILK EXCHANGES

One exchange of milk contains 12 g of carbohydrate, 8 g of protein, a trace of fat, and 80 kcal.

Non-Fat Fortified Milk

Skim or nonfat milk	1 cup
Powdered (nonfat dry, before adding liquid)	⅓ cup
Canned, evaporated skim milk	½ cup
Buttermilk made from skim milk	1 cup
Yogurt made from skim milk, (plain, unflavored)	1 cup

Low-Fat Fortified Milk

1% fat fortified milk (omit ½ fat exchange)	1 cup
2% fat fortified milk (omit 1 fat exchange)	1 cup
Yogurt made from 2% fortified milk (plain, unflavored) (omit 1 fat exchange)	1 cup

Whole Milk (omit 2 fat exchanges)

Whole milk	1 cup
Canned, evaporated whole milk	½ cup
Buttermilk made from whole milk	1 cup
Yogurt made from whole milk (plain, unflavored)	1 cup

FAT EXCHANGES

One exchange of fat contains 5 g of fat and 45 kcal.

Polyunsaturated		**Saturated**	
Margarine, soft, tub or stick*	1 tsp	Margarine, regular stick	1 tsp
Avocado (4″ diameter)†	⅛	Butter	1 tsp

*Made with corn, cottonseed, safflower, soy, or sunflower oil only.
†Fat content is primarily monounsaturated.

Polyunsaturated (cont.)		Saturated (cont.)	
Oil, corn, cottonseed,		Bacon fat	1 tsp
Safflower, soy,		Bacon crisp	1 strip
sunflower	1 tsp	Cream, light	2 tbsp
Oil, olive†	1 tsp	Cream, sour	2 tbsp
Oil, peanut†	1 tsp	Cream, heavy	1 tbsp
Olives†	5 small	Cream cheese‡	1 tbsp
Almonds†	10 whole	French dressing‡	1 tbsp
Pecans†	2 large whole	Italian dressing‡	1 tbsp
Peanuts, Spanish†	20 whole	Lard	1 tsp
Peanuts, Virginia†	10 whole	Mayonnaise‡	1 tsp
Walnuts	6 small	Salad dressing,	
Nuts, other†	6 small	mayonnaise-	
		type‡	2 tsp
		Salt pork	¾"
			cube

‡If made with corn, cottonseed, safflower, soy, or sunflower oil can be used on fat-modified diet.

GENERAL RULES

Free Foods	Foods to Avoid
Seasonings: Cinnamon, celery salt, garlic, garlic salt, lemon, mustard, ming, nutmeg, parsley, pepper, sugarless sweeteners, spices, vanilla, and vinegar.	Sugar, candy, honey, jam, jelly, marmalade, syrups, pie, cake, cookies, pastries, condensed milk, soft drinks, candy-coated gum; fried, scalloped or creamed foods; beer, wine, or other alcoholic beverages
Other foods: Coffee or tea (without sugar or cream), fat-free broth, bouillon, unflavored gelatin, sour or dill pickles, cranberries (without sugar)	

Source: The exchange lists are based on material in the *Exchange Lists for Meal Planning*, prepared by the Committees of the American Diabetes Association, Inc., and the American Dietetic Association in cooperation with the National Institute of Arthritis, Metabolism, and Digestive Diseases and the National Heart and Lung Institutes of Health, Public Health Service, U.S. Department of Health and Human Services.

Appendix C

INTERPRETING
NUTRITIONAL RESEARCH

The field of geriatric nutrition is rapidly evolving. Health care givers need to base their practice on current information. Obtaining that information often requires reviewing pertinent literature. The following will help you to do this.

Epidemiologic nutrition studies that are observational can establish associations between nutritional factors and disease in a population. They do not prove a cause-and-effect relationship. *Experimental* nutrition studies are clinical trials in which the investigator has direct control over the conditions making it possible to provide more proof of cause and effect. Because of ethical constraints, experimental studies done with humans are used only to test preventive or therapeutic measures (1).

Epidemiologic studies can be retrospective or prospective. Retrospective studies, also called case-controlled studies, begin after individuals have developed or failed to develop the disease that is being investigated. Prospective studies, also called cohort studies, begin before individuals have developed the disease in question. Efforts must be made to avoid selection bias. The sample must be representative of all individuals who could have been included. Recall error can be a problem when one group is more likely to recall events than the other group. Recall bias is more likely in those who have suffered subsequent traumatic events.

In ideal experimental studies individuals are assigned randomly and blindly either to the study or to the control group. Random assignment means that any one person has an equal chance of being assigned to either group. Double-blind assignment means that neither the participants nor the investigators know which group the participants have been assigned to (2).

The following guidelines will help you to evaluate research. One issue that is not addressed is: How certain should the data be before health care personnel utilize the findings when advising their patients? What is needed is the best available advice for a complex situation. For the question of modification of diet, it is better to suggest dietary changes that pose no risk based on incomplete evidence than to wait unnecessarily until the final word is in. "We would be remiss to withhold what can be useful because it is not perfect" (3).

GUIDELINES FOR INTERPRETING SCIENTIFIC RESEARCH*

These criteria apply to experimental studies as well as epidemiologic investigations.

1. There should be consistency in the data. If the substance seems to cause the given disease in some studies, but not in others, the matter is questionable and cannot yet be taken as fact. Other factors may be causing the differences in results.
2. The effect should be clear-cut. With borderline results, it is hard to tell whether the effect is real or whether it is just a matter of chance.
3. The more specific the effect, the better. If something seems to cause many different medical problems, but each only to a small degree, it probably really does not cause any of them.
4. The cause has to precede the effect, not the other way around.
5. The "route of administration" of the given substance is important since the many ways potentially harmful substances can work in the body are complex. If, for example, a dietary component were injected directly into the bloodstream instead of given orally as part of a complete diet, the results would be of limited value when trying to extrapolate to the human condition.
6. The results should be statistically significant. The smaller the p value, the smaller the probability that the results occurred by

*Adapted from *Does Everything Cause Something?*, Nutrition/Health Information Service, 99 Park Avenue, New York, New York 10016.

chance alone. A p value of 0.001 indicates that this result could have occurred by chance only once in 1000 times. $p = 0.05$ implies that the result has a 1 in 20 (5%) chance of occurring by happenstance alone. $p = 0.05$ is usually the maximum acceptable value for clinical studies. This means the effect reported in the test group is reliable.

7. Animal and human studies, ideally, should have a control group, similar in makeup except for exposure to the test substance.

8. If the population groups are very different in terms of age, socioeconomic status, education, work, or other factors, the resulting differences in disease may not be due to the test substance, but to one of these other factors.

9. Reports of a handful of cases or anecdotal evidence cannot be used to draw conclusions about large population groups. Those cases could be exceptions due to chances.

REFERENCES

1. Nutritional epidemiology, *Dairy Council Dig.* 53(4):1, July-Aug. 1982.
2. Riegelman, R., Studying a study, *Childbirth Educ.* 3:35, Fall 1983.
3. Grobstein, C., Should imperfect data be used to guide public policy? *Science* 83:18, 1983.

INDEX

Information provided in tables is indicated by the letter *t* following page numbers.

A

Abuse of elderly, 272–273
Acetylcholine, 199–200
Achlorhydria, 12
Acidifiers, 226
Acne rosacea, 232
Additives, 176
Aged, definition, 5
Aging, 7
  cardiovascular system, 8
  definition, 5
  endocrine system, 11
  energy needs, 44
  gastrointestinal system, 11
  glucose intolerance, 11
  immune system, 14
  nervous system, 10
  neuromuscular system, 10
  physiological changes, 8*t*
  renal system, 10
  respiratory system, 9
  skin, 13
Akinesia, 201
Alcohol, 77–87, 172, 191
  abuse, 77–78
  anemia and, 214
  in drugs, 83–84, 259–260
  drugs and, 83, 261–262
  effects of, 78–82
  hypoglycemia and, 124
  in long-term care, 84–85
  maldigestion and, 92
  in therapeutic diets, 85–87
  vitamins and, 81
  weight maintenance and, 80
Alcoholic hepatitis, 82
Alcoholism, 77
Alzheimer's Disease, 55, 198–200
  incidence, 198
Amebiasis, 91
Amenorrhea, 184

American Cancer Society Nutrition
Guidelines, 130*t*
American Diabetes Association, 120
American Heart Association,
162–163
Amphogel, 108
Ampicillin, 256
Amygdalin. *See* Laetrile
Anemia, 209–215
decubitus ulcers and, 234
Anorexia, 142–143
Antacids, 94–95, 190
Anticoagulants, 53
Aphasia, 70–71
Aphthous stomatitis. *See* Canker sores
Arm circumference, 25–26, 26*t*
Arthritis, 191–193
folk healing, 279
homemaking skills, 70
incidence, 191
Artificial sweeteners, 122
Ascites, 82
Ascorbic acid. *See* Vitamin C
Asian elderly, 68
Aspartame, 122
Aspirin
alcohol and, 83
nutrient deficiency and, 221
Assessment, 33–37, 137
weight and, 140
Atherosclerosis, 157–158
Aversions, food 147

B

Bacterial overgrowth, 91
Barbiturates, alcohol and, 83
Basal metabolic rate, 221
Bay leaf obstruction, 95
Bedridden, 207
Bedsores. *See* Decubitus ulcers
Beriberi, 230
Beta-carotene, 151
Bezoars, 90
Biliary obstruction, 91
Biotin, 55
Bistrain, Dr. Bruce, 220
Blind elderly, 71
Blood pressure, 9
Blood sugar level, 124
drugs and, 124

Blood urea nitrogen (BUN), 107, 109
BMR. *See* Basal metabolic rate
Body composition, 14, 15*t*
Body frame, 21
Bone loss, 14
Bone meal, 188
Bradykinesia, 201
Bronchitis, chronic, 248
BUN. *See* Blood urea nitrogen
Bureau of Labor Statistics, 268

C

Cachexia, 143
Caffeine, 191
Calciferol. *See* Vitamin D.
Calcium, 56, 185–188
balance, 186
carbonate, 188
food sources, 187*t*
gluconate, 188
intake, 185
kidney stones and, 112
supplements, 113
lactate, 188
phosphorus, 188
phosphorus ratio, 186
supplements, 188
Calorie requirements, in respiratory
disease, 245
Cancer, 129–152
anorexia in, 142
cachexia in, 143
feeding, 141–142
feeding problems, 143–147
feeding suggestions, 144–146
incidence, 129, 131, 135
localized effects, 132
malnutrition risk, 138–139
nutrition assessment, 137
weight in, 140*t*
protein requirements, 139–140
quackery, 150
risk, 130, 132
aging and, 130
diet and, 130
skin, 232
systemic effects, 132
treatment effects, 133
vitamin A and, 150–151
vitamin C and, 151

vitamin E and, 151
Canker sores, 230
Carbohydrates, 45–46, 198
  percent of diet as, 45
Cardiovascular disease, 157–179
  diet, 162
    garlic oil in, 170
    incidence, 157
    risk factors, 159–162
Cardiovascular system, 8–9
Casec, 236
Castor oil, 100
Catabolic stress index, 220
Cataracts, 97, 117
Cathartics, 92
Catholics, 279
Celiac sprue, 91
Chelation therapy, 170
Chemotherapy, 135
  agents, 136–137
  reactions, 136–137
Chenodeoxycholic acid, 100
Chlordiazepoxide. See Librium
Chlorine, 57
Chlorpropamide. See Diabinese
Cholecystitis, 99–100
Cholesterol, 159, 160, 162
Cholestyramine, 50, 92
Choline, 55
Chromium, 59
Chronic obstructive pulmonary
    disease, 243, 248–249
Cirrhosis, 82
Citymeals-on-wheels, 276
Clear-liquid diet, 284–286
Clinical examination, 28
Cobalamin. See Vitamin B_{12}
Colchicine, 92
Colonic irrigations, 150
Compliance, 163
Congregate meals, 274–275
Constipation, 100–102, 146,
    207
COPD. See Chronic obstructive
    pulmonary disease
Copper, 58, 192
Coumadin, 201, 256–257
Counseling, 65–70
  compliance, 65–71
    aging factors, 68–70
    physical limitations, 70–71
  techniques, 66–68

Cranberry juice, 226
Creatinine, 27–28, 107, 109

D

Decubitus ulcers, 232–240
  diet modifications for, 235–237
Dementia, 198–200, 203
Depression, 273–274
Dermatitis herpetiformis, 232
Desolates, 272
Diabetes mellitus, 115–125
  complications, 116–117
  diet in, 118
  liberalized diet in, 121
  in long term care, 121
  management, 117, 125
  obesity and, 118–119
  prevalence, 115
  skin changes and, 231
Diabetic exchange lists, 119–120,
    287–292, 287t
Diabetic foods, 123
Diabinese, 84
Dialysis, 109–111
  diet in, 110
Diarrhea, 97, 122, 145, 224–226
Diet assessment, 28, 31–40
Diet history, 31
Digestive disorders, 89–103
Digoxin, 256
Disaccharide deficiency, 92
Disordered behavior, 273–274
Disulfiramlike reaction, 84
Diverticulosis, 96
Diuretics, 175
Docosahexanoic acid (DHA), 165
Dolomite, 188
Domestic gas poisoning, 69–70
Drugs, 251–264
  adverse reactions, 251
  anemia and, 210, 214
  constipation caused by, 101
  maldigestion and, 92
  nutrient interactions, 252–255. See
    also Nutrient-drug interaction
  take on empty stomach, 257
  take with meals, 256
Dry mouth (xerostomia), 133, 144
Dumping syndrome, 92
Dysgeusia. See Mouth blindness

E

Economic status, 268
Educational status, 268–270
Eicosopentaenoic acid (EPA),
    165
Elderly
    definition, 5
    luncheon clubs, 276
    numbers of, 3, 4*t*
Emphysema, chronic, 248–249
End stage renal disease (ESRD), 107,
    109
Endocrine system, 11
Energy, 43–44
    need in infectious disease,
        221–222
Enteral feedings, ventilator-
    dependent patients, 245–246
Epidemiologic research studies,
    293
Ergocalciferol. *See* Vitamin D
Esophagitis, 93–95, 144
ESRD. *See* End stage renal
    disease
Estrogen, 184
Exercise, 15
Exfoliative dermatitis, 232
Experimental research studies,
    293–294

F

Fat, 46–47
    percent of diet as, 47
Fats, 159–169
    in foods, 166–169
Fatty acids, 164–165
Feeding devices, 71, 74–75,
    204
Fever, 218, 222–223
Fever blisters. *See* Herpes
    labialis
Fiber, 47–49, 100–101, 165
    crude fiber, 47
    dietary fiber, 47
    excess, 48
    fiber in foods, 48
    ideal level, 47
Fibrocystic breast disease, 53
Finite life span, 6

Fish oils, 165
Fluid requirement,
    ventilator-dependent patient,
        246
Fluoride, 188–189
Fluorine, 59
Fluorosis, 59
Folacin. *See* Folic acid
Folate. *See* Folic acid
Folk healing/medicine,
    278–279
Folic acid, 55
    food sources, 214–215
Food
    groups, 32
    habits, 277–278
        regional, 278
    as a positive social factor,
        274–277
    preferences, 267
    records, 31
    related behaviors, sexual differences
        in, 270–271
Food-borne disease, 69
Food-drug interaction. *See*
        Drug-nutrient interaction,
        Nutrient-drug interaction
Framingham Study, 161
Fructose, 122
    in diabetes, 122
Full-liquid diet, 283–286
Fulvicin, 256

G

Gag reflex, 200–201
Gallbladder disease, 99–100
Gallstones, 99–100
Gangrene, 117
Garlic oil, 170
Gas. see intestinal gas
Gastrectomy, 209
Gastroesophageal reflux. *See*
        Esophagitis
Gastrointestinal obstruction, 252,
    255
Gastrointestinal system, 11
Geophagia, 211
Giardiasis, 91–92
Gluconeogenesis, alcohol and,
    81–82

Glucose tolerance, 11
Glucose tolerance factor (GTF), 59
Glycemic index, 120
Goiter, 58
Goitrogens, 58
Gout, 190–191
  fasting and, 191
Grief, 274
GTF, *See* Glucose tolerance factor

H

Harris and Benedict equation, 221–222
Health belief system, 278–279
Hearing loss, 68–69
Heartburn. *See* Esophagitis
Height, 22
Height-Weight Tables, 20–23
Hemiplegia, 70
Hemochromatosis, 80–81
Hemoglobin levels, 210
Hepatic encephalopathy, 82
Herbal teas, 225
Herpes labialis, 232
Herpes zoster, 230
Hiatus hernia, 95
High blood pressure. *See* Hypertension
High carbohydrate, high fiber diets, 120
High-Density Lipoproteins (HDL), 161–162, 170
Home-delivered meals, 274–276
Hypercalcemia, 52, 188–189
Hypercalciuria, 189
Hypercapnia, 245
Hypercholesterolemia, 159
Hyperglycemia, decubitus ulcers and, 234
Hyperkalemia, 175
Hyperlipidemia, 159, 163
  diet for, 162
Hypertension, 170–173
  alcohol and, 172
  essential, 170
  hygienic treatment, 171–172
  incidence, 170
  nutrition and, 171
  salt and, 172

Hypervitaminosis, alcohol and, 81
Hypochondria, 270
Hypoglycemic reaction, 82
Hypokalemia, 80, 175
Hypophosphatemia, 56

I

IDDM. *See* Insulin Dependent Diabetes Mellitus
Immune function, 27
Impaired glucose tolerance, 115
Indigestion, 89–90
Infectious disease, 217–226
Infection, cultural
  practices and, 219
  nutritional requirements for, 220–222
INH. *See* Isoniazid
Insulin Dependent Diabetes Mellitus (IDDM), 115
Insulin requirements, 46
Interviewing, 32, 40
Intestinal gas, 97–99
Iodine, 58
Iron, 57
  alcohol and, 80–81
  food sources, 212
  supplemental forms, 211
Isoniazid, 230

J

Jewish Dietary Laws, 279–280

K

K-Phos, 226
Kasruth, 279–280
Kempner Rice-Fruit Diet, 172
Ketosis, 46
Kidney. *See also* Renal
  aging and, 105–106
  disease, 106
    in diabetes, 117
    nutritional intervention, 107
  function, 105
  loss of, 108

Kidney stones, 111–113, 188
    calcium and, 112
    oxylate and, 112–113
Kilocalories, 43
Kilojoules, 43
Kitchen safety, 70
Knee height, 25
Koilonychia, 230
Korsakoff's psychosis, 81
Kosher, 279

L

Lact-Aid, 97, 145, 146, 223
Lactose deficiency, 92
Lactose intolerance, 96–97, 223, 225
Laetrile, 149–150
Laradopa. *See* Levodopa
Lasix, 256
Levodopa, 202–203, 257, 259
Librium, alochol and, 83
Life expectancy, 5*t*
Light (lite) foods, 123
Linoleic acid, 46
Lipids. *See also* Fats, Fatty acids
Lipoproteins, 160–162
Liver
    damage, 81
    disease, 82–83, 102–103
Long-term care, 276, 277
Longevity, factors in, 6
Low-calorie foods, 123
Low-density lipoproteins, 161, 170
Low-fat diet, 163
Low Oxylate Diet Book, 113
Low purine diet, 191
Low-sodium diets, 173, 177–178
    urine testing in, 175
Lymphatic obstruction, 93

M

Macrocyctic anemia, 55
Macrominerals, 50
Magnesium, 56
    alcohol and, 80

Malabsorption, 90–93
Malnutrition
    clinical signs, 28, 29–30*t*
    skin changes and, 229–230
Manganese, 58
Mannitol, 122
    and diarrhea, 122
Mature adults, definitions, 5
MAOI. *See* Monoamine oxidase inhibitor
Meals-on-wheels, 275
Med Tymer, 263
Medications, 263. *See* Drugs. *See also* Compliance.
Medium-chain triglycerides, 91
Memory loss, 68, 198
Menopause, 184, 185
MCT. *See* Medium-chain triglycerides
Microminerals, 50
Mineral oil, 52, 92, 100
Minerals, 50–51
    calcium, 56
    chlorine, 57
    chromium, 59
    copper, 58
    fluorine, 59
    iodine, 58
    iron, 57
    magnesium, 56
    manganese, 58
    molybdenum, 59
    phosphorus, 56
    potassium, 57
    selenium, 59
    sodium, 57
    sulfur, 56
    zinc, 59
Mineral supplements, for decubitus ulcers, 238, 240
Molybdenum, 59
Monoamine oxidase inhibitor, 259
Monounsaturated fatty acids, 165
Mouth blindness, 133, 144
Mouthwash, 143
Movement disorders, 203–207
    feeding devices for, 204
    meal consistency, 204–205
Mylicon, 247
Myocardial infarction, 177–178

N

Naphthoquinones. *See* Vitamin K
NASA, 276
National Health Examination Survey, 171
Nausea, 145, 146
Neomycin, 92
Neoplastic disease. *See* Cancer
Neurologic disease, 197–207
Neuromuscular system, 10
Neurotransmitter, 200
Nervous system, 10
Niacin, 54
NIDDM. *See* Noninsulin dependent diabetes mellitus
Nitrogen balance, 45
Nitroglycerin, alcohol and, 83
Nocturia, 49, 108
Noninsulin Dependent Diabetes Mellitus, 115–116
    Diet Guidelines, 121*t*
Nonprescription medications. *See also* Over-the-counter medications
    sugar content of 263
Norwegian scabies, 230
Nutrient-drug interaction 255–259
Nutrient supplementation, 51
Nutrition education, 269–270
Nutrition misinterpretation, 149–152
Nutrition research, interpreting, 293–295
Nutritional deficiency, infection and, 219–220
Nutritional Side Effects of Cancer Treatment, 133–134*t*
NyQuil, 84

O

Obesity, 118–119
    decubitus ulcers and, 233–234
    skin changes and, 230
Older Americans Act, 274
Omega-3 fatty acids, 165
One, 25 dihydroxy vitamin D, 189
Osteoarthritis, 192
Osteomalacia, 190

Osteopenia, 184, 190
Osteoporosis, 183, 190
    in alcohol abusers 78
    in Blacks, 184
    calcium, 185–188
    dietary factors, 185–190
    fluoride, 188–189
    incidence, 184
    menopause and, 184
    smoking and, 185
    vitamin D, 189–190
Over-the-counter medications, 83–84, 259–263
Overnutrition, 274
Oxylate
    kidney stones and, 112–113
    foods high in, 112*t*

P

Pagophagia, 211
Pancreatic insufficiency, 91
Pancreatitis, 80
Pantothenic acid, Vitamin B$_3$, 55
Para-aminosalicyclic acid, 92
Parenteral nutrition, 139
Parkinson's Disease, 201–203, 257
    feeding disabilities, 201–202
    medication in, 202, 203*t*
Patient Aid
    A Guide to Good Nutrition During and After Chemotherapy and Radiation, 152
    A Word About Low-Sodium Diets, 179
    Are You at Risk for Bone Disease? 193
    Arthritis, Basic Facts that Can Help You. 193
    Grocery Guide: Tips on Wise Food Selection, 179
    Low Oxylate Diet Book, 113
    Managing Type II Diabetes, 125
    Nutrition and Chronic Respiratory Disease, 249
    Person to Person About Acid Reflux and Hiatål Hernia, 95
    Sodium: Facts for Older Citizens, 179

Patient Aid (*cont.*)
  Something's Got to Taste Good,
    The Cancer Patient's
    Cookbook, 152
  The Parkinson's Patient: What You
    and Your Family Should Know,
    207
  The Unseen Alcoholics—The
    Elderly, 87
  Using Your Medication Wisely:
    A Guide for The Elderly,
    264
  What Can Vitamins Do for Me
    Now?, 60
Penicillin G, 256
Pernicious anemia, 213–214
Peripheral parenteral nutrition (PPN),
    247
Peritoneal dialysis, 111
Pernicious anemia, 55
Personality change, 141,
    198
Phenytoin, 92
Phosphorous, 56, 186
Phytic acid, 186
Pica, 211
Polydextrose, 122
Polyunsaturated/Saturated Ratio. *See*
    P/S ratio
Polyunsaturates, 165
Potassium, 57, 175, 177
  in foods, 108
  overload, 108
PPN. See Peripheral parenteral
    nutrition
Pressure sores. *See* Decubitus ulcers
Pro-Banthine, 256
Progressive hospital diet,
    283–286
Protein, 44–45, 139–140
  percent of diet as, 45
Protein deficiency, decubitus ulcers
    and, 234
Protein requirement, in respiratory
    disease, 245
P/S ratio, 162–164
Psychosocial factors, in nutritional
    care, 267–268
Puerto Ricans, 279
Pureed food, 206
Pyridoxine, 257, 259. *See also*
    Vitamin B$_6$

R

Radioallergosorbent Test (RAST), 192
Radiation, 133–134
RDA. *See* Recommended Dietary
    Allowances
Recommended Dietary Allowances
    (RDA), 40
Recommended energy intake, 41
Reduced-calorie foods, 123
Reglan, 247
Regular diet, 283
Religious beliefs, 279–280
Renal. *See also* Kidney
  anemia and, 108
  failure, 107
  insufficiency, 107
  protein, 109
Renal system, 10
Reserve capacity, 7
Respiratory disease, 243–249
Respiratory system, 9
Resting metabolic expenditure,
    221–222
Retinol. *See* Vitamin A
Rheumatoid arthritis, 192
Riboflavin. *See* Vitamin B$_2$

S

Saccharin, 122
Saliva, thick, 144
Salt, 172
Saturated fat, 164
Seconal, 83
Selenium, 59, 151
Serum albumin, 139
Shingles, 230
Skin, aging, 229–232
Skin, testing, 27
Sinemet, 202
Smell acuity, 69–70
Social isolation, 271–273
Sodium, 57
  in additives, 176*t*
  in antacids, 94
  in foods, 174–175*t*
Soft diet, 204–205, 283–285
  foods in, 205*t*
Sorbitol, 122
  and diarrhea, 122

Soul food, 278
Southern blacks, 278
Spanish-speaking groups, 279
Stomatitis, 143, 144
Stroke, 200–201
  homemaking skills and, 70
Sucrose polyester, 170
Sulfur, 56
Sugar, in medications, 259,
  262–263
Sugar-free foods, 123
Surgery, 133–134
Sustacal, 286
Sympathomimetic amines, 258

T

Taste alterations, 147–149
Taste perception, 11–12, 69
Tetracycline, 256
TIBC. *See* Total iron binding
  capacity
Theobromine, 191
Theophylline, 191
Thiamin. *See* Vitamin B$_1$
Thirst, 226
Title III Nutrition Program, 274
Tocopherol. *See* Vitamin E
Tooth loss, 12, 90
Tophi, 190
Total iron binding capacity, 27
Total parenteral nutrition, 247
TPN. *See* Total parenteral nutrition
Triceps skinfold, 25–26, 26t
Triglycerides, 159, 160
Type I Diabetes, 115–116
Type II Diabetes, 115–117
Tryptophan, 54, 198
Tube feedings, lactose content, 97
Twenty-four hour recall, 31
  form, 38–39
Tyramine, 259
  food sources, 258

U

Ulcers, 99
Undernutrition, depression and,
  273–274
Uracid, 226

Uric acid, 190
  in alcohol use, 82
Urinalysis, 27–28
Urinary tract infection, 218, 226
Urine, 49
Urine glucose tests, 125
  drugs and, 125
Urine test, 175
UTI. *See* Urinary tract infection

V

Ventilator-dependent patients,
  244–248
Viokase, 91
Visual acuity, 68
Vitamin A, 150–151, 192
  analogs, 52
  retinol, 50, 52
Vitamin B$_1$ (thiamin), 50
Vitamin B$_2$ (riboflavin), 50, 54
Vitamin B$_6$. *See also* Pyridoxine. 54,
  202
  food sources, 258
Vitamin B$_{12}$, 55, 137, 197
  food sources, 213
Vitamin C, 50, 151, 192, 197
  antimicrobial activity, 221
  urinary acidifer, 226
Vitamin D (calciferol), 50, 52,
  189–190
  toxicity, 190
Vitamin D$_2$, 52
Vitamin D$_3$, 52
Vitamin E (tocopherol), 50, 53, 151,
  256
Vitamin K (naphthoquinones), 50,
  210, 256–257
  antagonists, 50
  food sources, 257
Vitamins, 50–51, 52t–55t
  A, 52
  B$_1$, 53
  B$_2$, 54
  B$_6$, 54
  B$_{12}$, 55
  biotin, 55
  C, 53
  choline, 55
  D, 52
  E, 53

Vitamins (*cont.*)
  fat soluble, 50
  folic acid, 55
  K, 53
  megadoses, skin changes and, 231
  niacin, 54
  pantothenic acid, 55
  supplementation, 51
  water soluble, 50
Vitamin supplements, for decubitus
    ulcers, 237
Vomiting, 145, 146, 223–224

W

Water, 49–50
  increased need for, 49
  optimal intake of, 50
Weight, 19–25

  and amputation, 25
Weight loss, 90–91, 119, 172
Wernicke's disease 81
Wheelchair homemaking skills and, 71

X

Xerostomia. *See* Dry mouth
Xylitol, 123
Xylose, 13
X rays, 184

Z

Zinc, 59, 192
  alcohol and, 80
  decubitus ulcers and, 238, 240
  food sources, 238–240